DATE DUE

The Sperm Cell

Production, Maturation, Fertilization, Regeneration

The Sperm Cell

Production, Maturation, Fertilization, Regeneration

Edited by

Christopher J. De Jonge
University of Minnesota
Minneapolis, MN, USA

and

Christopher L. R. Barratt
University of Birmingham
Birmingham, UK

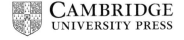
CAMBRIDGE
UNIVERSITY PRESS

CAMBRIDGE UNIVERSITY PRESS
Cambridge, New York, Melbourne, Madrid, Cape Town, Singapore, São Paulo

CAMBRIDGE UNIVERSITY PRESS
The Edinburgh Building, Cambridge CB2 2RU, UK

Published in the United States of America by Cambridge University Press, New York

www.cambridge.org
Information on this title: www.cambridge.org/9780521853972

First published 2006

Typeset by Charon Tec Ltd, Chennai, India
www.charontec.com

Printed in the United Kingdom at the University Press, Cambridge

A catalogue record for this publication is available from the British Library

ISBN-13 978-0-521-85397-2 hardback
ISBN-10 0-521-85397-4 hardback

Contents

v

Preface

In the past decade greater emphasis has been placed on investigation of the human male gamete. As a consequence many unique and revealing characteristics have been identified; providing greater insight and understanding regarding human sperm production, maturation, and function. However, there has not been a comprehensive book on these topics published for more than 8 years. The focus of this book will be on the human and where data is lacking non-human animal species will be substituted to serve as representative example.

The composition of the spermatozoon, always regarded as critical for successful fertilization, has gained even greater significance in the events post-fertilization. The fidelity of the genome in its composition and construction are known to significantly influence fertilization, embryogenesis and live birth. Several contributions to this book elegantly detail the overt and more subtle characteristics of both the competent and dysfunctional sperm genome complex.

Historically, the spermatozoon has somewhat been viewed as a typical single cell; meaning that its membranes, organelles and metabolic activities are all connected. Emerging data clearly demonstrates the uniqueness of the spermatozoon in that discrete compartments can be identified whose physiology and biochemistry are separable. Several of the chapters herein offer intriguing revelations in this regard.

The yin and yang image that forms the central core of the micrograph on the front of this book serves as a symbolic reflection of the book's subtitle: production, maturation, fertilization, regeneration. Indeed, the genomic and proteomic eras have heralded a new age for investigation of the spermatozoon and amazing results are being found. The ultimate chapter in this book details of how sperm are born and, yes, can be reborn from embryonic stem cell precursors.

It is our hope that this dynamic volume will serve as a cornerstone resource for all students and research workers whether new to the field or experienced. We believe it will serve as a key resource for and a reflection of the outstanding invigorated research activity taking place in this exciting field.

Christopher De Jonge
Christopher L.R. Barratt

List of contributors

R. John Aitken
ARC Centre of Excellence in Biotechnology
and Development, and Discipline of
Biological Sciences
University of Newcastle
University Drive
Callaghan, NSW
Australia

Liga Bennetts
Discipline of Biological Sciences
The University of Newcastle
Callaghan, NSW
Australia

Christopher L.R. Barratt
Reproductive Biology and
Genetics Group
Division of Reproductive and
Child Health
University of Birmingham
Edgbaston, Birmingham
England, UK

Assisted Conception Unit,
Birmingham Women's Hospital
Edgbaston, Birmingham
England, UK

Amander T. Clark
Program in Human Embryonic Stem Cell
Biology

Center for Reproductive Sciences
University of California
San Francisco, CA, USA

Departments of Obstetrics, Gynecology and
Reproductive Sciences, Physiology and
Urology
Programs in Developmental and Stem Cell
Biology and Human Genetics
University of California
San Francisco, CA, USA

Sarah J. Conner
Reproductive Biology and Genetics Group
Division of Reproductive and Child Health
University of Birmingham
Edgbaston, Birmingham
England, UK

Trevor G. Cooper
Institute of Reproductive Medicine of the
University
Münster
Germany

Christopher J. De Jonge
Department of Obstetrics, Gynecology and
Women's Health
Division of Reproductive Endocrinology
and Infertility
University of Minnesota
Minneapolis, MN, USA

Mark S. Fox
Program in Human Embryonic Stem Cell
Biology
Center for Reproductive Sciences
University of California
San Francisco, CA, USA

Departments of Obstetrics, Gynecology and
Reproductive Sciences, Physiology and
Urology
Programs in Developmental and Stem Cell
Biology and Human Genetics
University of California
San Francisco, CA, USA

Daniel Franken
Department of Obstetrics and Gynecology
Reproductive Biology Unit
Tygerberg Hospital
University of Stellenbosch
Capetown
Republic of South Africa

Bart M. Gadella
Department of Biochemistry and Cell
Biology, and Farm Animal Health
Faculty of Veterinary Medicine
Utrecht University
Yalelaan, Utrecht
The Netherlands

Claude Gagnon
Urology Research Laboratory, H 6.47
Royal Victoria Hospital
Montréal, Qué
Canada

Sophie La Salle
Department of Pharmacology and
Therapeutics
McGill University

Montreal Children's Hospital Research
Institute
Montreal, Quebec
Canada

Eve de Lamirande
Urology Research Laboratory
Royal Victoria Hospital and Faculty of
Medicine
McGill University, Montréal
Canada

Gaurishankar Manandhar
Division of Animal Sciences
University of Missouri–Columbia
Columbia, MO, USA

Sergio Oehninger
Department of Obstetrics and Gynecology
The Jones Institute for Reproductive Medicine
Eastern Virginia Medical School
Norfolk, VA, USA

Renee A. Reijo Pera
Program in Human Embryonic Stem Cell
Biology
University of California, San Francisco
San Francisco, CA, USA

Jeffrey A. Shaman
Department of Anatomy and
Reproductive Biology
Institute for Biogenesis Research
John A. Burns School of Medicine
University of Hawaii at Manoa
Honolulu, HI, USA

Shai Shefi
Department of Urology
University of California San Francisco
San Francisco, CA, USA

Peter Sutovsky
Division of Animal Sciences, and
Departments of Obstetrics and Gynecology
University of Missouri–Columbia
Columbia, MO, USA

Jacquetta M. Trasler
Departments of Pediatrics, Human Genetics
and Pharmacology and Therapeutics
McGill University
Montreal Children's Hospital Research
Institute
Montreal, Quebec
Canada

Paul J. Turek
Department of Urology
University of California San Francisco
San Francisco, CA, USA

Pablo E. Visconti
Department of Veterinary and Animal
Sciences
University of Massachusetts
Amherst, MA, USA

Peter H. Vogt
Section Molecular Genetics and Infertility
Department of Gynecology
Endocrinology and Reproductive
Medicine
University of Heidelberg
Heidelberg
Germany

W. Steven Ward
Department of Anatomy and Reproductive
Biology
Institute for Biogenesis Research
John A. Burns School of Medicine
University of Hawaii at Manoa
Honolulu, HI, USA

Ching-Hei Yeung
Institute of Reproductive Medicine
of the University
Münster
Germany

Mammalian spermatogenesis and sperm structure: anatomical and compartmental analysis

Peter Sutovsky[1,2] and Gaurishankar Manandhar[1]

[1]Division of Animal Sciences
[2]Departments of Obstetrics & Gynecology, University of Missouri–Columbia, Columbia, USA

Detailed theoretical analysis, using mathematical modeling, reveals that sex is a very inefficient way of reproducing. The inefficiency lies in making male offspring. In the majority of sexual species, only the female contributes energy and resources to the young. In contrast the males rarely contribute more than the minimum-a tiny sperm carrying genes, but devoid of other resources.

The Evolution of Life, edited by Linda Gamlin and Gail Vanes, Oxford University Press, New York, 1987

1.1 Introduction

What is said above argues that the male contribution at fertilization is restricted to one half of future embryonic chromosomes. Although inspired by general perception and often perpetuated by popular science, this assumption is incorrect. Besides being a launching pad for the remaining chapters of this tome, the goal of the present chapter is to demonstrate that the male germ cell, the spermatozoon, is well suited to make other important contributions to the zygote and embryo. Studying spermatogenesis allows us to show how the unique, paternally contributed resources are generated during the intricate and fascinating process of spermatogenesis. In a show of male vanity, we decided to take a somewhat unconventional approach to this treatise on spermatogenesis and sperm structure by putting the emphasis of paternal contributions made at fertilization. We thus focus mainly on the later stages of spermatogenesis, during which the haploid, somatic-cell like round spermatid is transformed into a specialized, nearly cytoplasm-free spermatozoon capable of acquiring progressive motility and fertilizing an ovum in the oviductal environment. During the ensuing fertilization and zygote development, the seemingly stripped-down spermatozoon contributes not only the paternal chromosomes, but also a centrosome, perinuclear material and perhaps even messenger ribonucleic acid (mRNA) to the zygote, and triggers oocyte activation, thus activating the maternal resources stored in the ooplasm. The differentiation of male and female germ cells results in the production of gametes that carry a reciprocal, non-overlapping complement of unique organelles and molecules not found in any other cell type. The purpose of selective elimination of certain cellular organelles and of the adaptation of other organelles during gametogenesis is to form two compatible cells with complementary endowments that, when brought together at fertilization, give rise to a zygote capable of developing into a new individual. Thus, the oocyte multiplies its cytoplasmic volume to accommodate a stockpile of mRNAs, proteins and other molecules required for zygote survival prior to oocyte-to-embryo transition and full activation of embryonic genome. The spermatozoon, in contrast, forfeits most of its cytoplasm and organelles to transform into a motile cell capable of surviving and functioning outside of the male reproductive system (Fig. 1.1).

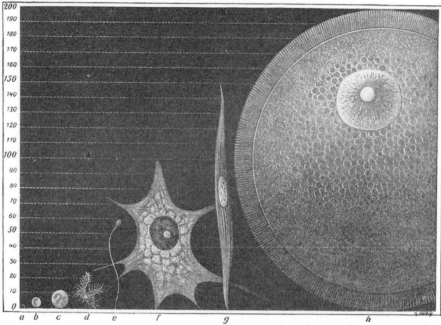

Aus Kahn, Leben des Menschen, Franckh'sche Verlagsbuchhandlung, Stuttgart

Abb. 19.

Figure 1.1   Illustration from an early 20th century book showing the comparison of cell size of a spermatozoon with that of an oocyte. The differentiation of male and female germ cells results in the production of gametes, highly specialized cells with unique features not found in any other cell type. The purpose of selective elimination of certain cellular organelles and of the adaptation of other organelles is to form two cells with complementary endowments that, when brought together at fertilization, give rise to a zygote capable of developing into a new individual. From *Wolf F (1928)*

Given the format and space limitations, this chapter is not intended to provide exhaustive information on mammalian spermatogenesis and sperm structure. For this purpose, we would like to refer the readers to a number of excellent monographies on this topic (e.g. Fawcett, 1975; Barth and Oko, 1989; Russell *et al.*, 1990; Hess and Moore, 1993; de Kretser and Kerr, 1994).

1.2 Structure and function of mammalian spermatozoon

To fully appreciate the mechanism of sperm biogenesis (i.e. spermatogenesis and spermiogenesis), it is important to briefly review the subcellular structure and function of the mammalian spermatozoon (reviewed by Fawcett, 1975). The spermatozoon (Fig. 1.2) is composed of a sperm head and sperm tail or flagellum. Both sperm head and sperm tail are covered by sperm plasma membrane, or plasmalemma. The rodent sperm head is hook-shaped (falciform), while ungulate, carnivore and primate sperm heads are spatula-shaped (spatulate). A major distinction between ungulate and rodent spermatozoon is the complete absence of a sperm centrosome and centrioles in the rodents, as opposed to a reduced form of centrosome with a single proximal centriole in the ungulates. As described below, all eutherian mammals share the other general features of the sperm head and sperm tail.

1.2.1 Sperm head

Progressing from inside-out, the sperm head is composed of a nucleus, in which the deoxyribonucleic acid (DNA) condensing core and linker histones have been partially replaced during spermiogenesis by protamines, positively charged DNA proteins that convey the hypercondensation of the sperm nucleus into a compact, hydrodynamic shape permissive of sperm motility and sperm penetration through egg vestments (Brewer *et al.*, 2002; Dadoune, 2003). The nucleus is covered by a reduced nuclear envelope (NE), from which the nuclear pore complexes (NPC) have been removed during spermiogenesis, except for some redundant NEs with NPC found in some species at the base of the sperm nucleus (Ho and Suarez, 2003). Protection is afforded to the sperm nucleus by the perinuclear theca (PT), sometimes referred to as 'perinuclear matrix,' forming a rigid shell composed of disulfide bond-stabilized structural proteins amalgamated with various other protein molecules (Oko, 1995), some of which function in cell signaling once they are released by PT dissolution into oocyte cytoplasm at fertilization (Sutovsky *et al.*, 2003). Sperm PT can be divided into three segments that mirror three major segments of the sperm head and serve unique functions during fertilization:
(1) Subacrosomal layer underlies the acrosomal segment of the sperm head and functions to anchor the acrosome, a Golgi-derived vesicle that forms a cap on the proximal hemisphere of the sperm head and harbors proteases and

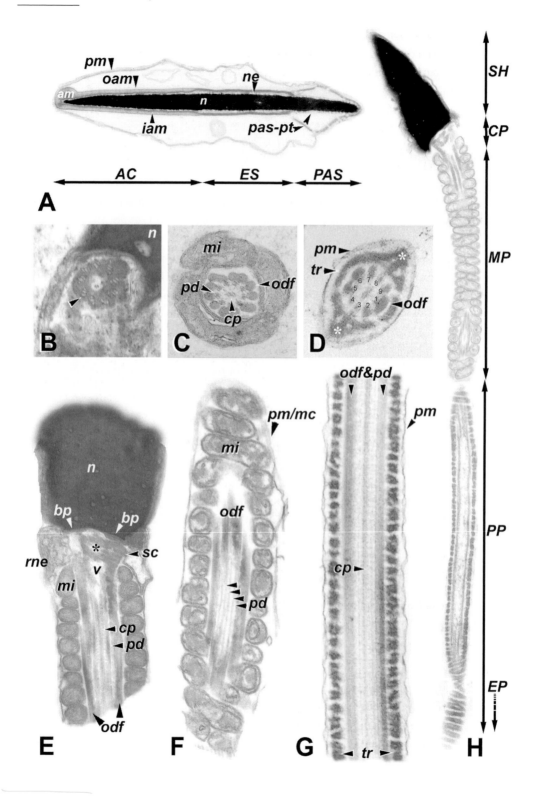

receptors required for sperm interaction with the zona pellucida of the oocyte. The inner and outer acrosomal membranes (IAM and OAM, respectively) are recognized, holding inside a dense acrosomal matrix containing the aforementioned proteases necessary for digesting a fertilization slit in the zona pellucida (ZP) (reviewed by Gerton, 2002; Yoshinaga and Toshimori, 2003). The subacrosomal PT is fused with the IAM and probably stabilizes receptor molecules on the IAM that are necessary for secondary binding of the sperm head to egg zona pellucida after acrosomal exocytosis. At fertilization, the IAM remains patent while the OAM is lost to vesiculation during acrosomal exocytosis induced by the binding of sperm plasmalemma/OAM complex to the ZP3 protein, the sperm receptor on egg zona pellucida (Fig. 1.2).

Figure 1.2   *Fine structure of the mammalian spermatozoon.* (A) Undulated sperm membranes after processing for transmission electron microscopy reveal fine structure of the mammalian sperm head in this sagittal section spanning all of equatorial segment (*ES*) and parts of the acrosomal region (*AC*) and postacrosomal sheath (*PAS*). Sperm head is covered by a plasma membrane (*pm*). In the *AC*, *pm* is closely associated with *oam* forming the acrosomal cap with acrosomal matrix (*am*) overlying the *iam*. The narrow space between the *iam* and *ne* in the *AC*, and between the *pm* and *ne* in all other segments of the sperm heads is occupied by *PT*, shown here in the post acrosomal sheath (*pas-pt*). Sperm nucleus (*n*) spans all three segments of the sperm head. (B–G) Cross-sections and longitudinal sections of the sperm tail connecting piece (B, E), midpiece (C, F) and principal piece (D, G). Connecting piece (B, E) harbors the proximal centriole (E; *) composed of nine microtubule triplets (B; arrowhead) and the empty vault (*v*) left after the degradation of the distal centriole during spermiogenesis. Neither centriole would be present in a cross-section of mouse spermatozoon, in which both centrioles are degraded during spermiogenesis. The proximal centriole is caged in the striated columns (*sc*) a direct continuation of outer dense fibers (*odf*) paralleled by peripheral microtubule doublets (*pd*) of the flagellar axoneme centered around a central pair (*cp*) of microtubules. This connecting piece structure is covered by redundant nuclear envelopes (*rne*) found proximally of the first mitochondria (*mi*) of the mitochondrial sheath. The midpiece (C, F) is wrapped in a helix of sperm *mi* covering the axoneme composed of nine *odf*, nine peripheral microtubule doublets (*pd*) and one central pair of microtubules (*cp*). This axonemal arrangement is retained distally in the principal piece (D, G) wherein it is covered by the fibrous sheath composed of two longitudinal columns (* in D) that run parallel to *odf* #3 and #8, as numbered counterclockwise in D. Longitudinal columns are interconnected by paired transversal ribs (*tr*) throughout the length of fibrous sheath. All sperm tail segments are covered by plasma membrane (*pm*). Sperm tail is connected to sperm head midpiece by the basal plate (*bp*) of the implantation fossa. (H) General structure of the spermatozoon is divided into five major parts: Sperm head (*SH*), and sperm tail connecting piece (*CP*), midpiece (*MP*), principal piece (*PP*) and end piece (*EP*)

(2) Equatorial segment is a folded-over complex of PT, OAM and IAM, that carries receptor molecules involved in the initial binding of the sperm head to egg plasma membrane, oolemma, once the fertilizing spermatozoon penetrates through the ZP and reaches the perivitelline space. Putative receptor molecules involved in sperm–oolemma binding, such as equatorin/MN9 (Toshimori *et al.*, 1992) are present in this region.

(3) Postacrosomal sheath (PAS) of the sperm PT is believed to harbor a complex of signaling proteins collectively referred to as SOAF, or the sperm borne, oocyte activating factors (reviewed by Sutovsky *et al.*, 2003). After sperm head fusion with the oolemma, some of the SOAF molecules disperse across the ooplasm to trigger the signaling pathway leading to oocyte activation and initiation of zygotic development, while other PAS-released molecules may remain associated with the sperm nucleus as it is transformed into a male pronucleus.

1.2.2 Sperm flagellum

The sperm tail or flagellum provides a motile force for the spermatozoon, which is based upon a unique 9 + 2 arrangement of microtubules within the sperm flagellar axoneme. The 9 + 2 arrangement refers to nine peripheral, symmetrically arranged microtubule doublets connected doublet-to-doublet by dynein arms and to the sheath of central pair of microtubules by radial spokes. The outer doublets, but not the central pair, are paralleled by nine outer dense fibers that provide flexible, yet firm support during flagellar movement. Topologically, the sperm tail can be divided into four major segments that share a common innermost structure of the microtubule-based axoneme paralleled by nine outer dense fibers, but differ in their external substructure. Progressing from proximal to distal end, these segments include:

(1) Connecting piece is composed of nine striated or segmented columns that are a direct continuation of the outer dense fibers in the other flagellar segments. Caged inside these nine columns is the dense mass of capitulum, which in most mammals, except rodents, contains the sperm (proximal) centriole, a remnant of the bi-centriolar centrosome found in early haploid spermatogenic cells. As we will discuss below, the complete degradation of both centrioles during spermiogenesis distinguishes rodents from ungulates, carnivores and primates. The basal plate provides the connection between the proximal terminus of the connecting piece and the implantation fossa of the sperm head.

(2) Midpiece is covered by the mitochondrial sheath in form of a helix of approximately 75–100 sperm mitochondria, which generate the energy for sperm flagellar motility. Each sperm mitochondrion carries multiple copies of the paternal mitochondrial genome. For reasons perhaps related to mutagenic oxidative stress encountered by the maturing and fertilization spermatozoon,

these paternal mitochondria with paternal mitochondrial DNA (mtDNA) appear to be eliminated by targeted proteolysis inside the fertilized ovum (reviewed by Sutovsky *et al.*, 2004b).

(3) Principal piece is separated from the midpiece by the annulus or Jensen's ring, a traverse ring of dense material found distal to the mitochondrial sheath. The principal piece is covered by the protective scaffold of fibrous sheath, composed of two longitudinal columns running parallel to outer dense fibers three and eight (see Fig. 1.2D), connected on both sides by a series of transverse ribs. The fibrous sheath provides support for the sperm axoneme. At the same time, proteins within the fibrous sheath seem to sequester protein kinases necessary for the process of sperm capacitation and hyperactivation prior to fertilization (Eddy *et al.*, 2003).

(4) End piece contains axonemal doublets and the ends of outer dense fibers and fibrous sheath.

1.3 Spermatogenesis

The purpose of spermatogenesis is to establish and maintain daily output of fully differentiated spermatozoa that in eutherian mammals ranges from >200 million in man to 2–3 billion in bull. This massive sperm production requires the unique architecture of the seminiferous epithelium, a self-contained system that is well-isolated from the blood stream, allowing only selective uptake of paracrine factors. Also unique to the reproductive system and germ line is that it is relatively quiescent and not fully differentiated prior to the onset of puberty.

1.3.1 Germ cell migration and establishment of seminiferous epithelium

The foundation of spermatogenesis is laid as early as day 7.5 *post coitum* in the mouse. At this time, the primordial germ cells (PGC) begin their migration from *epiblast* to the hind gut (Clark and Eddy, 1975). Once the PGCs colonize the genital ridge, they begin forming seminiferous cords that will eventually give rise to seminiferous tubules (Byskov and Høyer, 1994). In a fully differentiated testis, 12–20 seminiferous tubules form loops with both ends anchored in the rete testis of the testicular mediastinum. Coincident with mitotic arrest at birth, the PGCs within the seminiferous tubules became the non-proliferative A-type spermatogonia that are mitotically quiescent until the peri-pubertal period (Fig. 1.3). At that time, the increased production of gonadotropic hormones induces a massive mitotic proliferation of A-type spermatogonia, paralleled by testicular descent and the differentiation of A-type spermatogonia into B-type spermatogonia competent to enter meiosis. To sustain sperm production, spermatogenic stem cells undergo perpetual renewal. Thus an A-type spermatogonium could commit either to renewal or to

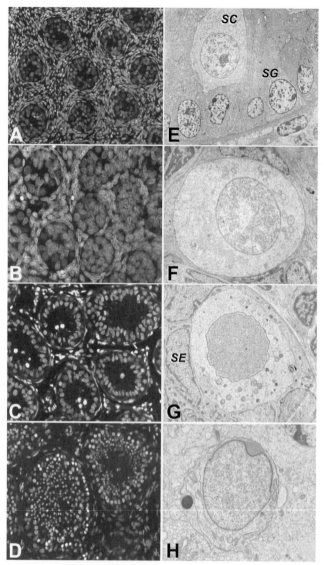

Figure 1.3   *Developmental, histological and ultrastructural study of spermatogenesis in the rhesus
monkey.* Fetal testis (A, B, E) shows large proportion of stromal cells and small seminiferous
tubules harboring mostly spermatogonia (*SG*), occasional pre-leptotene spermatocytes (*SC*)
and few Sertoli cells. Juvenile testis (C, F, G) contains enlarged seminiferous tubules with
occasional preleptotene spermatocytes (F, G) surrounded by *SG* and Sertoli cells (G, *SE*).
Adult testis shows large seminiferous tubules with all stages of spermatogenic cycle (D)
including the haploid spermatids (H). Panels A–D represent testicular tissue sections stained
with DNA-binding fluorochrome DAPI and viewed in epifluorescence microscope. Panels
E–H represent ultra-thin sections examined by transmission electron microscope. Necropsy
tissue specimens courtesy of Oregon National Primate Research Center, Beaverton, OR

differentiation. Continuous production of spermatozoa is maintained throughout the reproductive lifespan of eutherian mammals roughly at the rate of hundreds of millions per day. Such a massive proliferation and differentiation requires a certain degree of quality control that may be assured by programmed cell death, or apoptosis (Sinha-Hikim and Swerdloff, 1999).

1.3.2 Architecture of the seminiferous epithelium and blood-testis barrier

Unique architecture of the seminiferous tubule affords the seminiferous epithelium with both the influx of necessary nutrients and a relative autonomy from the body's immune defense, maintained by blood-testis barrier. Progressing from the outer diameter of the seminiferous tubule, enveloped in a basement membrane (BM), we observe A-type spermatogonia adjacent intimately to the BM, and B-type spermatogonia that sometime show only a small area of contact with the BM. This compartment also contains the basal pole of Sertoli cells and is referred to as the basal compartment. Moving towards the lumen, primary spermatocytes penetrate the blood-testis barrier formed by diverse cell–cell junctions between adjacent cytoplasmic projections of Sertoli cells (Johnson and Boekelheide, 2002a, b) and enter the adluminal compartment in which meiosis and spermiogenesis occur. This selective, semi-permeable barrier prevents immune system cells from infiltrating the lumen of seminiferous epithelium, which is considered an immune privileged site. Such an arrangement prevents the coating of highly antigenic sperm surface with antibodies that could hinder their function during sperm maturation, transit and fertilization.

1.3.3 Spermatogenic cycle of seminiferous epithelium

The cycle of seminiferous epithelium refers to synchronous evolution of one stage of spermatogenesis to the next (Barth and Oko, 1989), or a complete, ordered series of cell associations, stages, which occur in a given segment of a seminiferous epithelium over time (Russell *et al.*, 1990). Segment refers to a portion of seminiferous tubule occupied by one such association. Based on the type of spermatogenic cells present on a single cross-section of the seminiferous tubule at a given stage of the cycle of seminiferous epithelium (Fig. 1.4), individual authors recognize between 12–14 stages of seminiferous epithelium in rodents, 8 stages in carnivores, 12 stages in ungulates and 6–12 stages in primates. In human testis, six stages are recognized and in contrast to most animals, up to three distinct stages can be observed within the same cross-section of a human seminiferous tubule. Demarcation lines can be drawn to divide each cross-section into three distinct wedges, each containing one cellular association corresponding to one step of spermatogenesis. Roman numerals I–VI (I–XIV in other species) are assigned to these stages. Barth and Oko (1989) recognize four distinct types of A-spermatogonia (A_0, A_1, A_2, A_3), one intermediate

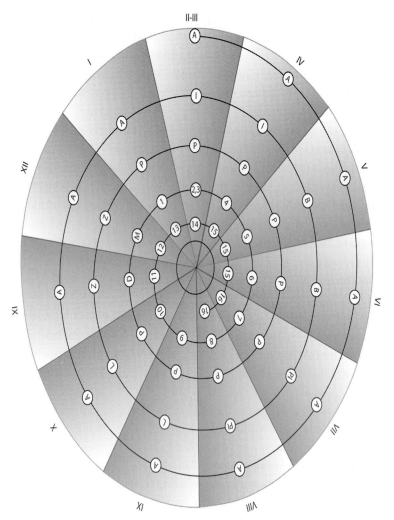

Figure 1.4   *Cycle of the seminiferous epithelium.* Mouse is shown as an example. Each of the
12 stages (I–XII) is characterized by unique association of diploid and haploid cells
progressing from the circumference of the circle, representing the basal compartment,
towards its center, representing the adluminal compartment of the seminiferous tubule
cross-section. A = A-type *SG*; I = intermediate type *SG*; B = B-type *SG*; Pl = pre-leptotene
spermatocytes; L = leptotene spermatocytes; Z = zygotene spermatocytes; P = pachytene
spermatocytes; D = diplotene; M = meiotic, dividing spermatocytes with fully condensed
chromosomes. Arabic numerals 1–16 refer to steps 1–16 of spermiogenesis in haploid
cells, spermatids. It is assumed that renewing spermatogenic stem cells are present at
all stages depicted here. The time length of different stages varies from species to
species, for example ranging from 7 hours (stages IX, X, XI) to 58 hours (stage VII) in rat
(Russell *et al.*, 1990)

type and two B-types (B$_1$ and B$_2$). Spermatocytes are dividend into preleptotene, leptotene, zygotene and pachytene primary spermatocytes, and secondary spermatocytes. This division is based on the position of spermatocytes within the seminiferous tubules and on the progression of meiotic prophase, as reflected by the presence of heterochromatin and synaptonemal complexes in sperm nuclei. The haploid stage of spermatogenesis is further divided into 14–19 steps, characterized by the advancement of sperm accessory structure biogenesis and progressive shedding of the redundant spermatogenic cytoplasm. At each given stage of spermatogenesis, a precisely defined association of haploid and diploid spermatogenic cells is present in a given cross-section of seminiferous tubule. For example, at stage VI of the spermatogenic cell cycle, the presence of B-type spermatogonia is associated with pachytene spermatocytes, step 6 round spermatids and step 15 elongating spermatids in mouse. To facilitate the recognition of individual stages, it is worth pointing that in mouse, stages II–VIII contain five different cell types including a spermatid of step 1–7 and an elongated spermatid of step 13–16. At the same time, stages I and IX–XII contain only four cell types including spermatogonia, spermatocytes and elongating spermatids (Fig. 1.4). Detailed description of seminiferous epithelium staging in mouse, rat and dog can be found in Russell *et al.* (1990). Bull spermatogenesis, in which stages I–VI contain five different cell types and stages VII–XII four cell types, is depicted in Barth and Oko (1989).

The unique architecture of seminiferous epithelium, based on the succession of spermatogonia, spermatocytes and spermatids from BM toward the lumen of seminiferous tubule is established in a stepwise manner during postnatal development. Subsequently, we can only find Sertoli cells, spermatogonia and preleptotene spermatocytes in a newborn mammal. Advanced spermatocytes (leptotene, zygotene, pachytene and dividing ones) and spermatids appear in the peri-pubertal and adult testis only (see Fig. 1.3). Such a succession greatly facilitates developmental expression profiling of sperm proteins. For example, in order to learn at which stage of spermatogenesis a particular protein is present, it would be necessary to harvest proteins or mRNAs from all appropriate stages of spermatogenic cell development. Instead of using labor intensive separation of individual spermatogenic cell types from an adult testis, one can simply harvest testicular tissue from young rodent animals at each week after birth up to day 35–42 and examine by subtractive analysis when the mRNA or protein in question first appears in the total testicular cell lysate by Southern blotting, hybridization *in situ* or Western blotting, respectively.

1.3.4 Spermatogenic wave of seminiferous epithelium

The wave of the seminiferous epithelium can be defined as the arrangement of the successive stages of cycle along the length of the seminiferous tubule. The progression of the spermatogenic cycle of the seminiferous epithelium is not synchronized along the length of the seminiferous tubule, but rather is distributed in distinct waves because each seminiferous tubule is a loop with both ends open to the rete testis. At each end, the order of segments starts at the highest stage and descends to stage I. Hence, the two descending orders have to meet somewhere in the middle of the loop. For example, if we start at in the segment of tubule displaying stage XII, the next stage along the length of tubule will be stage XI, then X, IX, etc., until we reach a cross-section displaying stage I. From this point, the stages will repeat this descending order starting by stage XII. However, this general rule is reversed in specific segments of seminiferous tubule in which the modulation of the wave occurs. This means that within the modulation segment, a stage of seminiferous tubule is flanked by stages of one order-up on both sides (e.g. XII, XI, X, XI, XII instead of XII, XI, X, IX, VIII). This assures an even distribution of all stages throughout the seminiferous epithelium and an uninterrupted, stable daily output of fully differentiated testicular spermatozoa.

1.3.5 Proliferative and meiotic phase of spermatogenesis

Spermatogenesis requires continuous differentiation and renewal of male germ cells. Successive mitotic divisions of the spermatogenic stem cells and spermatogonia, referred to as proliferative phase, assure renewal. This implies two distinct fates for a germ cell: either it undergoes mitosis to duplicate itself, or it enters meiosis to reduce in half its chromosomal complement and to differentiate into a spermatozoon. This later phase is referred to as the meiotic phase. Temporally, these two phases can either be viewed as concomitant (renewal and differentiation occurs at the same time within each segment of seminiferous tubule containing an association of four or five distinct germ cell types), or sequential (in time, proliferative phase is followed by meiotic phase in each individual germ cell). Spatially, the proliferative phase occurs in the nutrient rich basal compartment, while the differentiating cells within the adluminal compartment are sheltered from immune defense by the blood-testis barrier.

1.3.6 Haploid phase of spermatogenesis: spermiogenesis and spermiation

Haploid phase stands out within the context of spermatogenesis because this is when the somatic-cell like germ cells acquire unique sperm accessory structures that are necessary for the detachment of these cells from the seminiferous tubules, acquisition of fertilizing potential, transit through the female reproductive tract and fertilization of the oocyte. This last part of spermatogenesis can be divided into spermiogenesis, or spermatid elongation phase, during which the haploid spermatid generates sperm accessory structures, and spermiation, a process during which the remnants of germ cell cytoplasm are rejected and the fully differentiated spermatozoa detach from the seminiferous epithelium. Based on the biogenesis of individual sperm accessory structures and on the progression of sperm nuclear condensation, spermiogenesis can be divided into distinct steps, recognized by Arabic numerals. Individual authors distinguish up to 19 steps in rat, 16 steps in mouse, 14 steps in ungulates and in primates, and 12 steps in carnivores. Based on acrosomal biogenesis, Oko and Barth (1989) divide bull spermiogenesis into Golgi phase (step 1–3), acrosomal cap phase (step 4–7), acrosome phase (step 8–12) and maturation phase (steps 13 and 14).

During spermiogenesis, a somatic cell-like, but haploid round spermatid transforms into a highly specialized spermatozoon capable of acquiring progressive motility after epididymal sperm maturation and fertilizing potential after interacting with oviductal fluid and epithelia. Such an extensive remodeling process requires that the biogenesis of novel, transient or permanent accessory structures be synchronized with the remodeling, reduction or complete degradation of select spermatid organelles. This requires transcription, translation and post-translational modification of many constitutive and germ cell-specific gene products during the last outburst of transcriptional and translational activity during the early steps of spermiogenesis (Kleene et al., 1993; Eddy, 2002; Dadoune et al., 2004). At the organelle level, the formation of sperm accessory structures includes the derivation of acrosomal cap/acrosome from the Golgi (Moreno et al., 2000), the amalgamation of spermatid cytosol into sperm head skeleton, the PT (Oko, 1995), and the formation of the sperm axoneme with outer dense fibers and fibrous sheath (Oko, 1998). Sperm head shaping and sperm nuclear hypercondensation are achieved by the removal of histones, which includes their sequential displacement by transitional proteins and replacement by protamines (Meistrich et al., 2003). Concomitantly, the spermatid centrosome, composed of two perpendicularly apposed centrioles and a halo of microtubule-nucleating pericentriolar material, is reduced to a single, proximal centriole of a mature spermatozoon, embedded in a dense mass of capitulum (Sutovsky et al., 1999a). This is achieved by the degradation of the distal centriole once it helps growing the axonemal microtubule doublets (Manandhar et al., 1998). In mouse, both the proximal and the distal centrioles are degraded during spermatogenesis (Manandhar et al., 1998). Approximately one half of spermatid mitochondria are rejected during spermiogenesis while the other half acquires a reinforced outer mitochondrial membrane, the mitochondrial capsule (Cataldo et al., 1996), and are rearranged into a helical mitochondrial sheath. Similar to centrosome and mitochondria, the sperm NE is reduced rather than completely removed during spermiogenesis, as its NPC are removed during spermatid elongation (Sutovsky et al., 1999b).

Hardly could a more befitting description be found for the process of spermiogenesis than the epitome *Construction for the sake of destruction* (Glickman and

Chiechanover, 2002), providing a title of extensive review of the proteolytic ubiquitin system. During spermiogenesis, many organelles and proteins are recycled to
provide space and building blocks for the developing sperm accessory structures.
Ubiquitin-dependent proteolysis is indeed central to the process of spermiogenesis.
Ubiquitin is an evolutionarily conserved chaperone protein that binds covalently to
other proteins to mark them for proteolytic degradation by the 26 S proteasome, a
multi-subunit protease. Ubiquitin-substrate ligation and subsequent formation of
multi-ubiquitin chains are catalyzed by ubiquitin activating enzyme E1, ubiquitin
carrier E2 and a variety of substrate-specific ubiquitin ligases (E3 and E4 enzymes).
Proteasomal degradation of the ubiquitinated substrate is paralleled by the release
of polyubiquitin chains from which monoubiquitin is regenerated by ubiquitin
C-terminal hydrolases. Ubiquitin system and proteasomal subunits are expressed at
all stages in the male germ cell line (Agell and Mezquita, 1988; Wing *et al.*, 1996;
Baarends *et al.*, 1999; Wojcik *et al.*, 2000). In particular, ubiquitination and proteasomal degradation is instrumental in spermatid elongation (Kierszenbaum, 2002;
Escalier *et al.*, 2003), as also illustrated by ubiquitin-C promoter driven expression
of green fluorescence protein in the transgenic mouse testis (Color plate 1E).
Genetic ablation of ubiquitin-system enzymes at this phase of spermatogenesis
results in male infertility (Baarends *et al.*, 2003; Escalier *et al.*, 2003; Kwon *et al.*,
2003). Known ubiquitinated spermatid substrates include histones H2A and H3
(Chen *et al.*, 1998; Baarends *et al.*, 1999), which are degraded after being replaced in
the spermatid nucleus by protamines. Ubiquitination of the sperm mitochondrial
membrane protein prohibitin (Thompson *et al.*, 2003) may serve as a recognition
signal for the degradation of paternal mitochondria after fertilization. Other likely
ubiquitin-substrates at this stage are nucleolar ribonucleoproteins and NPC proteins,
nucleoporins that are removed from the spermatid NE (Sutovsky *et al.*, 1999b).

   Some unique structures and molecules appear transiently during spermiogenesis and disappear once the spermatozoon is fully differentiated. These include:

(1) Transitional proteins (TP1, TP2) that are intermediate DNA binding proteins
      during histone-protamine exchange in spermatid nucleus (Meistrich
      et al., 2003).

(2) Pro-acrosomal granules that are produced by the Golgi at step 1–3 of spermio-
      genesis and eventually docked to the apical surface of the sperm nucleus to form
      the nascent acrosomal granule and later acrosomal cap (Fig. 1.5).

(3) Caudal manchette (Plate 1A), a veil-like structure formed by microtubule
      nucleation around the nascent equatorial segment of step 7–12 spermatids
      (mouse).

The manchette is thought to contribute a mechanical force shaping the spermatid
nucleus into sperm nucleus and to shuttle newly synthesized proteins from the spermatid cytoplasmic lobe to the PAS where they are deposited into PT. The nuage or

chromatoid body, a dense homogeneous mass of unknown function found within the cytoplasmic lobe. Both the manchette and the chromatoid body harbor proteasomes, and thus could be degradation or repository sites for proteins removed from spermatid nucleus and NE during spermatid elongation (Kierszenbaum, 2002; Haraguchi *et al.*, 2005).

Throughout the process of spermiogenesis, the germ cells remain associated with Sertoli cells via cell–cell junctions and with each other via cytoplasmic bridges. Spermiogenesis is concluded at spermiation, when fully differentiated spermatozoa detach from each other and from the apical surface of seminiferous epithelium and travel through the lumen of the seminiferous tubule to the rete testis (Guraya, 1995). At this time, the cytoplasmic lobe is shed in the form of the residual body, leaving the last minute remnant of the spermatid cytoplasm, the cytoplasmic droplet (CD), wrapped around the sperm tail connecting piece. While the residual body is phagocytosed in the testis by Sertoli cells, the CD remains associated with the sperm tail connecting piece during sperm transit through rete testis and efferent ducts. This connecting piece-associated CD, composed mainly of Golgi-derived membranous vesicles and saccules (Oko *et al.*, 1993), is termed the proximal CD. During epididymal sperm maturation and passage of spermatozoa from caput to corpus epididymis, the CD slides down the midpiece to stop at the annulus, at which time it is referred to as the distal CD (reviewed by Cooper and Yeung, 1993). In most mammals, the CD is shed by the time spermatozoa reach the cauda epididymis, or shortly after ejaculation. Domestic boar semen often contains a large proportion of spermatozoa with CD, an occurrence that has an adverse effect on boar fertility (Kuster *et al.*, 2004).

1.3.7 Regulation of spermatogenesis

At the paracrine level, spermatogenesis is controlled by the secretion of hypothalamic gonadotropin releasing hormone (GnRH) that stimulates the secretion of follicle stimulating hormone (FSH) and luteinizing hormone (LH) from the pituitary gland (McLachlan, 2000). LH is though to be primarily responsible for stimulating the secretion of testosterone by Leydig cells located in the testicular stroma. Multiple intrinsic factor produced within the seminiferous epithelium (reviewed by Lacham-Kaplan, 2004) include, for example, stem cell renewal and sustenance factors such as c-kit tyrosine kinase receptor and its ligand, the stem cell factor produced mainly in the PGCs and spermatogonia (Sette *et al.*, 2000), tr-kit expressed in postmeiotic spermatids (Rosi *et al.*, 2000), BMP-4 (Ying and Zhao, 2001) and various transcription factors such as Creb/Crem (Don and Stelzer, 2004) and Oct3/4 (Yeom *et al.*, 1996). With regard to quality control, DNA repair molecules including E3-type ubiquitin ligase Hr6B (Baarends *et al.*, 2003), gonadotropin-regulated testicular ribonucleic acid (RNA) helicase GRTH/Ddx25 and DNA-repair protein Dmc1 (Tsai-Morris

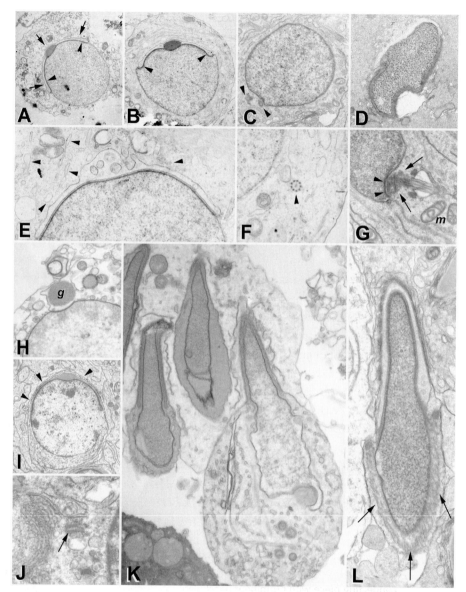

Figure 1.5 *Biogenesis of the sperm accessory structures during spermiogenesis.* Ultrathin sections of
rhesus monkey (A–G) and bull (H–L) testis were examined under transmission electron
microscope. (A, B) Floating and indented forms of acrosomal cap (arrows) in step 5–6
spermatids. Dark layer under the cap (arrowheads) is the nascent subacrosomal PT.
(C) Implantation of the nascent sperm tail (arrowheads) at the posterior pole of a step 7
spermatid nucleus. (D) Chromatin condensation in step 9–10 spermatid. Histone-
protamine exchange is in progress at this step. (E) Acrosomal cap in step 3 spermatid.
Acrosomal granule is not visible in this section capturing Golgi vesicles and stacks
(arrowheads) from which the membranes of the cap are derived. (F) Cross-section of the

et al., 2004), and apoptotic regulators such as Bax, Bcl-2, Fas/ FasL and various cas-pases (Sinha-Hikim *et al.*, 2003) are thought to be involved in spermatogenic qual-ity control and elimination of defective spermatogenic cells by apoptosis. In particular, *bcl-w* gene appears to have a role in somatic and germ cell survival in the testis but not in other tissues (Print *et al.*, 1998). Molecular chaperones (e.g. Hsp 70; Eddy, 1999) and substrate-specific proteases (26S proteasome) are prominently expressed in the testis (reviewed by Sutovsky, 2003). Cell–cell adhesion molecules that deter-mine cell polarity appear to be essential for normal spermiogenesis (Gliki *et al.*, 2004). Novel genes are continually being implicated in the control of spermatogenesis, among them the Y-chromosome associated genes/regions such as RNA-binding motif (*RBM*) and deleted in azoospermia (*DAZ*) (Cooke, 1999; Reijo-Pera, 2000).

1.3.8 Role of the testis in the sustenance of epididymal function

The role of the testis in the control of epididymal function is central to our under-standing of the mechanism of sperm production and epididymal sperm matura-tion. After being shed from the seminiferous epithelium, testicular spermatozoa are transported through rete testis and efferent ducts into the initial segment of the caput epididymis. Sperm transport into and through the epididymis is facilitated by the pressure from sperm mass produced in the testis, active fluid secretion from Sertoli cells and rete testis cells, contractions within testicular capsule and the myoid layer of the seminiferous tubule in the testis, and by the movement of cilia on the ciliated epithelial cells of the efferent ducts (Ilio and Hess, 1994). The mammalian epi-didymis evolved as a means of sperm storage and sustenance, facilitating the acqui-sition of fertilizing potential by the spermatozoa, sperm maturation, completion of sperm morphogenesis and removal of the CD (Bedford, 1979). In addition to sperm production, the mammalian testis exerts control over the sustenance and function-ing of the epididymis. The lumicrine hypothesis (Hinton *et al.*, 2000) postulates that testicular factors are necessary for the maintenance of normal epididymal

Caption for fig. 1.5 (*Cont.*)   nascent axoneme (arrowhead) with 9 + 2 doublets in a step 6–7 spermatid. The ODF and fibrous sheath are not yet developed at this step. (G) Nascent connecting piece with prominent basal plate (arrowheads) and connecting piece structure (arrows) in a step 12 spermatid. Mitochondria (*m*) already began their migration to the site of future mitochondrial sheath. (H) Attachment of the proacrosomal granule (*g*) to the nuclear indentation in the step 3 spermatid nucleus. (I) Step 8 spermatid with a prominent acrosomal cap reaching near the equator of the spermatid nucleus. Note a flattened smooth ER cistern (arrowheads) adjacent to the outer face of acrosomal cap. (J) A centriole (arrow) in the cytoplasm of step 3–4 spermatid. This centriole will later serve as a nucleation center for the polymerization of axonemal microtubules. (K) Step 11 spermatids. Uneven chromatin condensation may be a sign of testicular pathology. (L) Step 10 spermatid with a prominent caudal manchette (arrows)

structure and function. Control of epididymal function is exerted in part by androgens of testicular origin, and possibly by other, non-hormonal factors present in
rete testicular fluid. This hypothesis was tested by orchidectomy, which removes
testosterone and other factors of testicular origin, thus causing male infertility by
changing the architecture of proximal epididymal epithelia (Cyr, 2001). In contrast,
vasectomy does not alter the transmission of testis-secreted factors into epididymis
and, apart from possible induction of anti-sperm antibodies, has lesser effect on
testicular and epididymal function (Flickinger, 1982).

1.4 Changes to sperm structure during fertilization

The elaborate process of spermatogenesis and spermiogenesis, in particular, results
in the formation of specialized sperm accessory structures that afford the spermatozoon its motility and protect it from the environment encountered during sperm
transport through the female reproductive tract and interaction with egg vestments. To achieve motility, the spermatozoon must sacrifice most of its organelles
and most of its cytoplasmic volume. In a complementary manner, the oocyte cytoplasmic volume is multiplied, while some of the crucial components of cell cycle
machinery are reduced to avoid pathological parthenogenetic development.

1.4.1 Complementation of organelle reduction in male and female gametes

The ultimate purpose of spermatogenesis is to generate a vehicle for the transmission
of the paternal genome into the oocyte at fertilization. A remarkable mechanism is in
place, based on complementary, reciprocal reduction of organelles that are necessary
for the union of paternal and maternal genomes into one zygotic genome. Table 1.1
summarizes the biogenesis of sperm accessory structures and their fate after fertilization (reviewed by Sutovsky and Schatten, 2000). The sperm surface membranes,
including the plasma and acrosomal membranes are lost during sperm penetration
through the oocyte zona pellucida and during sperm–egg fusion. The sperm PT dis-
solves in the ooplasm to activate the oocyte. The smooth sperm NE is replaced by a
new, maternally derived NE perforated with NPC. Sperm nuclear protamines are
rapidly degraded and replaced by oocyte-derived histones. The zygotic centrosome is
reconstituted from maternal centrosomal proteins around the sperm-contributed
centriole. Finally, sperm mitochondria, axoneme and flagellar accessory structures
are degraded during preimplantation development.

1.4.2 Changes to sperm head structure during fertilization

The sperm acrosome is lost to exocytosis upon binding to sperm receptor on the
egg zona pellucida (ZP; Bleil and Wassarman, 1983; Gerton, 2002). Recent studies

Table 1.1. Biogenesis of sperm accessory structures and their fate after fertilization

Organelle	Sperm	Oocyte	Fate after fertilization
Nucleus	Hypercondensed, protamine-packed, transcriptionally silent homogeneous sperm chromatin	M-II plate of condensed chromosomes	Form pronuclei (PN), become apposed. Sperm protamines are replaced transiently by oocyte-specific histones at fertilization and permanently by maternal somatic histones after maternal-embryonic transition
Centrosome	One centriole devoid of pericentriolar material (PCM) or completely absent in rodents	A centriolar spindle poles made of PCM, with a pool of soluble PCM proteins in ooplasm	Sperm centriole attracts PCM from ooplasm and eventually duplicates, forming a zygotic centrosome. Zygotic centrosome duplicates one more time during first interphase, giving rise to two poles of the first mitotic spindle, each with a pair of centrioles surrounded by PCM
Nuclear envelope (NE)	Reduced, no NPC	None, but components are in a soluble ooplasmic pool	Sperm NE removed; new NEs with NPC are established in both male and female pronuclei
Microtubules	9 + 2 axoneme	Metaphase-II spindle microtubules	Sperm axoneme degraded/recycled after fertilization, oocyte spindle microtubules depolymerize and repolymerize into sperm aster microtubules organized by the sperm-released centriole
Signaling molecules	Sequestered in sperm PT	Soluble in ooplasm	Sperm borne SOAF triggers signaling cascade within ooplasm, induces oocyte activation, activates anti-polyspermy defense and initiates zygotic/embryonic development
mRNAs	Paternal transcriptome present, subcellular location not known. Perhaps in PT and/or residual cytoplasm	Large pool stored in ooplasm	Maternally stored mRNAs are translated or degraded prior to initiation of embryonic transcription; sperm borne paternal mRNAs are detectable inside the fertilized ovum, could be degraded, translated or regulating the translation of maternal mRNAs
Mitochondria & mtDNA	~1000 copies of mitochondrial genome in sperm mitochondria	~100,000 copies in oocyte mitochondria	Sperm mitochondria are degraded by ooplasmic proteasomes; maternal mtDNA is propagated clonally, resulting in uniparental, maternal inheritance of mitochondrial genes
Sperm accessory structures	Acrosome, ODF, FS	None	Lost during fertilization (acrosome) or degraded after fertilization in the ooplasm

indicate that zona penetration in mammalian fertilization might involve ubiquitin-proteasome system (Sutovsky et al., 2004a), as it is known to occur in Ascidians (Sawada et al., 2002). The outer face of the porcine oocyte zona pellucida contains ubiquitinated epitopes and the sperm acrosome possesses proteasomes (Sutovsky et al., 2004a). In somatic cells, the proteasomes degrade ubiquitinated proteins, a fundamental catabolic process that regulates a multitude of physiological processes such as the cell cycle, organelle degradation, signal transduction, etc. (reviewed by Glickman and Ciechanover, 2002). Diverse experimental evidence point out that proteasomes associated with the spermatozoa might interact and degrade the ubiquitinated substrates of the zona pellucida, thereby playing a crucial role in sperm ZP penetration. Anti-proteasomal antibodies and proteasomal inhibitors effectively block sperm penetration through the ZP but do not obstruct their acrosome reaction/exocytosis, zona binding or fusion with oolemma if the zona has been removed (Sutovsky et al., 2004a).

The equatorial (posterior) acrosome is a narrow membranous fold (~45 nm wide) surrounding the equatorial region of the sperm head. The composition of the equatorial acrosome is different from that of the anterior acrosome but is not yet fully characterized. One of the resident glycoproteins of equatorial acrosome is identified by monoclonal antibody MN9 as 38/48 kDa bands in mouse sperm extracts. The putative glycoprotein named as equatorin, is synthesized in the early spermiogenesis and becomes confined in this organelle originating from the anterior bulbous part or the acrosomal granule (Toshimori et al., 1992). After acrosomal exocytosis, the upper edge is opened from where equatorin is expelled out, while some of it remains adsorbed on the outer face of the equatorial plasma membrane (Manandhar and Toshimori, 2001). After ZP penetration, spermatozoa possess equatorin on the equatorial plasma membrane. Hence equatorin is latent in the intact spermatozoa and expressed on the equatorial membranes at the time when they are ready to interact with the oolemma. It might either directly participate in sperm–oocyte membrane fusion or modify the putative fusion molecules of the equatorial plasma membrane making them functional. The antibody MN9 blocks in vitro and in vivo fertilization without affecting other sperm functions (Toshimori et al., 1998; Yoshinaga et al., 2001). The residual equatorial acrosome and equatorin are incorporated into the zygote after fertilization and are detectable until the two cell embryo stage (Manandhar and Toshimori, 2001).

1.4.3 Sperm incorporation in the ooplasm, oocyte activation and zygotic development

The sperm plasma membrane is thought to be incorporated into the oocyte plasma membrane, oolemma, (Gundersen et al., 1986) during sperm–egg fusion mediated by adhesion molecules and receptors on the respective sperm and egg plasma membranes (Stein et al., 2004). Upon sperm–oolemma fusion, the equatorial and postacrosomal segments of the sperm head come in direct contact with the ooplasm and the underlying postacrosomal PT is rapidly eroded, releasing its content into the ooplasm (Sutovsky *et al.*, 1997, 2003; see Fig. 1.6). The sperm borne-oocyte activating factor (SOAF; Kimura *et al.*, 1998) is thought to be transmitted into ooplasm via this mechanism, inducing a full spectrum of events associated with oocyte activation. These include the completion of second meiotic division, induction of calcium transients across ooplasm, triggering of cortical granule exocytosis for defense against polyspermy, extrusion of second polar body and pronuclear development. The phospholipase C-zeta (PLCζ; Saunders *et al.*, 2002) appears to be the calcium oscillation-inducing component of SOAF (Saunders *et al.*, 2002), though a role in earlier events of fertilization has not been ruled out. Other PT proteins, including signaling molecules in various protein kinase pathways, transcriptional factors and structural proteins (reviewed by Mujica *et al.*, 2003; Sutovsky *et al.*, 2003) may contribute to the process of oocyte activation and to the early stages of pronuclear development. One striking feature of male pronuclear development is the reversal of spermatogenic histone-protamine exchange. After fertilization, protamines are rapidly removed from the decondensing sperm nucleus and replaced by oocyte-derived histones (Gao *et al.*, 2004). Similarly, the NPC-free sperm nuclear enveloped is removed and quickly replaced by a *de novo* formed NE with functional pore complexes (Sutovsky *et al.*, 1998). Recently, it was discovered that in addition to a complement of proteins required for fertilization and oocyte activation, mammalian spermatozoa carry their own complex and well conserved transcriptome (Ostermeier *et al.*, 2002). A possibility has been raised that some of those sperm contributed mRNAs could either be translated by the zygote or contribute to maternal mRNA silencing (Ostermeier *et al.*, 2004).

The sperm proximal centriole, devoid of pericentriolar material, is released from the complex structure of the sperm tail connecting piece to duplicate and form a zygotic centrosome, which is ultimately responsible for the formation of the sperm aster, and for pronuclear apposition (Navara *et al.*, 1994; Sutovsky *et al.*, 1996). Reciprocally, the oocyte centrosome does not contain centrioles, while the ooplasm is stocked with protein constituents of pericentriolar material and other proteins necessary for *de novo* centriole biogenesis. The sperm centriole thus attracts maternal pericentriolar material with microtubule nucleating proteins from the ooplasm. A notable exemption from this centrosomal rule is the mouse, in which the spermatid centrosome is not reduced, but degraded completely (Manandhar *et al.*, 1998), and pronuclear apposition relies exclusively on maternally-controlled asters. Sperm mitochondria are degraded by ooplasmic proteasomes, thus promoting maternal inheritance of mitochondria and mtDNA in mammals (Sutovsky *et al.*, 1999c, 2004b). Oocyte mitochondria contribute all energy and mitochondrial genes to the zygote, a strategy that may be advantageous due to

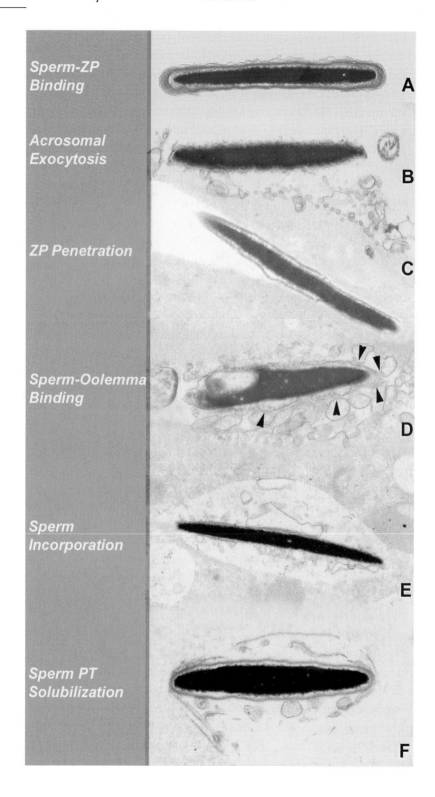

Sperm-ZP
Binding

Acrosomal
Exocytosis

ZP Penetration

Sperm-Oolemma
Binding

Sperm
Incorporation

Sperm PT
Solubilization

A

B

C

D

E

F

the volatile and potentially mutagenic environment to which paternal sperm mitochondria are exposed during sperm maturation, insemination and fertilization. Other sperm accessory structures such as outer dense fibers (ODF) and FS are not thought to have a role in zygotic development and are degraded after sperm tail incorporation into ooplasm. Some of the sperm-derived components are degraded very slowly and may persist until advanced stages of embryonic development (Gundersen and Shapiro, 1984; Sutovsky and Schatten, 2000).

1.5 Conclusions

Major progress has been achieved in spermatology in the last decade, including the successful transplantation of fresh (Brinster and Avarbock, 1994) and cryopreserved (Avarbock *et al.*, 1996) testicular tissues, reported production of spermatogenic cells from stem cells (Geijsen *et al.*, 2004; Toyooka *et al.*, 2003), production of transgenic animals (Yanagimachi, 2005) and routine use of intracytoplasmic sperm injection (ICSI) in clinical practice. However, many challenges remain, including the development of reliable conditions for spermiogenesis *in vitro*, the complete, repeatable profiling of the spermatogenic transcriptome and proteome, identification of all major genes involved in the control of spermatogenesis and gene therapy of human male infertility. The development of more accurate methods for assessing spermatogenesis and human semen quality remains a major challenge, given the variability of human sperm morphology (Fig. 1.7), increased enrollment of patients in assisted reproduction programs and paucity of objective markers of semen quality and male infertility.

Figure 1.6　*Irreversible changes of the sperm head structure during bovine fertilization.*
Cross-section of an intact sperm head (A) shows the structure of the acrosome, which becomes vesiculated after sperm binding to egg zona pellucida (B). Figure (C) shows sperm penetration slit with a sagital sperm head section revealing the IAM and part of the ES and PAS. The ES of the sperm head binds first to oocyte microvilli during sperm–oolemma fusion (arrowheads) in the perivitelline space (D). Sperm plasma membrane is removed during sperm incorporation into ooplasm (E), at which time the layers of equatorial and postacrosomal PT dissolve in the ooplasm (F) and release the sperm borne factors that induce oocyte activation. For the purpose of illustration, the images in this figure plate were edited by Adobe Photoshop tools and merged together, while the structural information from the original TEM negatives has been retained. The process of sperm-ZP penetration and sperm incorporation into ooplasm is completed in most ova with first 8 hours after sperm addition during bovine fertilization *in vitro*

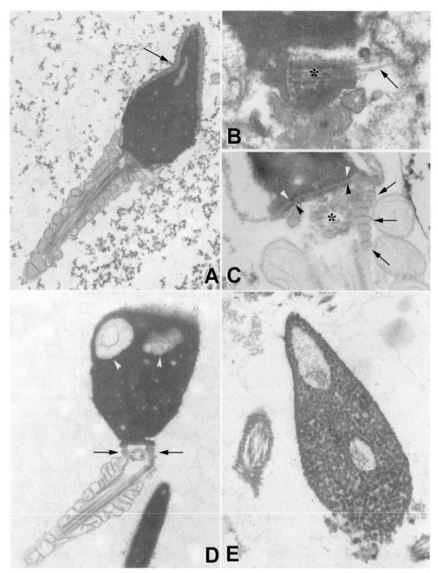

Figure 1.7   *Ultrastructure and pathology of the human spermatozoa.* (A) An unusual curvature of the
AC (arrow), perhaps a consequence of aberrant chromatin condensation in the
corresponding region of the nucleus, is observed in this otherwise normal spermatozoon.
(B) Longitudinal section of the proximal centriole (asterisk) and proximal centriolar
adjunct (arrow), an extension of the centriolar microtubule triplets often seen in human
spermatozoa. (C) Cross-section of basal plate (arrowheads), proximal centriole (asterisk)
and a striated column (arrows). (D) Abnormal spermatozoon with a connecting piece
defect (arrow) and prominent nuclear vacuoles (arrowheads), containing trapped
cytoplasm (see also Plate 1B). (E) Chromatin condensation defect combined with the
presence of nuclear vacuoles

Acknowledgments

We thank our collaborators Dr. Richard Oko, Dr. Ron Tovich and Dr. Antonio Miranda-Vizuete for the permission to include data from our collaborative research projects. We thank Kathryn Craighead for proofreading and Miriam Sutovsky and Nicole Leitman for the assistance with figure preparation. This work was in part supported by USDA-NRI Award #02069 and funding from the F21C program of the University of Missouri–Columbia.

REFERENCES

Agell N and Mezquita C (1988) Cellular content of ubiquitin and formation of ubiquitin conjugates during chicken spermatogenesis. *Biochem J* 250, 883–889.

Avarbock MR, Brinster CJ and Brinster RL (1996) Reconstitution of spermatogenesis from frozen spermatogonial stem cells. *Nat Med* 2, 693–696.

Baarends WM, van der Laan R and Grootegoed JA (2000) Specific aspects of the ubiquitin system in spermatogenesis. *J Endocrinol Invest* 23, 597–604.

Baarends WM, Hoogerbrugge JW, Roest HP, Ooms M, Vreeburg J, Hoeijmakers JH and Grootegoed JA (1999) Histone ubiquitination and chromatin remodeling in mouse spermatogenesis. *Dev Biol* 207, 322–333.

Baarends WM, Wassenaar E, Hoogerbrugge JW, van Cappellen G, Roest HP, Vreeburg J, Ooms M, Hoeijmakers JH and Grootegoed JA (2003) Loss of HR6B ubiquitin-conjugating activity results in damaged synaptonemal complex structure and increased crossing-over frequency during the male meiotic prophase. *Mol Cell Biol* 23, 1151–1162.

Barth AD and Oko RJ (1989) *Abnormal Morphology of Bovine Spermatozoa*. Ames: Iowa State University Press, 285 pp.

Bedford JM (1979) Evolution of the sperm maturation and sperm storage functions of the epididymis. In: *The spermatozoon*, eds DW Fawcett and JM Bedford, Baltimore–Munich: Urban & Schwarzenberg Inc., pp. 7–21.

Bleil JD and Wassarman PM (1983) Sperm–egg interactions in the mouse: sequence of events and induction of the acrosome reaction by a zona pellucida glycoprotein. *Dev Biol* 95, 317–324.

Brewer L, Corzett M and Balhorn R (2002) Condensation of DNA by spermatid basic nuclear proteins. *J Biol Chem* 277, 38895–38900.

Brinster RL and Avarbock MR (1994) Germline transmission of donor haplotype following spermatogonial transplantation. *Proc Natl Acad Sci USA* 91, 11303–11307.

Byskov AG and Høyer PE (1994) Embryology of mammalian gonads and ducts. In: *The Physiology of Reproduction*, eds E Knobil and JD Neill, 2nd edn. New York: Raven Press Ltd, pp. 487–540.

Cataldo L, Baig K, Oko R, Mastrangelo MA and Kleene KC (1996) Developmental expression, intracellular localization, and selenium content of the cysteine-rich protein associated with the mitochondrial capsules of mouse sperm. *Mol Reprod Dev* 45, 320–331.

Clark JM and Eddy E (1975) Fine structural observations on the origin and associations of primordial germ cells of the mouse. *Dev Biol* 47, 136–155.

Cooke HJ (1999) Y chromosome and male infertility. *Rev Reprod* 4, 5–10.

Cooper TG and Yeung CH (2003) Acquisition of volume regulatory response of sperm upon maturation in the epididymis and the role of the cytoplasmic droplet. *Microsc Res Tech* 61, 28–38.

Cyr DG (2001) Cell-cell interactions in the epididymis. In: *Andrology in the 21st Century*, eds B Robaire, H Chemes and CR Morales Englewood, NJ: Medimond Publishing Co, pp. 215–226.

Dadoune JP (2003) Expression of mammalian spermatozoal nucleoproteins. *Microsc Res Tech* 61, 56–75.

Dadoune JP, Siffroi JP and Alfonsi MF (2004) Transcription in haploid male germ cells. *Int Rev Cytol* 237, 1–56.

DeKretser DM and Kerr JB (1994) The cytology of testis. In: *The Physiology of Reproduction*, eds E Khobil and JD Neill, New York: Raven Press, pp. 1177–1290.

Don J and Stelzer G (2002) The expanding family of CREB/CREM transcription factors that are involved with spermatogenesis. *Mol Cell Endocrinol* 187, 115–124.

Eddy EM (1999) Role of heat shock protein HSP70-2 in spermatogenesis. *Rev Reprod* 4, 23–30.

Eddy EM (2002) Male germ cell gene expression. *Recent Prog Horm Res* 57, 103–128.

Eddy EM, Toshimori K and O'Brien DA (2003) Fibrous sheath of mammalian spermatozoa. *Microsc Res Tech* 61, 103–115.

Escalier D (2003) New insights into the assembly of the periaxonemal structures in mammalian spermatozoa. *Biol Reprod* 69, 373–378.

Fawcett D (1975) The mammalian spermatozoon. *Dev Biol* 44, 394–436.

Flickinger CJ (1985) The effects of vasectomy on the testis. *N Engl J Med* 313, 1283–1285.

Gao S, Chung YG, Parseghian MH, King GJ, Adashi EY and Latham KE (2004) Rapid H1 linker histone transitions following fertilization or somatic cell nuclear transfer: evidence for a uniform developmental program in mice. *Dev Biol* 266, 62–75.

Geijsen N, Horoschak M, Kim K, Gribnau J, Eggan K and Daley GQ (2004) Derivation of embryonic germ cells and male gametes from embryonic stem cells. *Nature* 427, 148–154.

Gerton G (2002) Function of the sperm acrosome. In: *Fertilization*, ed. D Hardy, San Diego: Academic Press, pp. 265–302.

Glickman MH and Ciechanover A (2002) The ubiquitin-proteasome proteolytic pathway: destruction for the sake of construction. *Physiol Rev* 82, 373–428.

Gliki G, Ebnet K, Aurrand-Lions M, Imhof BA and Adams RH (2004) Spermatid differentiation requires the assembly of a cell polarity complex downstream of junctional adhesion molecule-C. *Nature* 431, 320–324.

Gundersen GG and Shapiro BM (1984) Sperm surface proteins persist after fertilization. *J Cell Biol* 99, 1343–1353.

Gundersen GG, Medill L and Shapiro BM (1986) Sperm surface proteins are incorporated into egg membrane and cytoplasm after fertilization. *Dev Biol* 113, 207–217.

Guraya SS (1995) The comparative cell biology of accessory somatic (or Sertoli) cells in the animal testis. *Int Rev Cytol* 160, 163–220.

Haraguchi CM, Mabuchi T, Hirata S, Shoda T, Hoshi K, Akasaki K and Sadaki Y (2005) Chromatoid bodies: agresome-like characteristics and degradation sites for organelles of spermiogenic cells. *J Histochem Cytochem* 53, 455–465.

Hess RA and Moore BJ (1993) Histological methods for the evaluation of the testis. In: *Methods in Reproductive Toxicology*, eds RE Chapin and JJ Heindel, San Diego CA: Academic Press, pp. 52–85.

Hinton BT, Lan ZJ, Lye RJ and Labus JC (2000) Regulation of epididymal control by testicular factors: the lumicrine hypothesis. In: *The Testis: From Stem Cell to Sperm Function*, ed. E Goldberg Norwell, MA: Serono Symposia USA, pp.163–173.

Ho HC and Suarez SS (2003) Characterization of the intracellular calcium store at the base of the sperm flagellum that regulates hyperactivated motility. *Biol Reprod* 68, 1590–1596.

Ilio KY and Hess RA (1994) Structure and function of the ductuli efferentes: a review. *Microsc Res Tech* 29, 432–467.

Jiménez A, Zu W, Rawe VY, Pelto-Huikko M, Flickinger CJ, Sutovsky P, Gustafsson J-A, Oko R and Miranda-Vizuete A (2004) Spermatocyte/spermatid-specific thioredoxin-3, a novel Golgi apparatus-associated thioredoxin, is a specific marker of aberrant spermatogenesis. *J Biol Chem* 279, 34971–34982.

Johnson KJ and Boekelheide K (2002) Dynamic testicular adhesion junctions are immunologically unique. II. Localization of classic cadherins in rat testis. *Biol Reprod* 66, 992–1000.

Johnson KJ and Boekelheide K (2002) Dynamic testicular adhesion junctions are immunologically unique. I. Localization of p120 catenin in rat testis. *Biol Reprod* 66, 983–991.

Kierszenbaum AL (2002) Intramanchette transport (IMT): managing the making of the spermatid head, centrosome, and tail. *Mol Reprod Dev* 63, 1–4.

Kimura Y, Yanagimachi R, Kuretake S, Bortkiewicz H, Perry AC and Yanagimachi H (1998) Analysis of mouse oocyte activation suggests the involvement of sperm perinuclear material. *Biol Reprod* 58, 1407–1415.

Kleene KC (1993) Multiple controls over the efficiency of translation of the mRNAs encoding transition proteins, protamines, and the mitochondrial capsule selenoprotein in late spermatids in mice. *Dev Biol* 159, 720–731.

Kuster CE, Hess RA and Althouse GC (2004) Immunofluorescence reveals ubiquitination of retained distal cytoplasmic droplets on ejaculated porcine spermatozoa. *J Androl* 25, 340–347.

Kwon YT, Xia Z, An JY, Tasaki T, Davydov IV, Seo JW, Sheng J, Xie Y and Varshavsky A (2003) Female lethality and apoptosis of spermatocytes in mice lacking the UBR2 ubiquitin ligase of the N-end rule pathway. *Mol Cell Biol* 23, 8255–8271.

Lacham-Kaplan O (2004) *In vivo* and *in vitro* differentiation of male germ cells in the mouse. *Reproduction* 128, 147–152.

Manandhar G and Toshimori K (2001) Exposure of sperm head equatorin after acrosome reaction and its fate after fertilization in mice. *Biol Reprod* 65, 1425–1436.

Manandhar G, Sutovsky P, Joshi HC, Stearns T and Schatten G (1998) Centrosome reduction during mouse spermiogenesis. *Dev Biol* 203, 424–434.

McLachlan RI (2000) The endocrine control of spermatogenesis. *Baillieres Best Pract Res Clin Endocrinol Metab* 14, 345–362.

Meistrich ML, Mohapatra B, Shirley CR and Zhao M (2003) Roles of transition nuclear proteins in spermiogenesis. *Chromosoma* 111, 483–488.

Moreno RD, Ramalho-Santos J, Sutovsky P, Chan EK and Schatten G (2000) Vesicular traffic and Golgi apparatus dynamics during mammalian spermatogenesis: implications for acrosome architecture. *Biol Reprod* 63, 89–98.

Mujica A, Navarro-Garcia F, Hernandez-Gonzalez EO and De Lourdes Juarez-Mosqueda M (2003) Perinuclear theca during spermatozoa maturation leading to fertilization. *Microsc Res Tech* 61, 76–87.

Navara CS, First NL and Schatten G (1994) Microtubule organization in the cow during fertilization, polyspermy, parthenogenesis, and nuclear transfer: the role of the sperm aster. *Dev Biol* 162, 29–40.

Oko RJ (1995) Developmental expression and possible role of perinuclear theca proteins in mammalian spermatozoa. *Reprod Fertil Dev* 7, 777–797.

Oko R (1998) Occurrence and formation of cytoskeletal proteins in mammalian spermatozoa. *Andrologia* 30, 193–206.

Oko R, Hermo L, Chan PT, Fazel A and Bergeron JJ (1993) The cytoplasmic droplet of rat epididymal spermatozoa contains saccular elements with Golgi characteristics. *J Cell Biol* 123, 809–821.

Ostermeier GC, Dix DJ, Miller D, Khatri P and Krawetz SA (2002) Spermatozoal RNA profiles of normal fertile men. *Lancet* 360, 772–777.

Ostermeier GC, Miller D, Huntriss JD, Diamond MP and Krawetz SA (2004) Reproductive biology: delivering spermatozoan RNA to the oocyte. *Nature* 429, 154.

Print CG, Loveland KL, Gibson L, Meehan T, Stylianou A, Wreford N, de Kretser D, Metcalf D, Kontgen F, Adams JM and Cory S (1998) Apoptosis regulator bcl-w is essential for spermatogenesis but appears otherwise redundant. *Proc Natl Acad Sci USA* 95, 12424–12431.

Reijo-Pera RA (2000) The DAZ gene family and germ-cell development. In: *The Testis: From Stem Cell to Sperm Function*, ed. E Goldberg Norwell, MA: Serono Symposia USA, pp. 213–225.

Rossi P, Sette C, Dolci S and Geremia R (2000) Role of c-kit in mammalian spermatogenesis. *J Endocrinol Invest* 23, 609–615.

Russel LD, Ettin RA, Hikim APS and Clegg ED (1990) *Histological Pathological Evaluation of the Testis.* Clearwater FL: Cache River Press.

Saunders CM, Larman MG, Parrington J, Cox LJ, Royse J, Blayney LM, Swann K and Lai FA (2002) PLC zeta: a sperm-specific trigger of Ca(2+) oscillations in eggs and embryo development. *Development* 129, 3533–3544.

Sawada H, Sakai N, Abe Y *et al.* (2002) Extracellular ubiquitination and proteasome-mediated degradation of the ascidian sperm receptor. *Proc Natl Acad Sci USA* 99, 1223–1228.

Sette C, Dolci S, Geremia R and Rossi P (2000) The role of stem cell factor and of alternative c-kit gene products in the establishment, maintenance and function of germ cells. *Int J Dev Biol* 44, 599–608.

Sinha Hikim AP and Swerdloff RS (1999) Hormonal and genetic control of germ cell apoptosis in the testis. *Rev Reprod* 4, 38–47.

Sinha Hikim AP, Lue Y, Diaz-Romero M, Yen PH, Wang C and Swerdloff RS (2003) Deciphering the pathways of germ cell apoptosis in the testis. *J Steroid Biochem Mol Biol* 85, 175–182.

Stein KK, Primakoff P and Myles D (2004) Sperm–egg fusion: events at the plasma membrane. *J Cell Sci* 117, 6269–6274.

Sutovsky P (2003) Ubiquitin-dependent proteolysis in mammalian spermatogenesis, fertilization, and sperm quality control: killing three birds with one stone. *Microsc Res Tech* 61, 88–102.

Sutovsky P and Schatten G (2000) Paternal contributions to the mammalian zygote: fertilization after sperm–egg fusion. *Int Rev Cytol* 195, 1–65.

Sutovsky P, Oko R, Hewitson L and Schatten G (1997) The removal of the sperm perinuclear theca and its association with the bovine oocyte surface during fertilization. *Dev Biol* 188, 75–84.

Sutovsky P, Simerly C, Hewitson L and Schatten G (1998) Assembly of nuclear pore complexes and annulate lamellae promotes normal pronuclear development in fertilized mammalian oocytes. *J Cell Sci* 111, 2841–2854.

Sutovsky P, Manandhar G and Schatten G (1999a) Biogenesis of the centrosome during mammalian gametogenesis and fertilization. *Protoplasma* 206, 249–262.

Sutovsky P, Ramalho-Santos J, Moreno RD, Oko R, Hewitson L and Schatten G (1999b) On-stage selection of single round spermatids using a vital, mitochondrion-specific fluorescent probe MitoTracker™ and high resolution differential interference contrast (DIC) microscopy. *Human Reprod* 14, 2301–2312.

Sutovsky P, Moreno R, Ramalho-Santos J, Dominko T, Simerly C, and Schatten G (1999c) Ubiquitin tag for sperm mitochondria. *Nature* 402, 371–372.

Sutovsky P, Manandhar G, Wu A and Oko R (2003) Interactions of the sperm perinuclear theca with the oocyte: implications for oocyte activation, anti-polyspermy defense and assisted reproduction. *Microsc Res Tech* 61, 362–378.

Sutovsky P, Manandhar G, McCauley TC, Caamaño JN, Sutovsky M, Thompson WE and Day BN (2004a) Proteasomal interference prevents zona pellucida penetration and fertilization in mammals. *Biol Reprod* 71, 1625–1637.

Sutovsky P, van Leyen K, McCauley T, Day BN and Sutovsky M (2004b) Degradation of the paternal mitochondria after fertilization: implications for heteroplasmy, ART and mtDNA inheritance. *Reprod Biomed Online* 8, 24–33.

Thompson WE, Ramalho-Santos J and Sutovsky P (2003) Ubiquitination of prohibitin in mammalian sperm mitochondria: possible roles in the regulation of mitochondrial inheritance and sperm quality control. *Biol Reprod* 69, 254–260.

Toshimori K, Tanii I, Araki S and Oura C (1992) Characterization of the antigen recognized by a monoclonal antibody MN9: unique transport pathway to the equatorial segment of sperm head during spermiogenesis. *Cell Tissue Res* 270, 459–468.

Toshimori K, Saxena DK, Tanii I and Yoshinaga K (1998) An MN9 antigenic molecule, equatorin, is required for successful sperm–oocyte fusion in mice. *Biol Reprod* 59, 22–29.

Tovich PR, Sutovsky P and Oko RJ (2004) Novel aspect of perinuclear theca assembly revealed by immunolocalization of non-nuclear somatic histones during bovine spermiogenesis. *Biol Reprod* 71, 1182–1194.

Toyooka Y, Tsunekawa N, Akasu R and Noce T (2003) Embryonic stem cells can form germ cells *in vitro*. *Proc Natl Acad Sci USA* 100, 11457–11462.

Tsai-Morris CH, Sheng Y, Lee E, Lei KJ and Dufau ML (2004) Gonadotropin-regulated testicular RNA helicase (GRTH/Ddx25) is essential for spermatid development and completion of spermatogenesis. *Proc Natl Acad Sci USA* 101, 6373–6378.

Wing SS, Bedard N, Morales C, Hingamp P and Trasler J (1996) A novel rat homolog of the *Saccharomyces cerevisiae* ubiquitin-conjugating enzymes UBC4 and UBC5 with distinct biochemical features is induced during spermatogenesis. *Mol Cell Biol* 16, 4064–4072.

Wojcik C, Benchaib M, Lornage J, Czyba JC and Guerin JF (2000) Proteasomes in human spermatozoa. *Int J Androl* 23, 169–177.

Wolf F (1928) Die Natur as Artz und Helfer. Das Neue Naturärtzliche Hausbuch. Deutsche Verlags Stuttgart Berlin & Leipzig.

Yanagimachi R (2005) Intracytoplasmic injection of spermatozoa and spermatogenic cells: its biology and applications in humans and animals. *Reprod Biomed Online* 10, 247–286.

Yeom YI, Fuhrmann G, Ovitt CE, Brehm A, Ohbo K, Gross M, Hubner K and Scholer HR (1996) Germline regulatory element of *Oct-4* specific for the totipotent cycle of embryonic cells. *Development* 122, 881–894.

Ying Y and Zhao GQ (2001) Cooperation of endoderm-derived BMP2 and extraembryonic ectoderm-derived BMP4 in primordial germ cell generation in the mouse. *Dev Biol* 232, 484–492.

Yoshinaga K and Toshimori K (2003) Organization and modifications of sperm acrosomal molecules during spermatogenesis and epididymal maturation. *Microsc Res Tech* 61, 39–45.

Yoshinaga K, Saxena DK, Oh-oka T, Tanii I and Toshimori K (2001) Inhibition of mouse fertilization *in vivo* by intra-oviductal injection of an anti-equatorin monoclonal antibody. *Reproduction* 122, 649–655.

Sperm chromatin stability and susceptibility to damage in relation to its structure

Jeffrey A. Shaman and W. Steven Ward

Department of Anatomy and Reproductive Biology, Institute for Biogenesis Research, John A. Burns School of Medicine, University of Hawaii at Manoa, Honolulu, USA

2.1 Introduction: the malleable sperm genome

Over the last decade, our assumptions and ideas about the stability of the mammalian sperm genome have gone through a gentle and progressive change. Historically, we viewed the sperm genome as tightly packaged into a virtual crystalline state with very little biochemical accessibility. We now understand that in many cases of decreased male fertility sperm deoxyribonucleic acid (DNA) structure loses much of this inaccessibility and that the DNA is susceptible to damage. More recently, evidence has emerged from many different laboratories that spermatozoa contain nucleases that are capable of digesting their compact DNA. These data suggest that the sperm genome may be less stable than we thought and might even be flexible enough to regulate its own stability in a manner similar to somatic cells. In this review, we will explore the current status of the stability of the mammalian sperm genome in the context of what is known about sperm chromatin structure.

2.2 Sperm chromatin structure and fertility

Before discussing DNA damage as it relates to sperm chromatin structure we will briefly review those aspects of sperm chromatin, both known and suspected, that pertain to this discussion. During spermiogenesis the haploid sperm chromatin undergoes one of the most significant changes known in biology. All of the histones are replaced first by transition proteins, then by protamines (Meistrich et al., 2003). This condenses the sperm DNA so tightly that it is resistant to mechanical stresses such as sonication (Tateno et al., 2000) and even to boiling (Yanagida et al., 1991), both of which destroy the DNA in somatic cells. The major role of the spermatozoon is to deliver the paternal genome in pristine condition to the oocyte. The condensation of sperm DNA protects it during its transit from the male to the female in fertilization. It is important to understand, however, that the condensation of the haploid genome during spermiogenesis functions only for fertilization, and not for embryonic development. Yanagimachi and colleagues elegantly demonstrated this by injecting the nuclei of round spermatids into oocytes and showing that the resultant embryos developed into live pups at rates of 77% or more (Kimura and Yanagimachi, 1995; Ogura *et al.*, 1994). The chromatin of round spermatids is organized in the somatic fashion by histones (Meistrich *et al.*, 2003). So the condensation that occurs after this point is not necessary for the paternal genome to participate in embryogenesis.

Even with this high degree of sperm condensation, sperm DNA remains susceptible to damage, as discussed below. To begin to understand the mechanisms of this damage, it is important to know how the DNA is packaged and how this packaging differs from somatic cells. There are four major points to consider. The first is the mechanism of protamine binding. Protamines compact DNA very tightly by binding in the major groove of the DNA, end to end. This completely neutralizes the negative charges of the DNA double helix essentially transforming the DNA fiber into an uncharged polymer (Balhorn, 1982; Prieto *et al.*, 1997). Hud and Balhorn originally demonstrated that the major binding proteins of sperm chromatin, the protamines, fold the DNA into tightly packaged toroids each containing roughly 50 kb of DNA (Hud *et al.*, 1993, 1994) (Fig. 2.1). More recently, it has been shown that these toroids can form *in vitro* in a progressive manner when protamines are added to DNA (Brewer *et al.*, 1999, 2003). Mammalian protamines contain cysteines that have long been thought to stabilize sperm chromatin. This has recently been demonstrated in bull protamine *in vitro* (Vilfan *et al.*, 2004). When this structure of sperm chromatin is compared to that of somatic cells, which is bound to the relative open configuration of nucleosomes by histones (Ward and Ward, 2004), it becomes apparent that the protamine toroid provides the mechanisms for the added protection against mechanical and environmental DNA damaging agents. Figure 2.1 includes a cross section of the protamine toroid diagramming how most of the DNA is completely surrounded by other protamine-DNA strands.

The second point is that when DNA binds to protamines it is far less supercoiled than when it is bound to histones (Ward, 1993; Ward *et al.*, 1989). Supercoiling means coiling the double helix DNA strand upon itself. Histones coil the DNA once every 100 bp to wind the DNA into tight packages. But protamines coil the DNA an estimated once every 600 bp or so (Ward, 1993; Ward *et al.*, 1989) so the DNA is packaged more tightly but coiled less. This will become important later in this chapter when we discuss the role topoisomerase may play in the generation of single stranded nicks in sperm DNA. Topoisomerases may nick the DNA to allow it to uncoil for the protamines to replace the histones (Marcon and Boissonneault, 2004; McPherson and Longo, 1993).

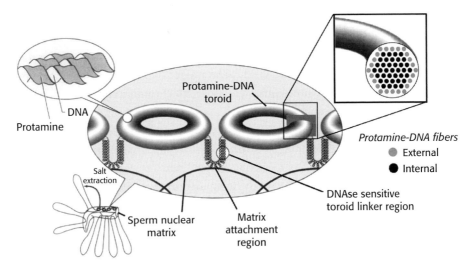

Figure 2.1   *Donut-Loop model for sperm chromatin structure.* This model was modified from (Sotolongo *et al.*, 2003) and reveals the internal structure of the protamine-DNA fibers within the toroid (inset)

The third important point to understand about sperm chromatin is that some histones do remain in the fully mature spermatozoon. Importantly, the positioning and the role of these histones is controversial. Some authors have demonstrated that in human spermatozoa some histone variants are located at the telomeres (Gineitis *et al.*, 2000; Zalensky *et al.*, 2002). Others have suggested that histone bound chromatin is located at the sites of DNA loop domain attachments, termed MARs (matrix attachment regions) (Pittoggi *et al.*, 2000; Wykes and Krawetz, 2003b). It is not clear what parts of the sperm chromatin remain bound to histones after the condensation process, but it is reasonable to argue that the replacement would not be complete. This is important because DNA that is bound to histones is much more susceptible to DNA damaging agents than DNA that is bound to protamines. Therefore, the sperm chromatin that is bound to histones would be candidate loci for sperm DNA damage.

The last point about sperm chromatin structure that we would like to present is what is known about the overall chromatin structure. Each mammalian sperm nucleus contains roughly three feet of DNA compacted into a small nucleus about 8 μm long, and about 1 μm thin (Ward and Coffey, 1991). There is not yet a model for how protamine toroids themselves condense into chromatin, and any such model would be speculative at this point. However, we do know that sperm chromatin is organized into loop domains by a sperm nuclear matrix, in a manner similar to that of somatic cells (Schmid *et al.*, 2001; Sotolongo and Ward, 2000; Ward *et al.*, 2000). These loop domains each contain roughly 50 kb (Ward *et al.*, 1989), which is the same size as a protamine toroid. We have proposed a model (Fig. 2.1) for sperm chromatin structure in which each protamine toroid is a single loop domain and provided experimental evidence to support it (McCarthy and Ward, 1999; Sotolongo *et al.*, 2003). The model suggests that each protamine toroid is connected by a toroid linker composed of chromatin that is more sensitive to damaging agents such as DNAse I. According to this model, the protamine linker regions would be a likely candidate for DNA damage in mature spermatozoa.

Understanding the structure of this compact sperm chromatin reveals several likely targets for DNA damage. We will next review the different chromatin structure assays that are currently being used to correlate human infertility with sperm DNA damage in the context of what we know about its structure.

2.3 Sperm DNA damage assays and human fertility

Many assays for sperm chromatin structure have been developed in an attempt to determine whether cases of idiopathic male infertility could be explained by the sperm DNA being damaged. The rationale is that DNA damage may not be reflected in the sperm morphology, motility, or even its ability to fertilize the oocyte. However, damaged sperm DNA would be expected to prevent or reduce the spermatozoon's potential to fertilize and/or inhibit embryo development. Several excellent reviews have recently been published that describe how the various techniques relate to each other and how they correlate with human fertility (Agarwal and Said, 2003; De Jonge, 2002; Evenson *et al.*, 2002; Sakkas *et al.*, 2003; Spano and Sakkas, 2005), and we will not attempt to review these clinical aspects. Instead, we will explore these assays in the context of our current model of sperm chromatin structure in an attempt to reveal new insights into their mechanisms.

There are two features we would like to consider: whether the assay detects single stranded (ss) or double stranded (ds) DNA breaks, and what level of accessibility to the sperm chromatin the assay provides. The differences between ss and ds DNA breaks are clear, but the latter point deserves some consideration with relation to our view of sperm chromatin. The Donut-Loop model (Fig. 2.1) predicts at least three separable levels of chromatin accessibility. The first and most open is the toroid linker region that contains the nuclear MAR. The toroid linkers are more sensitive to DNAse I than the protamine bound DNA (Sotolongo *et al.*, 2003). The chromatin structure of the toroid linkers is not known, but work by Krawetz and colleagues has shown that histone-bound DNA is associated with the nuclear matrix in human spermatozoa (Martins *et al.*, 2004; Wykes and Krawetz, 2003a). This suggests that the toroid linkers may be in the more open histone bound configuration. The second level of accessibility would be the chromatin fibers that are on the surface of the protamine toroid (Fig. 2.1). These fibers would be expected to

Table 2.1. Types of sperm chromatin structure assays (SCSAs) in order of increasing accessibility

Assay	Type of DNA break detected	Chromatin proteins removed
TUNEL	Accessible ds + ss DNA breaks	None
In situ translational	Accessible ss DNA breaks	None to few
SCSA	Non-toroidal ds + ss DNA breaks	Some histones
	(External toroidal ss + ds DNA breaks?)	(some external protamines?)
Neutral COMET	Most ds DNA breaks	ALL (histones + protamines)
Alkaline COMET	Most ds + ss DNA breaks	ALL (histones + protamines)

be accessible to enzymes, but the protamines that bind so completely to this DNA would probably severely, if not completely, inhibit the activity of DNA binding enzymes. The third level of sperm chromatin accessibility would be the majority of the chromatin fibers that are inside the toroid and completely covered by neighboring protamine-DNA strands (Fig. 2.1). These DNA strands are not accessible to any exogenous proteins while the toroids remain compact.

Let us now consider the different assays that are available to test for sperm DNA damage with respect to these three levels of DNA accessibility. One of the most common assays for the presence of DNA breaks in human spermatozoa is the TUNEL assay, or terminal deoxynucleotidyl transferase (TdT) mediated dUTP nick end labeling (Sgonc and Gruber, 1998). In this assay, the enzyme TdT is used to add labeled nucleotides to free 3' OH groups at the ends of DNA strands resulting in ss poly-U extensions. Therefore, TUNEL detects both ss and ds breaks. The labeled nucleotides that are thus incorporated into the DNA are detected with fluorescent antibodies. Most current protocols for sperm TUNEL assays do not include an extensive extraction procedure that would be expected to remove protamines or histones, except for the fixation procedure that includes ethanol and acetic acid that might remove some or all of the histones (Marcon and Boissonneault, 2004; Sakkas, et al., 2002). Indeed, this assay often depends on sperm nuclei remaining condensed so that they can be sorted by fluorescence activated cell sorting (FACS; Seli et al., 2004; Sun et al., 1997), confirming that most of the nuclear proteins remain *in situ*. The *in situ* translation assay also uses an enzymatic method to detect ss DNA breaks, but cannot detect ds breaks. These two assays have the least accessibility to sperm chromatin of all the assays described in this section (Table 2.1).

These facts suggest that most of the sperm DNA remains inaccessible to the TdT in the TUNEL assay because the protamine toroids remain largely intact and most of the DNA is localized within the toroid. Thus, we would predict that the major type of sperm chromatin that would be accessible to the TUNEL assay would be the toroid linker regions. We have shown that these regions are accessible to DNAse

I (Sotolongo *et al.*, 2003) and they should be accessible to the TdT that is used in the TUNEL assay. The second type of chromatin in which damage may be detected by this assay is the DNA that happens to be on the surface of the protamine toroids. We view this as less likely because the very high affinity that protamines have for DNA would probably prevent TdT binding to DNA. However, TUNEL may be able to detect these breaks since the TdT only adds to free 3′ OH ends. The third type would be severely damaged chromatin that has little or no protamines due to some type of chromatin defect (Fig. 2.2A, Color plate 2). Thus, the TUNEL assay is limited to

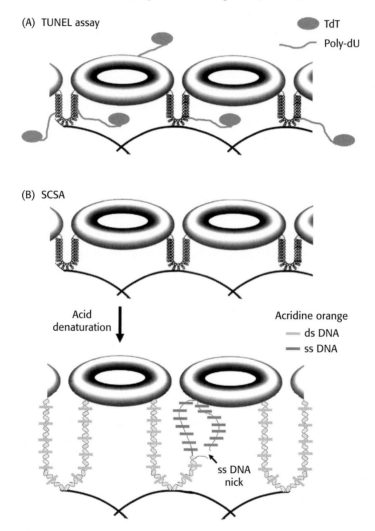

Figure 2.2   *The TUNEL assay and SCSA considered with respect to the Donut-Loop model.* (A) The TUNEL assay uses the enzyme TdT to add uridine residues to 3′ OH ends of nicked and broken DNA. (B) The SCSA assay denatures DNA that has nicks, then uses acridine orange to detect ss and ds DNA (see Color plate 2)

those areas of sperm chromatin that remain accessible to enzymatic modification. Because these areas may, in fact, be the most active sites during the first hours of fertilization when sperm chromatin is decondensed, this aspect may be why the TUNEL assay is more closely correlated with human infertility (Sakkas *et al.*, 2003; Spano and Sakkas, 2005) than, for example, the COMET assay that detects virtually all DNA breaks, as described below.

Another popular method of examining sperm DNA stability is the sperm chromatin structure assay (SCSA) developed by Don Evenson (Ballachey *et al.*, 1987; Larson-Cook *et al.*, 2003). In this assay, sperm samples are treated with mild acid to denature DNA that contains ss or ds nicks, but are otherwise not treated with conditions that are strong enough to extract the protamines. As in the TUNEL assay, the sperm nuclei remain condensed enough to be separable by flow cytometry. However, in the SCSA, no enzymes are required. The acid extracted sperm nuclei are stained with acridine orange, a DNA intercalating dye that stains ss DNA red and ds DNA green. The ratio of red to total staining (red/red + green) is called the DFI, or DNA fragmentation index. The DFI is therefore a measurement of the amount of sperm chromatin that can be denatured by mild acid or heat treatment. Because chromosomal DNA is tethered by attachments to the nuclear matrix every 50 kb or so (Ward *et al.*, 1989), and by the tight binding of the protamines (Fig. 2.1), it can only be denatured if there is a DNA break. Therefore, the SCSA can also infer ss or ds DNA breaks.

In the context of our model for sperm chromatin structure, we predict that most of the DNA breaks the SCSA identifies are located in the toroid linker regions (Fig. 2.2B). Acridine orange is a relatively small molecule when compared to the enzymes TdT and DNA polymerase, so access to the sperm chromatin should not be limiting. However, Evenson has suggested that condensed chromatin does not bind acridine orange well (Evenson and Jost, 2000) and it may be that the protamines prevent the actual intercalation of the dye into the ds DNA. Intercalating agents extend the DNA and can distort it so much that histones can no longer bind it. It is possible that protamines, which are linked by covalent intermolecular disulfides, cannot be displaced by intercalators and actually inhibit their binding. Regardless of whether acridine orange can bind to the protamine-bound DNA, it is clear that protamine-bound DNA will not denature even if ss DNA nicks are present. Given these facts, we predict that the SCSA would have a similar accessibility in detecting ss and ds DNA breaks as the TUNEL assay (Fig. 2.2B, Color plate 2).

The last assay that we will discuss is the COMET assay. This assay is unique in that all the protamines and histones are extracted by high salt and disulfide reducing reagents (McVicar *et al.*, 2004; Tomsu *et al.*, 2002). Spermatozoa are embedded in agarose on a glass slide so that when the proteins are extracted the chromosomal DNA remains localized. The extraction procedures used with the COMET assay

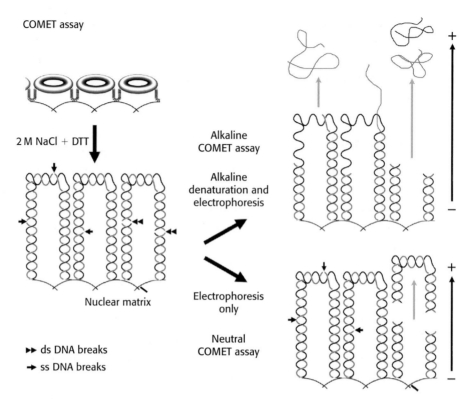

COMET assay

2 M NaCl + DTT

Alkaline
COMET assay

Alkaline
denaturation and
electrophoresis

Nuclear matrix

Electrophoresis
only

▸▸ ds DNA breaks

Neutral
COMET assay

➤ ss DNA breaks

Figure 2.3   *The neutral and alkaline COMET assays and the nuclear matrix.* Both COMET assays
extract the histones and protamines with high salt, so that the Donut-Loop model is not
relevant in this assay. The attachment sites of the DNA to the nuclear matrix, however,
would remain intact in this assay. Note that DNA double-helices depicted in the extracted
loop diagrams are not drawn to scale, but are shown as shorter segments for clarity (see
Color plate 3)

are consistent with the formation of nuclear halos, in which naked loops of DNA
of about 50 kb in length, are attached at their bases to the sperm nuclear matrix
(Nadel *et al.*, 1995; Ward *et al.*, 1989) (Fig. 2.1.) The DNA is then denatured by base
(alkaline COMET assay) or kept at neutral pH (neutral COMET assay) and subjected to an electric current. Those fragments of DNA that are free of the sperm
nuclear matrix migrate towards the positive electrode, creating a comet-like
appearance (Fig. 2.3, Color plate 3). According to this view of the COMET assay, ss
DNA breaks would only be freed from the sperm nucleus if two ss DNA breaks are
present on the same strand of DNA within one loop (Fig. 2.3). Likewise, ds DNA
breaks would only be detected if two ds DNA breaks occurred in one loop. Finally,
if some patients had sperm nuclear matrix aberrations (Barone *et al.*, 2000) the
COMET assay might identify more DNA breaks.

If the models shown in Figures 2.2 and 2.3 for understanding SCSAs are correct, we may conclude that the TUNEL, SCSA, and *in situ* translation assays primarily detect the toroid linker regions, while the COMET assays detect many more DNA breaks per sperm cell, but without any distinction for their chromosomal localization.

2.4 Sperm apoptosis

The TUNEL assay described above was originally used to measure apoptosis in somatic cells. The association of positive TUNEL assay results (i.e., DNA strand breaks) in ejaculated sperm led to the idea that mature sperm cells may possess the ability to go through apoptosis. That this is a controversial proposal is not surprising – the sperm cell is the protector and deliverer of the embryo's paternal compliment of DNA; the last thing one expects are apoptotic nucleases to be present. However, current data suggest that these nucleases do exist in some ejaculated spermatozoa.

Apoptosis is a strictly regulated programmed cell death (Kerr *et al.*, 1972) utilized by somatic cells for proper development, homeostasis, and removal of damaged or dangerous cells. It is marked by chromatin condensation, plasma membrane blebbing, nucleosome-sized as well as a high molecular weight (50–100 kb) DNA fragmentation, the externalization of certain inner-membrane constituents, and cell fragmentation into compact membrane-enclosed structures termed apoptotic bodies which contain cytosol, the condensed chromatin, and organelles. Apoptosis has also been suggested to play key roles in adjusting the appropriate number of proliferating germ cells associated with Sertoli cells, removing abnormal sperm, and in other normal spermatogenic processes (Berensztein *et al.*, 2002; Billig *et al.*, 1995; Blanco-Rodriguez, 1998; Furuchi *et al.*, 1996; Knudson *et al.*, 1995; Print and Loveland, 2000). The apoptotic machinery is also implicated in the selective depletion of unneeded portions of cytoplasm during *Drosophila* (Arama *et al.*, 2003) and rat (Blanco-Rodriguez and Martinez-Garcia, 1999) spermiogenesis into cytoplasmic masses dubbed 'residual bodies'. And while apoptotic markers including DNA nicks, caspases and other proteins, and phosphatidylserine (PS) translocation have been observed in ejaculated spermatozoa, it is unclear whether they are residues of an abortive apoptotic process started before ejaculation (Sakkas *et al.*, 1999b), an anomaly of sperm production, or signs of apoptosis initiated post-ejaculation.

Do mature spermatozoa have the ability to go through apoptosis? This is a more difficult question to answer. The presence of DNA strand breaks and spontaneous DNA fragmentation in ejaculated spermatozoa has led to much speculation. Hypotheses of the reasons for their existence in mature spermatozoa include the failure to repair naturally induced nicks during chromatin remodeling, fragmentation due to reactive oxygen species (ROS) (Aitken *et al.*, 1998; Muratori *et al.*, 2003), endogenous nucleases that can be activated under certain conditions (Maione *et al.*, 1997; Sotolongo and Ward, 2000; Sotolongo *et al.*, 2003), and actual apoptotic DNA cleavage. And while some apoptotic markers positively correlate with infertility in humans, a causative effect has yet to be seen (Oehninger *et al.*, 2003).

As mentioned above, there exists a major topological problem in going from histone-bound to protamine-bound DNA. Histones coil DNA more than protamines, and thus when protamines replace histones, these supercoils must be removed. To remove these supercoils, nicks must be introduced into the DNA by a nuclease. Topoisomerase has been implicated in this process (McPherson and Longo, 1993) as it allows for controlled nicking, increase in linking number and subsequent DNA relaxation, and religation of the DNA. DNA nicks can be seen, *in situ*, using the TUNEL assay to detect DNA strand breaks in the early stages of spermatogenesis. DNA nicks are maximally seen during the transition from round to elongated spermatids in the testis and visualized in close to 100% of the cells (Marcon and Boissonneault, 2004). These nicks are nearly absent once packaging is complete. A positive correlation has been seen between topoisomerase presence and DNA strand breaks; topoisomerases have been identified in spermatogonia, spermatocytes, and round and early-elongating spermatids (Chen and Longo, 1996) while few people report their localization in mature spermatozoa (St Pierre *et al.*, 2002). Some spontaneous DNA fragmentation has been observed post-ejaculation and increases with glutathione peroxidase inhibitor treatment. This suggests an involvement of ROS as a possible cause of DNA fragments in mature sperm (Muratori *et al.*, 2003). Finally, nucleases have been found in the lumen of the cauda epididymides of bull, boar, rabbit, and rat (reviewed in Jones, 2004).

Apoptotic markers seen in ejaculated spermatozoa include Bcl-xl (Cayli *et al.*, 2004; Sakkas *et al.*, 2002), caspase-3, -8, and -9, Fas receptors (Paasch *et al.*, 2003; Sakkas *et al.*, 1999b, 2002; Wang *et al.*, 2003; Weng *et al.*, 2002), PARP (Blanc-Layrac *et al.*, 2000), as well as the externalization of the normally membrane-internal PS by Annexin V binding (Paasch *et al.*, 2003; Weng *et al.*, 2002), and DNA strand breaks (Aravindan *et al.*, 1997; Evenson *et al.*, 1999; Gorczyca *et al.*, 1993; Sakkas *et al.*, 2002; Van Kooij *et al.*, 2004).

There has also been seen an increase in caspase enzyme activity in men with decreased sperm cell motility, but also in motile fractions from sub fertile patients (Taylor *et al.*, 2004). Samples with lower sperm concentration and poor morphology correlated with increased TUNEL staining and Fas and p53 expression (Sakkas *et al.*, 2002), and with increased immature sperm concentration and Bcl-xl expression (Cayli *et al.*, 2004; Sakkas *et al.*, 2002). However, TUNEL positive cells and apoptotic markers are not always found together (Sakkas *et al.*, 2002).

The prevailing idea is that apoptosis does not occur in mature spermatozoa, rather that apoptotic markers exist in immature spermatogenic cells that were not selected against during spermiogenesis. DNA fragmentation as detected by the TUNEL assay can be caused by topoisomerase during the change from histone- to protamine-bound DNA or by ROS (Aitken *et al.*, 1998; Muratori *et al.*, 2003; Wang *et al.*, 2003). The protein markers can be leftover from abortive apoptosis, cells that should have been removed from the mature sperm population but were not, or from normal spermiogenic occurrences such as cytoplasmic depletion. Membrane phosphotidyl serine translocation, while seen in sperm in different experimental conditions, could be related to positive functional changes in sperm such as capacitation (de Vries *et al.*, 2003; Gadella and Harrison, 2002) and in cryopreserved sperm is likely due to membrane damage (Guthrie and Welch, 2005). In fact, in experiments where mature sperm are incubated for 24 h, necrosis rather than apoptosis is detected even though there is a significant decrease in cell motility (Lachaud *et al.*, 2004). In an experiment where apoptosis was activated in sperm cells, betulinic acid was used to induce apoptosis and it was detected by mitochondrial transmembrane potential disruption and activation of caspases-9 and -3 (Paasch *et al.*, 2004). Nevertheless, naturally induced apoptosis has yet to be fully described or accurately detected in mature spermatozoa.

2.5 Sperm nucleases

While a nuclease could be detrimental to the integrity of the paternal genome, they are necessary for proper spermatogenesis. As discussed earlier, negative supercoils must be removed from the DNA when histones are replaced by protamines during spermiogenesis. To remove these supercoils, nicks must be introduced into the DNA by a nuclease, at specific stages of spermiogenesis, as discussed above (Marcon and Boissonneault, 2004). Topoisomerase has been implicated in this process as it allows for controlled nicking, increase in linking number and subsequent DNA relaxation, and religation of the DNA. The TUNEL assay does detect *in situ* DNA strand breaks in the early stages of spermatogenesis (Marcon and Boissonneault, 2004). However, the lack of proper elimination of errant cells during spermatogenesis could allow cells with DNA strand breaks to continue along the maturation pathway thus causing positive TUNEL assays in epididymal and ejaculated sperm.

The studies described above provide evidence for nucleolytic activity by topoisomerases during spermiogenesis, but at least three separate laboratories have shown that mature spermatozoa may also have active nucleases. Spadaforra and colleagues suggested that the mouse spermatozoon digests a discrete portion of its histone-bound DNA when challenged with exogenous DNA (Maione *et al.*, 1997). A portion of exogenous DNA is internalized into the nuclei triggering nuclease(s) that cleave the exogenous and the genomic DNA. The nuclease response requires challenges with much higher DNA concentrations in ejaculated sperm compared to that in epididymal spermatozoa, eventually leading to cell death in both groups (Spadafora, 1998). Yanagimachi and colleagues have shown that ethylene diamine tetracetic acid (EDTA) and ethylene glycol bis-2-aminoethyl ether-N,N′,N″, n′-tetraacetic acid (EGTA) treatment of spermatozoa prior to intracytoplasmic sperm injection can prevent paternal chromosomal damage (Kaneko *et al.*, 2003; Kusakabe *et al.*, 2001; Tateno *et al.*, 2000), suggesting that some endogenous nuclease does exist in spermatozoa. Finally, our laboratory has shown that fully mature spermatozoa from hamster, mouse, and human have the ability to digest their DNA into loop-sized fragments of 50 kb or so (Sotolongo *et al.*, 2003, 2005). More recent, unpublished data from our laboratory suggests that these nucleases are associated with the sperm nuclear matrix, and can be activated even more completely than we have previously shown. These data suggest that mature spermatozoa do contain some type of nuclease. We propose that these will be similar to the apoptotic related nucleases in somatic cells, including topoisomerase II, but that they might not necessarily function for that purpose. Just as the proteolytic apoptotic machinery was 'borrowed' for normal spermiogenesis functions in *Drosophila* (Arama *et al.*, 2003), so might the nucleolytic functions be used for processes other than classical apoptosis in spermatozoa.

2.6 Conclusions

There is now no doubt that the chromatin of mature mammalian spermatozoa which we once viewed as almost impenetrable to DNA damaging agents can, and often does, contain both ss and ds DNA breaks. Understanding the mechanisms surrounding the generation of sperm chromatin breaks has clinical significance in humans, as the presence of this DNA damage often correlates with male infertility. Several recent reviews presenting hypotheses for the generation of these breaks have been published. The possibilities include abortive apoptosis of spermatogenic cells (Sakkas *et al.*, 2003), incomplete repair of topoisomerase-induced nicks during histone replacement by protamines (Marcon and Boissonneault, 2004; Sakkas *et al.*, 1999a), and the generation of ROS that cause DNA nicks in mature spermatozoa (Aitken *et al.*, 2003). Our recent work has demonstrated that mammalian spermatozoa also contain endogenous nucleases that are capable of digesting all the sperm chromatin (Sotolongo *et al.*, 2003, 2005). Much work remains to be done to understand the origins of DNA damage in the tightly packed sperm chromatin, but it is clear that it has a significant clinical impact.

In this chapter, we have explored the various current SCSAs in light of our models for sperm DNA packaging. Our major conclusion is that the assays that seem to be more correlative with human infertility, specifically the TUNEL and SCSA, probably detect only a subset of sperm DNA damage. This damage is located in those chromatin foci that are in the most open configuration – the toroid linker regions that contain the nuclear matrix attachment sites and the sperm DNA that is most susceptible to exogenous nucleases. Both the alkaline and neutral COMET assays detect virtually all ss and/or ds DNA breaks without regard to the different types of chromatin structure that histones and protamines confer on sperm DNA. In a model that is similar to our Donut-Loop structure, Spadafora has proposed that sperm chromatin contains active sites that are associated with the sperm nuclear matrix (Spadafora, 1998). These active sites would correlate to protamine linker regions. Regardless of whether such active sites exist in spermatozoa, current models of somatic cell chromatin structure suggest that virtually all types of DNA function occur at the sites where the DNA is attached to the nuclear matrix (Pienta *et al.*, 1991). Thus, we have suggested that these same sites in sperm nuclei serve as the nucleation sites for pronuclear DNA replication (Sotolongo and Ward, 2000). If these hypotheses are correct, it seems predictable that SCSAs that focus on these toroid linker sites would be more clinically useful than assays that are not able to distinguish them from the rest of the sperm chromatin.

Of course, it is not yet clear how much of what we have proposed in this work will be modified as research on sperm chromatin structure progresses. However, considering the current sperm DNA assays in the context of our Donut-Loop model predicts the clinical correlations that have been observed to date. We anticipate that further research on how sperm chromatin is packaged will contribute both to a better understanding of the clinical assays that detect sperm DNA damage, and the biological significance of these DNA breaks.

REFERENCES

Agarwal A and Said TM (2003) Role of sperm chromatin abnormalities and DNA damage in male infertility. *Human Reprod Update* 9, 331–345.

Aitken RJ, Gordon E, Harkiss D, Twigg JP, Milne P, Jennings Z and Irvine DS (1998) Relative impact of oxidative stress on the functional competence and genomic integrity of human spermatozoa. *Biol Reprod* 59, 1037–1046.

Aitken RJ, Baker MA and Sawyer D (2003) Oxidative stress in the male germ line and its role in the aetiology of male infertility and genetic disease. *Reprod Biomed Online* 7, 65–70.

Arama E, Agapite J and Steller H (2003) Caspase activity and a specific cytochrome c are required for sperm differentiation in *Drosophila*. *Dev Cell* 4, 687–697.

Aravindan GR, Bjordahl J, Jost LK and Evenson DP (1997) Susceptibility of human sperm to in situ DNA denaturation is strongly correlated with DNA strand breaks identified by single-cell electrophoresis. *Exp Cell Res* 236, 231–237.

Balhorn R (1982) A model for the structure of chromatin in mammalian sperm. *J Cell Biol* 93, 298–305.

Ballachey BE, Hohenboken WD and Evenson DP (1987) Heterogeneity of sperm nuclear chromatin structure and its relationship to bull fertility. *Biol Reprod* 36, 915–925.

Barone JG, Christiano AP and Ward WS (2000) DNA organization in patients with a history of cryptorchidism. *Urology* 56, 1068–1070.

Berensztein EB, Sciara MI, Rivarola MA and Belgorosky A (2002) Apoptosis and proliferation of human testicular somatic and germ cells during prepuberty: high rate of testicular growth in newborns mediated by decreased apoptosis. *J Clin Endocrinol Metab* 87, 5113–5118.

Billig H, Furuta I, Rivier C, Tapanainen J, Parvinen M and Hsueh AJ (1995) Apoptosis in testis germ cells: developmental changes in gonadotropin dependence and localization to selective tubule stages. *Endocrinology* 136, 5–12.

Blanc-Layrac G, Bringuier AF, Guillot R and Feldmann G (2000) Morphological and biochemical analysis of cell death in human ejaculated spermatozoa. *Cell Mol Biol (Noisy-le-grand)* 46, 187–197.

Blanco-Rodriguez J (1998) A matter of death and life: the significance of germ cell death during spermatogenesis. *Int J Androl* 21, 236–248.

Blanco-Rodriguez J and Martinez-Garcia C (1999) Apoptosis is physiologically restricted to a specialized cytoplasmic compartment in rat spermatids. *Biol Reprod* 61, 1541–1547.

Brewer LR, Corzett M and Balhorn R (1999) Protamine-induced condensation and decondensation of the same DNA molecule. *Science* 286, 120–123.

Brewer L, Corzett M, Lau EY and Balhorn R (2003) Dynamics of protamine 1 binding to single DNA molecules. *J Biol Chem* 278, 42403–42408.

Cayli S, Sakkas D, Vigue L, Demir R and Huszar G (2004) Cellular maturity and apoptosis in human sperm: creatine kinase, caspase-3 and bcl-xl levels in mature and diminished maturity sperm. *Mol Hum Reprod* 10, 365–372.

Chen JL and Longo FJ (1996) Expression and localization of DNA topoisomerase ii during rat spermatogenesis. *Mol Reprod Dev* 45, 61–71.

De Jonge C (2002) The clinical value of sperm nuclear DNA assessment. *Human Fertil (Camb)* 5, 51–53.

de Vries KJ, Wiedmer T, Sims PJ and Gadella BM (2003) Caspase-independent exposure of aminophospholipids and tyrosine phosphorylation in bicarbonate responsive human sperm cells. *Biol Reprod* 68, 2122–2134.

Evenson D and Jost L (2000) Sperm chromatin structure assay is useful for fertility assessment. *Methods Cell Sci* 22, 169–189.

Evenson DP, Jost LK, Marshall D, Zinaman MJ, Clegg E, Purvis K, de Angelis P and Claussen OP (1999) Utility of the sperm chromatin structure assay as a diagnostic and prognostic tool in the human fertility clinic. *Human Reprod* 14, 1039–1049.

Evenson DP, Larson KL and Jost LK (2002) Sperm chromatin structure assay: its clinical use for detecting sperm DNA fragmentation in male infertility and comparisons with other techniques. *J Androl* 23, 25–43.

Furuchi T, Masuko K, Nishimune Y, Obinata M and Matsui Y (1996) Inhibition of testicular germ cell apoptosis and differentiation in mice misexpressing bcl-2 in spermatogonia. *Development* 122, 1703–1709.

Gadella BM and Harrison RA (2002) Capacitation induces cyclic adenosine $3',5'$-monophosphate-dependent, but apoptosis-unrelated, exposure of aminophospholipids at the apical head plasma membrane of boar sperm cells. *Biol Reprod* 67, 340–350.

Gineitis AA, Zalenskaya IA, Yau PM, Bradbury EM and Zalensky AO (2000) Human sperm telomere-binding complex involves histone h2b and secures telomere membrane attachment. *J Cell Biol* 151, 1591–1598.

Gorczyca W, Traganos F, Jesionowska H and Darzynkiewicz Z (1993) Presence of DNA strand breaks and increased sensitivity of DNA *in situ* to denaturation in abnormal human sperm cells: analogy to apoptosis of somatic cells. *Exp Cell Res* 207, 202–205.

Guthrie HD and Welch GR (2005) Impact of storage prior to cryopreservation on plasma membrane function and fertility of boar sperm. *Theriogenology* 63, 396–410.

Hud NV, Allen MJ, Downing KH, Lee J and Balhorn R (1993) Identification of the elemental packing unit of DNA in mammalian sperm cells by atomic force microscopy. *Biochem Biophys Res Commun* 193, 1347–1354.

Hud NV, Milanovich FP and Balhorn R (1994) Evidence of novel secondary structure in DNA-bound protamine is revealed by raman spectroscopy. *Biochemistry* 33, 7528–7535.

Jones R (2004) Sperm survival versus degradation in the mammalian epididymis: a hypothesis. *Biol Reprod* 71, 1405–1411.

Kaneko T, Whittingham DG and Yanagimachi R (2003) Effect of ph value of freeze-drying solution on the chromosome integrity and developmental ability of mouse spermatozoa. *Biol Reprod* 68, 136–139.

Kerr JF, Wyllie AH and Currie AR (1972) Apoptosis: a basic biological phenomenon with wide-ranging implications in tissue kinetics. *Br J Cancer* 26, 239–257.

Kimura Y and Yanagimachi R (1995) Mouse oocytes injected with testicular spermatozoa or round spermatids can develop into normal offspring. *Development* 121, 2397–2405.

Knudson CM, Tung KS, Tourtellotte WG, Brown GA and Korsmeyer SJ (1995) Bax-deficient mice with lymphoid hyperplasia and male germ cell death. *Science* 270, 96–99.

Kusakabe H, Szczygiel MA, Whittingham DG and Yanagimachi R (2001) Maintenance of genetic integrity in frozen and freeze-dried mouse spermatozoa. *Proc Natl Acad Sci USA* 98, 13501–13506.

Lachaud C, Tesarik J, Canadas ML and Mendoza C (2004) Apoptosis and necrosis in human ejaculated spermatozoa. *Human Reprod* 19, 607–610.

Larson-Cook KL, Brannian JD, Hansen KA, Kasperson KM, Aamold ET and Evenson DP (2003) Relationship between the outcomes of assisted reproductive techniques and sperm DNA fragmentation as measured by the sperm chromatin structure assay. *Fertil Steril* 80, 895–902.

Maione B, Pittoggi C, Achene L, Lorenzini R and Spadafora C (1997) Activation of endogenous nucleases in mature sperm cells upon interaction with exogenous DNA. *DNA Cell Biol* 16, 1087–1097.

Marcon L and Boissonneault G (2004) Transient DNA strand breaks during mouse and human spermiogenesis new insights in stage specificity and link to chromatin remodeling. *Biol Reprod* 70, 910–918.

Martins RP, Ostermeier GC and Krawetz SA (2004) Nuclear matrix interactions at the human protamine domain: a working model of potentiation. *J Biol Chem* 279, 51862–51868.

McCarthy S and Ward WS (1999) Functional aspects of mammalian sperm chromatin. *Human Fertil* 2, 56–60.

McPherson SM and Longo FJ (1993) Nicking of rat spermatid and spermatozoa DNA: possible involvement of DNA topoisomerase ii. *Dev Biol* 158, 122–130.

McVicar CM, McClure N, Williamson K, Dalzell LH and Lewis SE (2004) Incidence of fas positivity and deoxyribonucleic acid double-stranded breaks in human ejaculated sperm. *Fertil Steril* 81 (Suppl 1), 767–774.

Meistrich ML, Mohapatra B, Shirley CR and Zhao M (2003) Roles of transition nuclear proteins in spermiogenesis. *Chromosoma* 111, 483–488.

Muratori M, Maggi M, Spinelli S, Filimberti E, Forti G and Baldi E (2003) Spontaneous DNA fragmentation in swim-up selected human spermatozoa during long term incubation. *J Androl* 24, 253–262.

Nadel B, de Lara J, Finkernagel SW and Ward WS (1995) Cell-specific organization of the 5s ribosomal rna gene cluster DNA loop domains in spermatozoa and somatic cells. *Biol Reprod* 53, 1222–1228.

Oehninger S, Morshedi M, Weng SL, Taylor S, Duran H and Beebe S (2003) Presence and significance of somatic cell apoptosis markers in human ejaculated spermatozoa. *Reprod Biomed Online* 7, 469–476.

Ogura A, Matsuda J and Yanagimachi R (1994) Birth of normal young after electrofusion of mouse oocytes with round spermatids. *Proc Natl Acad Sci USA* 91, 7460–7462.

Paasch U, Agarwal A, Gupta AK, Sharma RK, Grunewald S, Thomas Jr., AJ and Glander HJ (2003) Apoptosis signal transduction and the maturity status of human spermatozoa. *Ann N Y Acad Sci* 1010, 486–488.

Paasch U, Grunewald S, Dathe S and Glander HJ (2004) Mitochondria of human spermatozoa are preferentially susceptible to apoptosis. *Ann N Y Acad Sci* 1030, 403–409.

Pienta KJ, Getzenberg RH and Coffey DS (1991) Cell structure and DNA organization. *Crit Rev Eukaryot Gene Expr* 1, 355–385.

Pittoggi C, Zaccagnini G, Giordano R, Magnano AR, Baccetti B, Lorenzini R and Spadafora C (2000) Nucleosomal domains of mouse spermatozoa chromatin as potential sites for retroposition and foreign DNA integration. *Mol Reprod Dev* 56, 248–251.

Prieto MC, Maki AH and Balhorn R (1997) Analysis of DNA-protamine interactions by optical detection of magnetic resonance. *Biochemistry* 36, 11944–11951.

Print CG and Loveland KL (2000) Germ cell suicide: new insights into apoptosis during spermatogenesis. *Bioessays* 22, 423–430.

Sakkas D, Mariethoz E, Manicardi G, Bizzaro D, Bianchi PG and Bianchi U (1999a) Origin of DNA damage in ejaculated human spermatozoa. *Rev Reprod* 4, 31–37.

Sakkas D, Mariethoz E and St John JC (1999b) Abnormal sperm parameters in humans are indicative of an abortive apoptotic mechanism linked to the fas-mediated pathway. *Exp Cell Res* 251, 350–355.

Sakkas D, Moffatt O, Manicardi GC, Mariethoz E, Tarozzi N and Bizzaro D (2002) Nature of DNA damage in ejaculated human spermatozoa and the possible involvement of apoptosis. *Biol Reprod* 66, 1061–1067.

Sakkas D, Manicardi GC and Bizzaro D (2003) Sperm nuclear DNA damage in the human. *Adv Exp Med Biol* 518, 73–84.

Schmid C, Heng HH, Rubin C, Ye CJ and Krawetz SA (2001) Sperm nuclear matrix association of the prm1→prm2→tnp2 domain is independent of alu methylation. *Mol Hum Reprod* 7, 903–911.

Seli E, Gardner DK, Schoolcraft WB, Moffatt O and Sakkas D (2004) Extent of nuclear DNA damage in ejaculated spermatozoa impacts on blastocyst development after *in vitro* fertilization. *Fertil Steril* 82, 378–383.

Sgonc R and Gruber J (1998) Apoptosis detection: an overview. *Exp Gerontol* 33, 525–533.

Sotolongo B and Ward WS (2000) DNA loop domain organization: the three dimensional genomic code. *J Cell Biochem* 35, 23–26.

Sotolongo B, Lino E and Ward WS (2003) Ability of hamster spermatozoa to digest their own DNA. *Biol Reprod* 69, 2029–2035.

Sotolongo B, Huang TF, Isenberger E and Ward WS (2005) An endogenous nuclease in hamster, mouse and human spermatozoa cleaves DNA into loop-sized fragments. *J Androl* 26, 272–280.

Spadafora C (1998) Sperm cells and foreign DNA: a controversial relation. *Bioessays* 20, 955–964.

Spano M and Sakkas D (2005) The significance of sperm nuclear DNA strand breaks on reproductive outcome. Current Opinions in Obstetrics and Gynecology *In Press.*

St Pierre J, Wright DJ, Rowe TC and Wright SJ (2002) DNA topoisomerase ii distribution in mouse preimplantation embryos. *Mol Reprod Dev* 61, 335–346.

Sun JG, Jurisicova A and Casper RF (1997) Detection of deoxyribonucleic acid fragmentation in human sperm: Correlation with fertilization *in vitro. Biol Reprod* 56, 602–607.

Tateno H, Kimura Y and Yanagimachi R (2000) Sonication per se is not as deleterious to sperm chromosomes as previously inferred. *Biol Reprod* 63, 341–346.

Taylor SL, Weng SL, Fox P, Duran EH, Morshedi MS, Oehninger S and Beebe SJ (2004) Somatic cell apoptosis markers and pathways in human ejaculated sperm: potential utility as indicators of sperm quality. *Mol Human Reprod* 10, 825–834.

Tomsu M, Sharma V and Miller D (2002) Embryo quality and ivf treatment outcomes may correlate with different sperm comet assay parameters. *Human Reprod* 17, 1856–1862.

Van Kooij RJ, de Boer P, De Vreeden-Elbertse JM, Ganga NA, Singh N and Te Velde ER (2004) The neutral comet assay detects double strand DNA damage in selected and unselected human spermatozoa of normospermic donors. *Int J Androl* 27, 140–146.

Vilfan ID, Conwell CC and Hud NV (2004) Formation of native-like mammalian sperm cell chromatin with folded bull protamine. *J Biol Chem* 279, 20088–20095.

Wang X, Sharma RK, Sikka SC, Thomas Jr., AJ, Falcone T and Agarwal A (2003) Oxidative stress is associated with increased apoptosis leading to spermatozoa DNA damage in patients with male factor infertility. *Fertil Steril* 80, 531–535.

Ward MA and Ward WS (2004) A model for the function of sperm DNA degradation. *Reprod Fertil Dev* 16, 547–554.

Ward WS (1993) Deoxyribonucleic acid loop domain tertiary structure in mammalian spermatozoa. *Biol Reprod* 48, 1193–1201.

Ward WS and Coffey DS (1991) DNA packaging and organization in mammalian spermatozoa: comparison with somatic cells. *Biol Reprod* 44, 569–574.

Ward WS, Partin AW and Coffey DS (1989) DNA loop domains in mammalian spermatozoa. *Chromosoma* 98, 153–159.

Ward WS, Kishikawa H, Akutsu H, Yanagimachi H and Yanagimachi R (2000) Further evidence that sperm nuclear proteins are necessary for embryogenesis. *Zygote* 8, 51–56.

Weng SL, Taylor SL, Morshedi M, Schuffner A, Duran EH, Beebe S and Oehninger S (2002) Caspase activity and apoptotic markers in ejaculated human sperm. *Mol Hum Reprod* 8, 984–991.

Wykes SM and Krawetz SA (2003a) Conservation of the prm1→prm2→tnp2 domain. *DNA Seq* 14, 359–367.

Wykes SM and Krawetz SA (2003b) The structural organization of sperm chromatin. *J Biol Chem* 278, 29471–29477.

Yanagida K, Yanagimachi R, Perreault SD and Kleinfeld RG (1991) Thermostability of sperm nuclei assessed by microinjection into hamster oocytes. *Biol Reprod* 44, 440–447.

Zalensky AO, Siino JS, Gineitis AA, Zalenskaya IA, Tomilin NV, Yau P and Bradbury EM (2002) Human testis/sperm-specific histone h2b (htsh2b). Molecular cloning and characterization. *J Biol Chem* 277, 43474–43480.

Genomic and proteomic approaches to defining sperm production and function

Sarah J. Conner[1] and Christopher L.R. Barratt[1,2]

[1]Reproductive Biology and Genetics Group, Division of Reproductive and Child Health, University of Birmingham;
[2]Assisted Conception Unit, Birmingham Women's Hospital, Edgbaston, Birmingham, England, UK

3.1 Introduction

The purpose of this chapter is to provide the reader with an insight into potential new developments in male infertility; specifically, sperm development and function, concentrating on the technologies of gene expression, proteomics and use of gene knock out experiments. We initially discuss the future of traditional semen analysis, as a baseline to describing new technologies. The overall objective is to stimulate the reader to find out more about these developments and to provide some guidance on how the information can be used to develop more effective diagnostic tools for the future. It is our premise that a more detailed understanding of the physiology of both the normal and pathological cell is central to developing rational, non-assisted reproductive technology (non-ART) therapy.

3.2 How useful is a semen assessment for the diagnosis and prognosis of male infertility?

The value of traditional semen parameters (concentration, motility and morphology) in the diagnosis and prognosis of male infertility has been debated for almost 60 years and, perhaps not surprisingly, the debate continues (see Björndahl et al., 2005). There are many difficulties in the design of studies to assess the value of traditional semen parameters, for example number of semen samples to assess, relevance of different outcomes (in vitro fertilisation (IVF) versus in vivo conception) etc., but one of the most significant variables is the degree of quality control (QC) measures in place to ensure the assessment is valid. The majority of studies that have concluded that traditional semen parameters have limited or no value in the diagnosis/prognosis of male infertility do not provide any (or very limited) information on QC procedures and thus it is difficult to determine the relevance of their findings. For example, if the methods cannot detect a difference of 25% on sperm concentration it is not surprising that sperm concentration is not significantly related to fertility (e.g. Polansky and Lamb, 1988). More recent publications, with better-defined populations, and an improved awareness of the need for QC (Björndahl *et al.*, 2005; De Jonge and Barratt, 1999; WHO, 1999) have shown that traditional semen parameters do provide some degree of prognostic and diagnostic information for the infertile couple (Bonde *et al.*, 1998; Larsen *et al.*, 2000; Tomlinson *et al.*, 1999). However, even with rigorous QC procedures in place, it is only at the lower ranges of the spectrum that these parameters are most useful (Comhaire, 2000) and, even then they can only be used as guidance for couples and do not represent absolute values.

Traditional semen analysis will therefore only be a limited first line tool in the diagnosis of male infertility. Consequently, andrologists have focused on developing simple, robust and effective tests of sperm function. However, despite the plethora of potential assays available, results have been very disappointing (ESHRE, 1996; Muller, 2000). In fact, assessing the current data, it is difficult to see that there are more effective methods to assess sperm function than perhaps the most simple (and oldest) sperm function assay – penetration of spermatozoa into human cervical mucus (or artificial substitutes) (Aitken *et al.*, 1992; Ivic *et al.*, 2002). One exception, and potential assay on the horizon, is the assessment of the DNA integrity of the spermatozoon however, recent data questions the preliminary favourable results (Bungum *et al.*, 2004; Gandini *et al.*, 2004). Comprehensive studies are required to see whether this assay lives up to its initial promise and stands the test of time or, as with many of the other putative sperm function assays, dies a slow and painful death.

While the paucity of robust assays of sperm function is surprising, frustrating and disappointing it does allow clinical and research andrologists to re-evaluate and formulate more sophisticated strategies to guide the field into the next generation of functional assays.

3.3 The sperm and testis transcriptome

3.3.1 Sperm mRNA

Following considerable debate, it has now been established that human sperm contain complex populations of RNA. There have been a number of studies using sperm RNA as a template to successfully determine the presence of targets of interest, for example L type calcium channels (Goodwin *et al.*, 2000) and oestrogen receptor alpha and beta (Aquila *et al.*, 2004). In addition, using cDNA microarrays, the possibility of the sperm RNA profile as an indication of male fertility has been suggested. A rigorous study by Ostermeier and colleagues (2002) documented sperm RNA profiles of fertile men. Comparisons were made with gene expression in the testis and lymphocyte controls. Intriguingly, there was minimal overlap with the lymphocyte profile suggesting an essentially pure population of sperm RNA. Additionally, one individual ejaculate contained almost all the unique expressed sequence tags (ESTs) as were detected in the pooled fertile controls. Concordance between testicular and the sperm profiles supported the view that sperm RNA can be used to monitor past events during spermatogenesis. This study paves the way for the more detailed molecular examination of sperm dysfunction and may represent a powerful non-biased systematic approach. Surprisingly, to date, no study has compared these normal profiles ('molecular signatures' Miller *et al.*, 2005) with those from men with defined sperm dysfunction to try and address possible differences that may be related to function. One specific case would be to compare those men with poor sperm hyperactivation and determine if the transcripts for the reported calcium entry and activation channels are present (e.g. the CatSper family). An obvious advantage of sperm microarrays, which are non-invasive, is that testicular biopsies, which can be very difficult to obtain, may become redundant as a material for gene expression. It remains to be seen if this will happen.

The functional significance of RNA in sperm is still a matter of debate. Comparison of sperm RNA populations with those in the early zygote and the unfertilised egg show that there is a population of RNAs in both the early zygote and sperm that are not present in the unfertilised human egg (Ostermeier *et al.*, 2002, 2004). At least six candidate mRNAs have been identified including clusterin and protamine 2, although the exact function and critical importance of these sperm specific mRNAs has yet to be established. In a recent review, David Miller (Miller *et al.*, 2005) suggests that the RNA may have a role in selective chromatin repackaging and possibly in mediating specific imprinting events at fertilisation. The latter is a fascinating concept. Additionally, micro RNAs (miRNAs) and silencing RNAs (siRNAs) have also been detected in human spermatozoa and these may also play a role in early fertilisation events (Ostermeier *et al.*, 2005).

3.3.2 The transcriptome of the testis

There have been a large number of publications using microarray analysis to study the transcriptome of the animal testis. A variety of approaches have been developed ranging from relatively simple methods examining a very limited gene set, to more sophisticated techniques developing subtracted cDNA libraries. The widespread use of gene expression array technology to assess global transcription represents a very powerful tool to study a plethora of exciting developments in sperm production such as profiling the specific stages of gene expression in spermatogenesis (Shima *et al.*, 2004; Small *et al.*, 2005), examining the effect of androgens on gene expression (Zhou *et al.*, 2005) and obtaining expression profiles of isolated germ cells (Hofmann *et al.*, 2005).

In order to exploit the wealth of information that is generated from microarray experiments, Primig and colleagues (Wrobel and Primig, 2005) have developed a unique interactive web-based resource on germ cell expression data (www. germonline.org). This provides a novel cross species knowledge base that has numerous features including graphical displays for expression signals and contains the latest available microarray data allowing direct access by researchers thus permitting up to date information to be readily available (see Wiederhehr et al., 2004; Wrobel and Primig, 2005). Importantly, it also allows the comparison of data from different organisms (e.g. *Saccharomyces cerevisiae*), thus facilitating the potential to understand fundamental developmental processes (e.g. meiosis).

Ellis and colleagues (2004) described the construction and validation of a comprehensive subtractive cDNA microarray covering approximately 2000 testicular genes that are strongly representative of genes expressed in meiosis and post-meiotic stages. The objective was to determine the transcriptional profile of the first wave of spermatogenesis in the mouse and compare the results to a variety of models of male infertility: (1) $XXSxr^b$ (few if any germ cells); (2) *mshi* homozygotes (reduced numbers of spermatogonia and no progression beyond the meiotic stages); (3) *Bax* $(-/-)$ (atypical pre-meiotic cells and depleted post-meiotic stages); (4) *bs* homozygotes (failure of post-meiotic acrosome assembly leading to reduced sperm numbers); (5) *azh* (teratozoospermia and subfertility); (6) *bcl-w*. Their detailed analysis demonstrated clustering of gene expression at different stages and different days during the first wave of spermatogenesis (56dpp). The post-meiotic gene cluster (spermatid associated clusters) had the highest proportion of uncharacterised genes (of unknown function) highlighting our limited understanding of this complex period of cell development (see also Schultz et al., 2003). In comparisons between controls and the $XXSxr^b$ mouse there was low-level somatic expression of genes in germ cell types. In comparison with *mshi* and *Bax* there was near normal levels of early onset transcripts (early germ cell stages) but a relative absence of genes in the latter stages of spermatogenesis. Interestingly, while the testicular histology of the *azh* and *bcl-w* mutants were different from that found in normal animals, few transcriptional differences were detected in the mutants as compared to normal mice. The failure to detect difference in the *azh* model may be due to the fact that there is no expression of mRNA in the latter stages of spermatogenesis (during chromatin repackaging) where the transcripts are believed to be pre-expressed and stored.

Schultz et al. (2003) used an Affymetrix mouse (U74 v2) oligonucleotide array set analysing approximately 20,000 genes to study the germ cell-enriched gene expression profile from post-partum day 1 to adult mice. There were a significant number of testis-specific transcripts identified coincident with or after meiosis – approximating to 4% of the mouse genome. These data provided a large number of candidate genes for contraceptive targeting as well as a number of proteins that may be involved in fertilisation. When Schultz et al. compared specific post-meiotic gene transcripts to the literature databases approximately 50% of the genes lead to complete loss of fertility in knockout animals. These results encourage examination of late/post-meiotic transcripts to assess their potential as contraceptive targets.

In addition to examining expression profiles for male fertility there is likely to be an increased use of microarray technology in toxicology studies. For example, Aguilar-Mahecha and colleagues (2002) examined the effect of chronic cyclophosphamide on gene expression in the rat using 216 cDNAs. Cyclophosphamide treatment led to a substantial decrease in gene expression: decreased levels of gene expression in pachytene spermatocytes (34% of genes studied), round spermatids (29% of genes studied) and elongating spermatids (4% of genes studied). In elongating spermatids only, drug treatment increased expression in 8% of genes studied (Aguilar-Mahecha et al., 2002). In contrast to the chronic exposure results, acute exposure caused increased gene expression in all the cell types examined (Aguilar-Mahecha et al., 2001). Future toxicological research should benefit greatly with the development of more advanced microarrays that can screen the whole genome.

The advent of microarrays to scan the genome makes it now possible to study human spermatogenesis in normal and subfertile populations. In conjunction with non-invasive fine needle aspirations of the testis we are likely to see a number of studies of human expression profiles associated with male fertility. One interesting example would be to study the expression profile of men with high levels of sperm aneuploidy in an attempt to determine the genes involved in this condition.

3.3.3 The sperm proteome

Comprehensive and systematic identification and quantification of proteins expressed in cells and tissues are providing important and fascinating insights into the dynamics of cell function. For example, there has been a wealth of detailed proteomic studies to identify molecular signatures of disease states (e.g. phosphoprotein networks in cancer cells (Irish et al., 2004)).

Rapid technological advances facilitate faster and more accurate revelations of cell function, for example comprehensive proteomic mapping of the lung endothelial cell surface (Durr et al., 2004). Complementing the growth in technology and the number of pathologies subject to diagnosis, there has been an expansion in the variety of bioinformatics approaches to study protein–protein interaction networks (Papin et al., 2005). Additionally, there have been important developments in mathematical computing/prediction (e.g. Baysian networks), to try and determine the complex stochastic non-linear interactions between signalling molecules in cells (Sachs et al., 2005).

Spermatozoa would appear ideal to study from a proteomic perspective because they are transcriptionally inactive. However, there have been relatively few studies examining the proteome of human spermatozoa. Studies have used antisperm antibody sera in an attempt to detect potential sperm targets for male contraception. This is a logical approach because antisperm antibodies are associated with sterility, albeit in a very limited number of cases. Unfortunately, however, this rational approach has met with limited success (see Naaby-Hansen *et al.*, 1997; Shetty *et al.*, 1999; Shibahara *et al.*, 2002) with very few robust candidate proteins being identified (see for review Bohring and Krause, 2003). For example, Bohring *et al.* (2001) have identified six potential candidates (HSP 70, HSP70-2, disulphide isomerase ER60, the inactive form of caspase 3 and two subunits of the proteosome complex) but there has been a paucity of data on the relevance of these candidates as potential contraceptive targets, and the identification of new ones.

There are two main difficulties with using antisperm antibodies to identify protein targets. Firstly, the nature of the antisperm antibody response in the infertile patient is very poorly understood. Secondly, as a result of this, our techniques/assays to detect functional antisperm antibodies is limited (see for review Chiu and Chamley, 2004). However, with improved diagnosis of immune infertility and rapid developments in proteomic technology, specifically identification of membrane proteins, this strategy is likely to lead to the discovery of some interesting contraceptive candidates.

Other than the above, there have been very few studies that have employed proteomic approaches to examine male infertility. A small number of studies have attempted initial characterisation of the sperm plasma membrane (Shetty *et al.*, 2001). Further studies have examined specific processes, for example calcium-binding proteins and proteins that are tyrosine phosphorylated (Ficarro *et al.*, 2003; Naaby-Hansen *et al.*, 2002). Interestingly, it is over 10 years since the discovery of tyrosine phosphorylation as a putative marker of capacitation yet the role of the proteins and their sequence of activation is very sketchy and, with the exception of the A-kinase anchoring proteins (AKAPs) (AKAP3 and AKAP4), only a small number of candidate proteins have been identified (see Naz and Rajesh, 2004). However, some progress is being made. For example, Gary Olson has identified the phospholipid hydroperoxide glutathione peroxidase in hamster sperm as being phosphorylated on tyrosine residues during capacitation (Nagdas *et al.*, 2005). However, we are still a long way from obtaining even a minimal 'picture' of events.

The slow progress/application of the proteomic revolution in human spermatozoa contrasts markedly with other fields. A relevant example is the large-scale proteomic studies on human cilia (e.g. Ostrowski *et al.*, 2002). Estimates from *Chlamydomonas* suggest there are at least 250 flagellar proteins. In close agreement, Ostrowski and colleagues were able to identify 200 ciliary axonemal proteins, some of which were sperm/testis specific (e.g. Sp17). Using the aforementioned as a foundation, more detailed and efficient studies of human sperm are likely.

Table 3.1. Assessment of variation of the sperm proteome by automated gel analysis

Experimental comparison	Total number of spots detected in reference gel	Number of spots with increased or decreased expression on one gel compared to the other (percentage of total spot number)	Number of spots absent from one gel compared to the other (percentage of total spot number)
Same ejaculate	1087	58 (5.3)	14 (1.3)
Different ejaculates			
Same donor	1175	84 (7.1)	16 (1.4)
Different donors	882	67 (7.6)	16 (1.8)
Fertile donor and	963	36 (4.0)	48 (5.0)
patient A			(28 unique to control; 20 unique to patient)

Experimental, intra-donor, inter-donor and patient versus control variation was assessed by gel analyses of four gel pairs using Phoretix Evolution software. Increased and decreased expression was defined as a greater than 4-fold difference in spot intensity between the two gels.
Adapted from Pixton *et al.* (2004).

In our laboratory we have been using proteomic strategies to identify defects in sperm function responsible for fertilisation (Lefievre *et al.*, 2003, 2004; Pixton *et al.*, 2004). Specifically we are interested in identifying differences in sperm protein expression between control (fertile) men and patients with spermatozoa that failed to fertilise oocytes *in vitro*. Our initial studies have focused on a 2D gel-based approach and developing a series of fertile controls (with several ejaculates) in order to determine if any differences observed in the patient samples are real. Initial results are interesting. To our surprise, there was relatively little intra-donor and inter-donor variation (1.4% and 1.8% of the total number of spots identified, respectively) (see Table 3.1). However, differences between gels do occur and when accounting for this, we have categorised one man (Pixton *et al.*, 2004) where we have identified 20 differences between the control that we are confident represent true differences.

However, our approach is very limited. A combination of proteomic approaches is required. For example, Ostrowski and colleagues (2002) only identified 38 potential proteins using 2D PAGE. A number of proteins were not resolved (e.g. dynein heavy chains which have a large molecular mass) and complementary approaches were needed to provide a detailed picture. 1D gels identified another 110 proteins. A second approach involved isolated axonemes, followed by digestion and analysis directly by liquid chromatography with tandem mass spectrometry (LC/MS/MS) or multi-dimensional LC/MS/MS. This led to the identification of a further 66 proteins. In conclusion, more than one proteomic strategy needs to be employed.

In studies we have performed on the human zona pellucida, we had to try several different methods to definitively identify ZP1 as a fourth zona protein. The most successful approach used trypsin digestion followed by direct MS/MS (Conner *et al.*, 2005; Lefievre *et al.*, 2004). A further difficulty in comparing sperm samples (e.g. patient versus control), is exactly how to do this. Our initial studies have used gel-based software. While impressive (see Fig. 2 Pixton *et al.*, 2004) what is really required is comparison between the samples run and analysed simultaneously (i.e. internal controls). Such proteomic technologies now exist. Interestingly, Baker and colleagues (2005) analysed post-translational modifications occurring during sperm maturation in the rat using differences in two-dimensional gel electrophoresis (DIGI). This used resolvable cyanine dyes to compare samples. Eight unambiguous proteins were identified and one (β subunit of the mitochondrial F1ATPase) was shown to be serine phosphorylated as sperm transit the epididymis.

There have been several proteomic studies to determine the content of seminal plasma (Starita-Geribaldi *et al.*, 2003a, b). In addition to the obvious application in the diagnosis of prostate cancer (Fung *et al.*, 2004), the seminal plasma proteome may provide an additional tool in the diagnosis of spermatogenesis defects (Pointis *et al.*, 2003) and, changes in profile associated with genito–urinary tract infections.

3.4 Mouse models for male infertility: the role of knockout mice

Mouse models with an infertility phenotype are being published with increased frequency. These numbered over 200 in 2002 and are described in a excellent comprehensive review by Matzuk and Lamb (2002). Genotypes affecting fertility are also being reported in on-line databases, for example see The Jackson Laboratories Reproductive Genomics: Mutant Mouse Models of Infertility (http://reprogenomics.jax.org/) or http://www.germonline.org.

In this section we discuss in greater detail a selection of these gene products and their associated phenotypes that impact on sperm function. We concentrate particularly on those proteins that are affecting sperm transport, capacitation and initial interaction with the egg vestments (see Fig. 3.1).

3.4.1 Akap4

The *Akap4* gene encodes an AKAP and is only expressed in spermatogenic cells. AKAPs are associated with the regulatory domains of cAMP-dependent kinases (protein kinase A, PKA) and AKAP4 is the major fibrous sheath protein of the principal piece. It is thought that the AKAP4 protein has a role in the recruitment of PKA to the fibrous sheath where it regulates flagellar function through localised phosphorylation (Miki and Eddy, 1998, 1999).

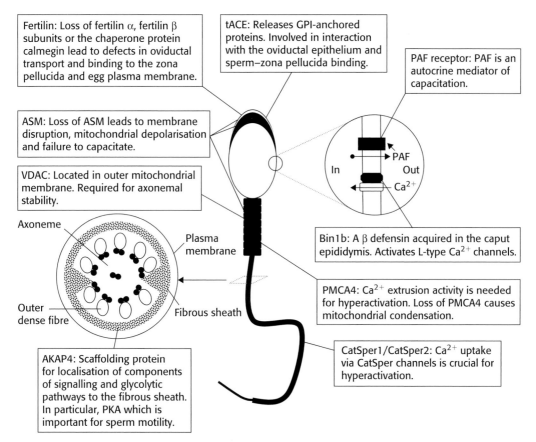

Fertilin: Loss of fertilin α, fertilin β subunits or the chaperone protein calmegin lead to defects in oviductal transport and binding to the zona pellucida and egg plasma membrane.

tACE: Releases GPI-anchored proteins. Involved in interaction with the oviductal epithelium and sperm–zona pellucida binding.

PAF receptor: PAF is an autocrine mediator of capacitation.

ASM: Loss of ASM leads to membrane disruption, mitochondrial depolarisation and failure to capacitate.

VDAC: Located in outer mitochondrial membrane. Required for axonemal stability.

Axoneme

Plasma membrane

PAF

In   Out

Ca^{2+}

Bin1b: A β defensin acquired in the caput epididymis. Activates L-type Ca^{2+} channels.

Outer dense fibre

Fibrous sheath

PMCA4: Ca^{2+} extrusion activity is needed for hyperactivation. Loss of PMCA4 causes mitochondrial condensation.

AKAP4: Scaffolding protein for localisation of components of signalling and glycolytic pathways to the fibrous sheath. In particular, PKA which is important for sperm motility.

CatSper1/CatSper2: Ca^{2+} uptake via CatSper channels is crucial for hyperactivation.

Figure 3.1   A schematic diagram of a spermatozoon illustrating the location and effect of gene deletion experiments in the mouse. Particular emphasis is placed on the process of sperm capacitation and transport in the female tract and interaction with the egg vestments

Disruption of the *Akap4* gene therefore provides an alternative method for studying the role of PKA in spermatozoa as well as the function of the AKAP4 protein itself. *Akap4* gene knockout mice are infertile; although they produce normal sperm numbers they are all immotile (Miki *et al.*, 2002). Fibrous sheath formation does not go to completion, resulting in sperm with a reduced principal piece diameter and a shortened flagellum. A redistribution of and a reduction in the amount of PKA were also suggested to be a factor in the loss of sperm motility in the mutant mice. A further study (Huang *et al.*, 2005) examined the effect of the *Akap4* null mutation on intracellular distribution of a number of signalling proteins suggested to interact with AKAP4. In the mutant mice there was disruption of the distribution of PKA (both regulatory and catalytic subunits), phosphatidylinositol 3-kinase (PI 3-kinase) and sperm autoantigenic protein 17 (SP17) suggesting that these proteins are associated with the fibrous sheath. Whilst the subcellular distribution of the gamma catalytic subunit of protein phosphatase 1 (PPIγ2) was unchanged, a decrease in the phosphorylation of the protein and an increase in PPIγ2 activity were observed. The authors postulate that the decrease in the phosphorylation of PPIγ2 may reflect the lower ATP levels observed in the *Akap4* knockout mice. A number of glycolytic enzymes are anchored to the fibrous sheath (Eddy *et al.*, 2003; Miki *et al.*, 2002) and it is therefore probable that in the mutant mice the process of glycolysis is disrupted which is known to have an impact on sperm function.

It is clear that the fibrous sheath has more than a structural role. The effects of disrupting the *Akap4* gene suggest that AKAP4 positions PKA in proximity to its target protein and also anchors a number of signal transduction proteins and components of the glycolytic pathway that are essential for sperm function.

3.4.2 Vdac3

Voltage-dependent anion channels (VDACs) are found in the outer mitochondrial membrane of all eukaryotes. They are small (30 kDa) channel proteins that are involved in the translocation of metabolites and are sometimes also referred to as mitochondrial porins. There are three mammalian *Vdac* genes encoding VDAC1-3 proteins (Decker *et al.*, 1999; Sampson *et al.*, 1997). Targeted mutation of *Vdac3* causes male infertility (Sampson *et al.*, 2001). Normal numbers of spermatozoa are produced but motility is decreased (approximately 25% of wild type). The mutant mice also have defects in oxidative phosphorylation in skeletal muscle. Electron microscopy revealed structural defects in two thirds of the sperm axonemes; often the loss of a single microtubule doublet. The defect was rarely observed in testicular sperm but developed with maturation of the sperm in the epididymis. These mice demonstrate that functional mitochondria are required for the correct formation of the axonemes with resultant effects on sperm motility and fertility.

3.5 Sperm transit in the female tract

Following ejaculation spermatozoa have to traverse the female tract to bind and fertilise the ovulated oocyte – a journey that we know almost nothing about (review De Jonge, 2005). An important factor in this migration is sperm motility and the subsequent development of hyperactivation.

3.5.1 Angiotensin-converting enzyme

The Angiotensin-converting enzyme (ACE) is an upregulator of blood pressure through its peptidase activity (Hooper, 1994; Turner and Hooper, 2002). A testis-specific isoform of the enzyme exists that is found in both spermatids and spermatozoa. The male testis specific ACE-null mouse (*tACE*) was found to have reduced fertility (Hagaman *et al.*, 1998). The somatic ACE isoform appears to have no negative effect on sperm function. Sperm from the tACE mutant mice show defective transport through the female tract despite having normal motility, sperm numbers and morphology. Additionally, binding to the zona pellucida was also impaired.

The tACE is a membrane-bound protein and is lost from the membrane during capacitation (Kohn *et al.*, 1995). This is as a result of proteolytic cleavage leaving a specific vestige on the sperm surface (Ehlers *et al.*, 1996; Ramchandran *et al.*, 1994). It has been suggested that this loss of tACE may be important for the release of sperm from the oviductal epithelium. Interestingly, the *tACE* knockout mouse presents with a similar phenotype to null-mutations of cyritestin (Shamsadin *et al.*, 1999), fertilin β (Cho *et al.*, 1998) and calmegin (Ikawa *et al.*, 2001). These mutant mice may all have a common as yet undiscovered defect in the capacitation process.

ACE has recently been shown to have an additional activity as a glycosyl-phospatidylinositol (GPI)-anchored protein-releasing enzyme (GPIase) (Kondoh *et al.*, 2005). Comparison of immunoblots of sperm from wild type and ACE null mice identified two GPI-anchored proteins (Tesp5 and Ph-20) that are released from sperm. In the mutant mice these proteins are no longer released from the sperm membrane, implying that ACE acts to convert these proteins to their soluble form. Addition of ACE or peptidase-inactivated ACE to sperm from the *ACE*-null mice restored sperm–zona pellucida binding resulting in the birth of normal Ace +/− pups. These results imply that the release of GPI-anchored proteins is important for sperm–zona binding; this may involve a sperm protein that becomes functional following its release from its GPI-anchor or the unmasking of a zona-binding protein.

3.5.2 Fertilin and calmegin

Fertilin is a sperm surface protein member of the ADAM family comprising an α (ADAM1) and β (ADAM2) subunit. Members of the ADAM family are proposed to have cell adhesion properties, protease activity or both (Blobel, 1997). Disruption of the fertilin β (*Ftnb*) gene had no effect on sperm number, morphology or motility; and mutant sperm were able to undergo capacitation and spontaneous acrosome reaction. The fertilin α subunit of fertilin was also found to be absent from mature sperm in the fertilin β knockout mouse meaning that the results obtained cannot be attributed to the loss of fertilin β alone (Cho *et al.*, 2000). Binding to the zona pellucida was completely diminished in these mice and binding of *Ftnb*-null sperm to zona-free eggs was reduced. Although the loss of fertilin α and fertilin β is clearly important for the adhesion of sperm to the egg plasma membrane, the inhibition is not total (Cho *et al.*, 1998, 2000). Sperm from the knockout mice were also found to be defective in their migration into the oviduct.

Calmegin is a testis-specific molecular chaperone protein homologous to the ubiquitous calnexin (Watanabe *et al.*, 1994). Male calmegin–null male mice have greatly reduced fertility even though spermatogenesis is morphologically normal (Ikawa *et al.*, 1997). Since calmegin is not present after the final stages of spermatogenesis it cannot be directly participating in fertilisation events (Watanabe *et al.*, 1992; Yoshinaga *et al.*, 1999) and is likely to act as a chaperone for essential sperm proteins.

In vitro, mutant sperm do not bind to the zona pellucida but can fertilise eggs where the zona has been partially dissected, albeit at lower rates than wild type, suggesting that calmegin functions as a chaperone for the sperm surface proteins that mediate the interactions between sperm and egg. Further investigation of sperm function in the calmegin knockout mice showed that the sperm were also defective in migrating into the oviducts and in binding but not fusing to the egg plasma membrane (Ikawa *et al.*, 2001), a phenotype closely resembling the fertilin β knockout mouse. Immunoprecipitation showed that calmegin bound to fertilin α and fertilin β during spermatogenesis. In the calmegin–null mice fertilin α and fertilin β were unable to undergo heterodimerisation and fertilin β was undetectable in the mature sperm. Similar effects of disrupting a chaperone protein on it's substrate proteins have been observed when the loss of a functional calnexin lead to failure of the insulin receptor to homerdimerise and the loss of the receptor from the cell surface (Bass *et al.*, 1998). The calmegin/fertilin mutant animals will provide an excellent tool to improve our understanding of the molecular nature of sperm transport to and within the oviduct.

3.6 Capacitation and hyperactivation

3.6.1 Platelet activating factor

Platelet activating factor (PAF) or 1-O-alkyl-2-acetyl-sn-glyceryl-3-phosphocholine is a signalling phospholipid involved in diverse events (see for review Prescott *et al.*, 2000). PAF is hydrolysed by a specific phospholipase, PAF-acetylhydrolase. It comprises two catalytic domains (α1 and α2) and a LIS1 domain. Mutant mice with targeted disruption of the catalytic domains both individually and together have been generated (Koizumi *et al.*, 2003). α1-deficient mice are indistinguishable from wild type, whilst α2-deficient mice are infertile with disruption of early spermiogenesis (Yan *et al.*, 2003). The double knockout mice were infertile with a significant loss of germ cells early in spermatogenesis. Levels of LIS1 were also decreased in the double mutant.

PAF has also been implicated later in the reproductive process as a possible autocrine mediator of capacitation (Wu *et al.*, 2001). PAF is present in spermatozoa and is released during *in vitro* capacitation (Angle *et al.*, 1991; Wu *et al.*, 2001). A PAF receptor has been found in sperm of all mammalian species studied, including human (Angle *et al.*, 1991). Importantly, the addition of PAF significantly improves success at IUI although the mechanisms of this are as yet unknown (Roudebush *et al.*, 2004).

A PAF receptor knockout mouse was created by homologous recombination that had greatly reduced rates of capacitation as assessed by the rate of spontaneous acrosome reaction but was still capable of *in vivo* fertilisation (Ishii *et al.*, 1998). However, sperm from the null mouse had much lower *in vitro* fertilisation success than wild-type sperm.

3.6.2 Acid sphingomyelinase

Mutations in the acid sphingomyelinase (ASM) gene cause Niemann–Pick disease (NPD). ASM breaks down sphingomyelin to ceramide and phosphorylcholine. Disruption of the ASM gene in mice causes a number of defects in the spermatozoon (Butler *et al.*, 2002). Sperm plasma, mitochondrial and acrosomal membranes are disrupted, with elevated levels of sphingomyelin and cholesterol and mitochondrial membrane depolarisation. This lipid accumulation leads to morphological abnormalities in the flagellum with consequent effects on motility. Also, the sperm also fail to complete capacitation. It is known that loss of cholesterol from the sperm plasma membrane is a key process during capacitation (Cross, 1998) and also that the levels of sphingomyelin in the membrane can affect the rate of capacitation (Cross, 2000).

3.6.3 CatSper1/CatSper2

Spermatozoa contain several Ca^{2+} permeable channels however only one family has unequivocally been shown to be required for male fertility; the CatSper-channels are localised to the plasma membrane of the principal piece of the flagellum. CatSper1 (Ren *et al.*, 2001) and CatSper2 (Quill *et al.*, 2001, 2003) are both sperm-specific. They are characterised by six membrane-spanning regions, similar to the voltage-dependent K^+ channels, but with a pore region and overall homology more like the voltage-dependent Ca^{2+} channels (Ren *et al.*, 2001).

Both Catsper1 and CatSper2 have been the subject of targeted disruption to generate knockout mice (Carlson *et al.*, 2003; Quill *et al.*, 2003; Ren *et al.*, 2001). CatSper mutant mice have normal spermatogenesis, sperm concentration and sperm morphology. Although mutant sperm are capable of undergoing capacitation and acrosome reaction they are unable to undergo hyperactivation. Consistent with this, the null sperm were able to fertilise zona-free but not zona-intact eggs *in vitro*. These results support the hypothesis that the Ca^{2+} entry crucial for the control of hyperactivation of motility is control by the CatSper channels. It is tempting to suggest that the CatSper proteins interact to form a channel but there is presently no evidence to support this. The two proteins do not co-precipitate, nor do they co-localise in the flagellum and they are expressed at different times during spermatogenesis (Quill *et al.*, 2001; Ren *et al.*, 2001; Schultz *et al.*, 2003).

Although it is possible to 'routinely' record channels from the human sperm head (Gu *et al.*, 2004), it is currently not technically possible to directly measure ion channels on the principal piece. Several groups have attempted heterologous expression of Catsper1 and Catsper2 but have been unable to detect currents, even when the two proteins are co-expressed, perhaps indicating that there are other components to the channel or accessory proteins (Quill *et al.*, 2001; Ren *et al.*, 2001).

3.6.4 PMCA4

Plasma membrane Ca^{2+}-ATPases (PMCA) are Ca^{2+} extrusion pumps involved in the regulation of intracellular Ca^{2+} levels (Carafoli and Chiesi, 1992; Garcia and Strehler, 1999). In mammals four distinct genes encode four isoforms of the protein. PMCA1 and PMCA4 are expressed in most adult tissues and both have been the subject of targeted mutation to generate knockout mice (Okunade *et al.*, 2004; Schuh *et al.*, 2004). Disruption of *Pmca1* was embryo lethal, indicative of an essential housekeeping or developmental function. Loss of PMCA4 resulted in male infertility with very low numbers of sperm successfully traversing the female tract (Schuh *et al.*, 2004). Under non-capacitating conditions, sperm from the *Pmca4*-null mice resembled wild type sperm. However under capacitating conditions these sperm were found to be incapable of undergoing hyperactivation. The sperm had increased mitochondrial condensation suggestive of Ca^{2+} overload (Wennemuth *et al.*, 2003) and also had a 2.5-fold increase in resting $[Ca^{2+}]_i$. PMCA4 is localised mainly to the principal piece of the flagellum placing it in close proximity to the CatSper proteins, which also function in sperm motility (see above).

3.7 Sperm–zona pellucida interaction

Many sperm proteins have been proposed as candidates for the zona pellucida receptor. A number of mutant mouse lines with deficient zona pellucida binding have been produced that have other sperm defects, for example ACE, calmegin, ADAM2 (see above).

3.7.1 Phospholipase Cδ4

Phospholipase C (PLC) catalyses the hydrolysis of phosphatidylinositol-4,5-bisphosphate to 1,4,5-triphosphate and diacylglycerol. Of the 11 mammalian PLC homologues identified, PLCδ4 is evolutionarily the most primitive. In sperm, PLCδ4 is localised to the anterior acrosome of the head. Targeted disruption of the PLCδ4 gene primarily affects male fertility (Fukami *et al.*, 2001, 2003). Spermatogenesis and other sperm parameters appear normal but homozygous-null males produced fewer and smaller litters *in vivo* and, *in vitro*, fewer eggs were fertilised. The majority of sperm from the PLCδ4-null mice could not fuse with zona-free eggs but fertilisation was achieved by intracytoplasmic sperm injection (ICSI). Fukami and colleagues (2003) showed that the defect in PLCδ4 knockout animals related to defective influx of calcium and abnormal mobilisation of calcium stores. In addition, the spatio-temporal dynamics were also impaired. Barratt and Publicover (2001) outlined the similarity between the pathology (and putative signalling mechanisms) of these mice and those in men with defective zona-induced acrosome reactions, however as yet no detailed studies have been performed.

3.8 Translating mouse models to the human: how do we go from knockout to diagnosis of male fertility

It would appear easy to screen men with specific phenotypes of infertility for genes that have been knocked out in mice and show male subfertility. Technically it is not difficult. Why then don't we have a plethora of genetic defects being reported? The reasons are multi-factorial and include (1) differences in gene function between mouse and man, (2) the mode of inheritance does not follow traditional genetic pathways and (3) redundancy of the reproductive process. In addition to this there are specific issues that make the translation of information from the knockout to human challenging. To illustrate this we use the example of globozoospermia.

Globozoospermia (round headed spermatozoa) is a well known but extremely rare condition. The majority of men have almost normal sperm concentrations with a relatively high proportion of motile spermatozoa; however, abnormalities in sperm binding to the egg vestments necessitate the use of ICSI to achieve conception. To date, there is no clear explanation for the underlying cause(s). Although not a frequent observation, globozoospermia has been reported to occur within families (Kilani et al., 2004) and, as with some other severe forms of teratozoospermia there is a suggested higher incidence in families with consanguinity (Baccetti et al., 2001; Pirrello et al., 2005).

There are examples of knockout animals with severe teratozoospermia, which may provide clues to the genetic origin of globozoospermia. Mice lacking the casein kinase II α[1] catalytic subunit are infertile and have sperm morphology similar to that manifested in globozoospermia (Xu et al., 1999). Several other knockout mice have also been reported that demonstrate a similar phenotype, for example Golgi-associated PDZ- and coiled-coil motif-containing protein (GOPC) (Yao et al., 2002) and Hrb (Kang-Decker et al., 2001). So what complicates the identification of genes causing globozoospermia if we have three candidate genes?

Firstly, globozoospermia is not a single pathology, as different men with the condition can show a wide spectrum of phenotypes. For example, some reports describe clear abnormalities in the nucleus, presumably in chromatin packaging (Vicari et al., 2002), while others do not (Larson et al., 2001). Even in siblings with globozoospermia, there can be very significant differences. For example, in a case study of two brothers with globozoospermia, Carrell and colleagues noted profound differences in cytoplasmic organisation, aneuploidy rates and nuclear protein extracts (Carrell *et al.*, 1999). Additionally, some studies report globo- zoospermia with 100% of the spermatozoa with round heads, while other studies report globozoospermia when only a majority have round heads. There is also variation over the presence of an acrosome or at least the remnants of an acrosome. The variety in pathology may be reflective of the different underlying causes, which may manifest themselves in the varying success at ICSI. However, what is clear is that a strategy to screen for gene(s) that reportedly are manifested as globozoospermia in mice is not likely to be translatable to human, where screening more than one man with globozoospermia is absolutely required to obtain very detailed profiles.

Secondly, more detailed studies of the nature of the defect in the mouse are required. These are now appearing. The Hrb$^{-/-}$ mouse actually shows a multitude of sperm morphology defects including multi-flagellation, super-numerary centri- oles and multi-nucleation (Juneja and van Deursen, 2005). Studies of the GOPC$^{-/-}$ mouse have examined the failure in spermatids to form perinuclear structures (Ito *et al.*, 2004) and how defects in the posterior ring lead to the expression of coiled tails that are manifested in the epididymis (Suzuki-Toyota *et al.*, 2004). Clearly, referring to these mice as having a globozoospermia phenotype is too simplistic.

Perhaps not surprisingly in view of the above, examination of men with globo- zoospermia for mutations in casein kinase IIά (encoded by Csnk2a2 gene) have not been fruitful. Pirrello examined for mutations in both Csnk2a2 and Csnk2b genes in six patients with globozoospermia and 10 controls (Pirrello *et al.*, 2005). No mutations were identified. Consequently, if screening subfertile men for genes that have been knocked out in mice is to be more successful there needs to be rigorous study of both the mouse and human phenotype.

Successful examples of identifying gene defects in subfertile men by screening for genes knocked out in mice have been reported. The null mutation for *SYCP3* that encodes a component of the synaptonemal complex is manifested as azoospermia with meiotic arrest. Miyamoto and colleagues screened 19 azoospermic patients with meiotic arrest and azoospermia (Miyamoto *et al.*, 2003). In two patients a 1 bp deletion that resulted in a premature stop codon and truncated protein was identi- fied. This was the first autosomal gene previously show to be targeted mutation in mice that has been identified with male infertility.

3.9 What's the future for the diagnosis of sperm dysfunction and male infertility?

There are three platforms for progress. Firstly, a comprehensive high quality semen assessment is the cornerstone of male infertility assessment and all efforts should be made to improve standards of semen assessments. Secondly, global co-ordinated gene expression and proteomic studies are timely and now required. The information gained from such projects will be overwhelming and it is essential that integrated web-based programmes continue to evolve to assist the researcher in understanding the broader context of their findings. Thirdly, rapid developments in chip (microarray and proteomic) based diagnostics will be made but their use must be rigorously tested in the clinical environment. Male infertility has suffered too long from trials of new diagnostics that have little or no power to answer the question.

In conclusion, the diagnosis and treatment of male infertility is at a very exciting stage. The prophesied molecular revolution (see Cram and De Kretser, 2002) has now arrived and andrology will be a very different field in 5 years time.

Acknowledgements

The authors are grateful to all members of our laboratory (past and present) as well as the staff at the Assisted Conception Unit, Birmingham Women's Hospital, Birmingham, England.

Work in the author's laboratory is supported by the MRC, Wellcome Trust, Lord Dowding Fund and BBSRC.

REFERENCES

ESHRE (European Society of Human Reproduction and Embryology) Andrology Special Interest Group (1996) Consensus workshop on advanced diagnostic andrology techniques. *Human Reprod* 11, 1463–1479.

Aguilar-Mahecha A, Hales BF and Robaire B (2001) Acute cyclophosphamide exposure has germ cell specific effects on the expression of stress response genes during rat spermatogenesis. *Mol Reprod Dev* 60, 302–311.

Aguilar-Mahecha A, Hales BF and Robaire B (2002) Chronic cyclophosphamide treatment alters the expression of stress response genes in rat male germ cells. *Biol Reprod* 66, 1024–1032.

Aitken RJ, Bowie H, Buckingham D *et al.* (1992) Sperm penetration into a hyaluronic acid polymer as a means of monitoring functional competence. *J Androl* 13, 44–54.

Angle MJ, Tom R, Khoo D *et al.* (1991) Platelet-activating factor in sperm from fertile and subfertile men. *Fertil Steril* 56, 314–318.

Aquila S, Sisci D, Gentile M *et al.* (2004) Estrogen receptor (ER) alpha and ER beta are both expressed in human ejaculated spermatozoa: evidence of their direct interaction with phosphatidylinositol-3-OH kinase/Akt pathway. *J Clin Endocrinol Metab* 89, 1443–1451.

Baccetti B, Capitani S, Collodel G *et al.* (2001) Genetic sperm defects and consanguinity. *Human Reprod* 16, 1365–1371.

Baker MA, Witherdin R, Hetherington L *et al.* (2005) Identification of post-translational modifications that occur during sperm maturation using difference in two-dimensional gel electrophoresis. *Proteomics* 5, 1003–1012.

Barratt CL and Publicover SJ (2001) Interaction between sperm and zona pellucida in male fertility. *Lancet* 358, 1660–1662.

Bass J, Chiu G, Argon Y *et al.* (1998) Folding of insulin receptor monomers is facilitated by the molecular chaperones calnexin and calreticulin and impaired by rapid dimerization. *J Cell Biol* 141, 637–646.

Björndahl L and Barratt CL (2005) Semen analysis: setting standards for the measurement of sperm numbers. *J Androl* 26, 11.

Björndahl L, Tomlinson MJ and Barratt CLR(2004) Raising standards in semen analysis: professional and personal responsibility. *J Androl* 25, 862–863.

Bohring C and Krause W (2003) Immune Infertility: towards a better understanding of sperm (auto)- immunity. The value of proteomic analysis. *Human Reprod* 18, 915–924.

Bohring C, Krause E, Habermann B *et al.* (2001) Isolation and identification of sperm membrane antigens recognized by antisperm antibodies and their possible role in immunological infertility disease. *Mol Human Reprod* 7, 113–118.

Bonde JP, Ernst E, Jensen TK *et al.* (1998) Relation between semen quality and fertility: a population-based study of 430 first-pregnancy planners. *Lancet* 352, 1172–1177.

Bungum M, Humaidan P, Spano M *et al.* (2004) The predictive value of sperm chromatin structure assay (SCSA) parameters for the outcome of intrauterine insemination IVF and ICSI. *Human Reprod* 19, 1401–1408.

Butler A, He X, Gordon RE *et al.* (2002) Reproductive pathology and sperm physiology in acid sphingomyelinase-deficient mice. *Am J Pathol* 161, 1061–1075.

Carafoli E and Chiesi M (1992) Calcium pumps in the plasma and intracellular membranes. *Curr Top Cell Regul* 32, 209–241.

Carlson AE, Westenbroek RE, Quill T *et al.* (2003) CatSper1 required for evoked Ca^{2+} entry and control of flagellar function in sperm. *Proc Natl Acad Sci USA* 100, 14864–14868.

Carrell DT, Emery BS and Liu L (1999) Characterisation of aneuploidy rates, protamine levels, ultrastructure, and functional ability of round-headed sperm from two siblings and implications for intracytoplasmic sperm injection. *Fertil Steril* 71, 511–516.

Chiu WW and Chamley LW (2004) Clinical associations and mechanisms of action of antisperm antibodies. *Fertil Steril* 82, 529–535.

Cho C, Bunch DO, Faure JE *et al.* (1998) Fertilization defects in sperm from mice lacking fertilin beta. *Science* 281, 1857–1859.

Cho C, Ge H, Branciforte D *et al.* (2000) Analysis of mouse fertilin in wild-type and fertilin beta(−/−) sperm: evidence for C-terminal modification alpha/beta dimerization and lack of essential role of fertilin alpha in sperm-egg fusion. *Dev Biol* 222, 289–295.

Comhaire F (2000) Clinical andrology: from evidence-base to ethics The 'E' quintet in clinical andrology. *Human Reprod* 15, 2067–2071.

Conner SJ, Lefievre L, Hughes DC *et al.* (2005) Cracking the egg: increased complexity in the zona pellucida. *Human Reprod* 20, 1148–1152.

Cram D and de Kretser DM (2002) Genetic diagnosis: the future. In: Assisted Reproductive Technologies: Accomplishments & New Horizons, eds CJ de Jonge and CLR Barratt. Cambridge: Cambridge University Press, pp. 186–205.

Cross NL (1998) Role of cholesterol in sperm capacitation. *Biol Reprod* 59, 7–11.

Cross NL (2000) Sphingomyelin modulates capacitation of human sperm *in vitro*. *Biol Reprod* 63, 1129–1134.

De Jonge CJ (2005) Biological basis for human capacitation. *Human Reprod Update* 11, 205–214.

De Jonge CJ and Barratt CL (1999) WHO manual who should care? *Human Reprod* 14, 2431–2433.

Decker WK, Bowles KR, Schatte EC *et al.* (1999) Revised fine mapping of the human voltage-dependent anion channel loci by radiation hybrid analysis. *Mamm Genome* 10, 1041–1042.

Durr E, Yu J, Krasinska KM *et al.* (2004) Direct proteomic mapping of the lung microvascular endothelial cell surface *in vivo* and in cell culture. *Nat Biotechnol* 22, 985–992.

Eddy EM, Toshimori K and O'Brien DA (2003) Fibrous sheath of mammalian spermatozoa. *Microsc Res Tech* 61, 103–115.

Ehlers MR, Schwager SL, Scholle RR *et al.* (1996) Proteolytic release of membrane-bound angiotensin-converting enzyme: role of the juxtamembrane stalk sequence. *Biochemistry* 35, 9549–9559.

Ellis PJ, Furlong RA, Wilson A *et al.* (2004) Modulation of the mouse testis transcriptome during postnatal development and in selected models of male infertility. *Mol Human Reprod* 10, 271–281.

Ficarro S, Chertihin O, Westbrook VA *et al.* (2003) Phosphoproteome analysis of capacitated human sperm evidence of tyrosine phosphorylation of a kinase-anchoring protein 3 and valosin-containing protein/p97 during capacitation. *J Biol Chem* 278, 11579–11589.

Fukami K, Nakao K, Inoue T *et al.* (2001) Requirement of phospholipase Cdelta4 for the zona pellucida-induced acrosome reaction. *Science* 292, 920–923.

Fukami K, Yoshida M, Inoue T *et al.* (2003) Phospholipase Cδ4 is required for Ca^{2+} mobilization essential for acrosome reaction in sperm. *J Cell Biol* 161, 79–88.

Fung KY, Glode LM, Green S *et al.* (2004) A comprehensive characterization of the peptide and protein constituents of human seminal fluid. *Prostate* 61, 171–181.

Gandini L, Lombardo F, Paoli D *et al.* (2004) Full-term pregnancies achieved with ICSI despite high levels of sperm chromatin damage. *Human Reprod* 19, 1409–1417.

Garcia ML and Strehler EE (1999) Plasma membrane calcium ATPases as critical regulators of calcium homeostasis during neuronal cell function. *Front Biosci* 4, D869–D882.

Goodwin LO, Karabinus DS, Pergolizzi RG *et al.* (2000) L-type voltage-dependent calcium channel alpha-1C subunit mRNA is present in ejaculated human spermatozoa. *Mol Human Reprod* 6, 127–136.

Gu Y, Kirkman-Brown JC, Korchev Y, Barratt CLR and Publicover SJ (2004) Multi-state, 4-aminopyridine-sensitive ion channels in human spermatozoa. *Dev Biol* 274, 308–317.

Hagaman JR, Moyer JS, Bachman ES *et al.* (1998) Angiotensin-converting enzyme and male fertility. *Proc Natl Acad Sci USA* 95, 2552–2557.

Hofmann MC, Braydich-Stolle L and Dym M (2005) Isolation of male germ-line stem cells; influence of GDNF. *Dev Biol* 279, 114–124.

Hooper NM (1994) Families of zinc metalloproteases. *FEBS Lett* 354, 1–6.

Huang Z, Somanath PR, Chakrabarti R *et al.* (2005) Changes in intracellular distribution and activity of protein phosphatase PP1gamma2 and its regulating proteins in spermatozoa lacking AKAP4. *Biol Reprod* 72, 384–392.

Ikawa M, Wada I, Kominami K *et al.* (1997) The putative chaperone calmegin is required for sperm fertility. *Nature* 387, 607–611.

Ikawa M, Nakanishi T, Yamada S *et al.* (2001) Calmegin is required for fertilin alpha/beta heterodimerization and sperm fertility. *Dev Biol* 240, 254–261.

Irish JM, Hovland R, Krutzik PO *et al.* (2004) Single cell profiling of potentiated phosphoprotein networks in cancer cells. *Cell* 118, 217–228.

Ishii S, Kuwaki T, Nagase T *et al.* (1998) Impaired anaphylactic responses with intact sensitivity to endotoxin in mice lacking a platelet-activating factor receptor. *J Exp Med* 187, 1779–1788.

Ito C, Suzuki-Toyota F, Maekawa M *et al.* (2004) Failure to assemble the peri-nuclear structures in *GOPC* deficient spermatids as found in round-headed spermatozoa. *Arch Histol Cytol* 67, 349–360.

Ivic A, Onyeaka H, Girling A *et al.* (2002) Critical evaluation of methylcellulose as an alternative medium in sperm migration tests. *Human Reprod* 17, 143–149.

Juneja SC and van Deursen JM (2005) A mouse model of familial oligoasthenoteratozoospermia. *Human Reprod* 20, 881–893.

Kang-Decker N, Mantchev GT, Juneja SC, McNiven MA and Van Deursen JM (2001) Lack of acrosome formation in Hrb-deficient mice. *Science* 294, 1531–1533.

Kilani Z, Ismail R, Ghunaim S, Mohamed H, Hughes DC, Brewis IA and Barratt CLR (2004) Evaluation and treatment of familial globozoospermia: a study of five brothers. *Fertil Steril* 85, 1436–1439.

Kohn FM, Miska W and Schill WB (1995) Release of angiotensin-converting enzyme (ACE) from human spermatozoa during capacitation and acrosome reaction. *J Androl* 16, 259–265.

Koizumi H, Yamaguchi N, Hattori M *et al.* (2003) Targeted disruption of intracellular type I platelet activating factor-acetylhydrolase catalytic subunits causes severe impairment in spermatogenesis. *J Biol Chem* 278, 12489–12494.

Kondoh G, Tojo H, Nakatani Y *et al.* (2005) Angiotensin-converting enzyme is a GPI-anchored protein releasing factor crucial for fertilization. *Nat Med* 11, 160–166.

Larsen L, Scheike T, Jensen TK *et al.* (2000) Computer-assisted semen analysis parameters as predictors for fertility of men from the general population The Danish First Pregnancy Planner Study Team. *Human Reprod* 15, 1562–1567.

Larson KL, Brannian JD, Singh NP, Burbach JA, Jost LK, Hansen KP *et al.* (2001) Chromatin structure in globozoospermia: a case report. *J Androl* 22, 424–431.

Lefièvre L, Barratt CL, Harper CV *et al.* (2003) Physiological and proteomic approaches to studying prefertilization events in the human. *Reprod Biomed Online* 7, 419–427.

Lefièvre L, Conner SJ, Salpekar A *et al.* (2004) Four zona pellucida glycoproteins are expressed in the human. *Human Reprod* 19, 1580–1586.

Matzuk MM and Lamb DJ (2002) Genetic dissection of mammalian fertility pathways. *Nat Cell Biol* 4 (Suppl) s41–s49.

Miki K and Eddy EM (1998) Identification of tethering domains for protein kinase A type I alpha regulatory subunits on sperm fibrous sheath protein FSC1. *J Biol Chem* 273, 34384–34390.

Miki K and Eddy EM (1999) Single amino acids determine specificity of binding of protein kinase A regulatory subunits by protein kinase A anchoring proteins. *J Biol Chem* 274, 29057–29062.

Miki K, Willis WD, Brown PR *et al.* (2002) Targeted disruption of the Akap4 gene causes defects in sperm flagellum and motility. *Dev Biol* 248, 331–342.

Miller D, Ostermeier GC and Krawetz SA (2005) The controversy potential and roles of spermatozoal RNA. *Trend Mol Med* 11, 156–163.

Muller CH (2000) Rationale, interpretation, validation and uses of sperm function tests. *J Androl* 21, 10–30.

Naaby-Hansen S, Flickinger CJ and Herr JC (1997) Two-dimensional gel electrophoretic analysis of vectorially labelled surface proteins of human spermatozoa. *Biol Reprod* 56, 771–787.

Naaby-Hansen S, Mandal A, Wolkowicz MJ *et al.* (2002) CABYR a novel calcium-binding tyrosine phosphorylation-regulated fibrous sheath protein involved in capacitation. *Dev Biol* 242, 236–254.

Nagdas SK, Winfrey VP and Olson GE (2005) Tyrosine phosphorylation generates multiple isoforms of the mitochondrial capsule protein phospholipid hydroperoxide glutathione peroxidase (PHGPx) during hamster sperm capacitation. *Biol Reprod* 72, 164–171.

Naz RK and Rajesh PB (2004) Role of tyrosine phosphorylation in sperm capacitation/acrosome reaction. *Reprod Biol Endocrinol* 2, 75.

Okunade GW, Miller ML, Pyne GJ *et al.* (2004) Targeted ablation of plasma membrane Ca^{2+}-ATPase (PMCA) 1 and 4 indicates a major housekeeping function for PMCA1 and a critical role in hyperactivated sperm motility and male fertility for PMCA4. *J Biol Chem* 279, 33742–33750.

Ostermeier GC, Dix DJ, Miller D *et al.* (2002) Spermatozoal RNA profiles of normal fertile men. *Lancet* 360, 772–777.

Ostermeier GC, Miller D, Huntriss JD *et al.* (2004) Reproductive biology: delivering spermatozoan RNA to the oocyte. *Nature* 429, 154.

Ostermeier GC, Goodrich RJ, Moldenhauer JS *et al.* (2005) A suite of novel human spermatozoal RNAs. *J Androl* 26, 70–74.

Ostrowski LE, Blackburn K, Radde KM *et al.* (2002) A proteomic analysis of human cilia: identification of novel components. *Mol Cell Proteomics* 1, 451–465.

Papin JA, Hunter T, Palsson BO *et al.* (2005) Reconstruction of cellular signalling networks and analysis of their properties. *Nat Rev Mol Cell Biol* 6, 99–111.

Pirrello O, Machey N, Schmidt F, Terriou P, Menezo Y and Viville S (2005) Search for mutations involved in human globozoospermia. *Human Reprod* 20, 1314–1318.

Pixton KL, Deeks ED, Flesch FM *et al.* (2004) Sperm proteome mapping of a patient who experienced failed fertilization at IVF reveals altered expression of at least 20 proteins compared with fertile donors: case report. *Human Reprod* 19, 1438–1447.

Polansky FF and Lamb EJ (1988) Do the results of semen analysis predict future fertility? A survival analysis study. *Fertil Steril* 49, 1059–1065.

Prescott SM, Zimmerman GA, Stafforini DM *et al.* (2000) Platelet-activating factor and related lipid mediators. *Ann Rev Biochem* 69, 419–445.

Quill TA, Ren D, Clapham DE *et al.* (2001) A voltage-gated ion channel expressed specifically in spermatozoa. *Proc Natl Acad Sci USA* 98, 12527–12531.

Quill TA, Sugden SA, Rossi KL *et al.* (2003) Hyperactivated sperm motility driven by CatSper2 is required for fertilization. *Proc Natl Acad Sci USA* 100, 14869–14874.

Ramchandran R, Sen GC, Misono K *et al.* (1994) Regulated cleavage-secretion of the membrane-bound angiotensin-converting enzyme. *J Biol Chem* 269, 2125–2130.

Ren D, Navarro B, Perez G *et al.* (2001) A sperm ion channel required for sperm motility and male fertility. *Nature* 413, 603–609.

Roudebush WE, Toledo AA, Kort HI, Mitchell-Leef D, Elsner CW and Massey JB (2004) Platelet-activating factor significantly enhances intra uterine insemination pregnancy rates in non-male factors infertility. *Fertil Steril* 82, 52–56.

Sachs K, Perez O, Pe'er D *et al.* (2005) Causal protein-signalling networks derived from multi-parameter single-cell data. *Science* 308, 523–529.

Sampson MJ, Lovell RS and Craigen WJ (1997) The murine voltage-dependent anion channel gene family conserved structure and function. *J Biol Chem* 272, 18966–18973.

Sampson MJ, Decker WK, Beaudet AL *et al.* (2001) Immotile sperm and infertility in mice lacking mitochondrial voltage-dependent anion channel type 3. *J Biol Chem* 276, 39206–39212.

Schuh K, Cartwright EJ, Jankevics E *et al.* (2004) Plasma membrane Ca^{2+} ATPase 4 is required for sperm motility and male fertility. *J Biol Chem* 279, 28220–28226.

Schultz N, Hamra FK and Garbers DL (2003) A multitude of genes expressed solely in meiotic or postmeiotic spermatogenic cells offers a myriad of contraceptive targets. *Proc Natl Acad Sci USA* 100, 12201–12206.

Shamsadin R, Adham IM, Nayernia K *et al.* (1999) Male mice deficient for germ-cell cyritestin are infertile. *Biol Reprod* 61, 1445–1451.

Shetty J, Naaby-Hansen S, Shibahara H *et al.* (1999) Human sperm proteome: immunodominant sperm surface antigens identified with sera from infertile men and women. *Biol Reprod* 61, 61–69.

Shetty J, Diekman AB, Jayes FC *et al.* (2001) Differential extraction and enrichment of human sperm surface proteins in a proteome: identification of immunocontraceptive candidates. *Electrophoresis* 22, 3053–3066.

Shibahara H, Sato I, Shetty J *et al.* (2002) Two-dimensional electrophoretic analysis of sperm antigens recognized by sperm immobilizing antibodies detected in infertile women. *J Reprod Immunol* 53, 1–12.

Shima JE, McLean DJ, McCarrey JR *et al.* (2004) The murine testicular transcriptome: characterizing gene expression in the testis during the progression of spermatogenesis. *Biol Reprod* 71, 319–330.

Small CL, Shima JE, Uzumcu M *et al.* (2005) Profiling gene expression during the differentiation and development of the murine embryonic gonad. *Biol Reprod* 72, 492–501.

Starita-Geribaldi M, Roux F, Garin J, Chevallier D, Fenichael P and Pointis G (2003a) Development of narrow immobilized pH gradients covering one pH unit for human seminal plasma proteomic analysis. *Proteomics* 3, 1611–1619.

Starita-Geribaldi M, Poggioli S, Zucchini M, Garin J, Chevallier D, Fenichael P and Pointis G (2003b) Mapping of seminal plasma proteins by 2-dimensional gel electrophoresis in men with normal and impaired spermatogenesis. *Mol Human Reprod* 7, 715–722.

Suzuki-Toyota F, Ito C, Toyama Y *et al.* (2004) The coiled tail of the round-headed spermatozoa appears during epididymal passage in *GOPC*-deficient mice. *Arch Histol Cytol* 67, 361–371.

Tomlinson MJ, Kessopoulou E and Barratt CL (1999) The diagnostic and prognostic value of traditional semen parameters. *J Androl* 20, 588–593.

Turner AJ and Hooper NM (2002) The angiotensin-converting enzyme gene family: genomics and pharmacology. *Trends Pharmacol Sci* 23, 177–183.

Vicari E, Perdichizzi A, De Palma A, Burrello N, D'Agata R and Calogero AE (2002) Globozoospermia is associated with chromatin structure abnormalities: case report. *Human Reprod* 17, 2128–2133.

Watanabe D, Sawada K, Koshimizu U *et al.* (1992) Characterization of male meiotic germ cell-specific antigen (Meg 1) by monoclonal antibody TRA 369 in mice. *Mol Reprod Dev* 33, 307–312.

Watanabe D, Yamada K, Nishina Y *et al.* (1994) Molecular cloning of a novel Ca(2+)-binding protein (calmegin) specifically expressed during male meiotic germ cell development. *J Biol Chem* 269, 7744–7749.

Wennemuth G, Babcock DF and Hille B (2003) Calcium clearance mechanisms of mouse sperm. *J Gen Physiol* 122, 115–128.

Wiederkehr C, Basavaraj R, Sarrausted M *et al.* (2004) Database model and specification of GermOnline Release 20 a cross-species community annotation knowledgebase on germ cell differentiation. *Bioinformatics* 20, 808–811.

World Health Organization (WHO) (1999) *WHO Laboratory Manual for the Examination of Human Semen and Sperm-Cervical Mucus Interaction*. Cambridge, UK Cambridge University Press.

Wrobel G and Primig M (2005) Mammalian male germ cells are fertile ground for expression profiling of sexual reproduction. *Reproduction* 129, 1–7.

Wu C, Stojanov T, Chami O *et al.* (2001) Evidence for the autocrine induction of capacitation of mammalian spermatozoa. *J Biol Chem* 276, 26962–26968.

Xu X, Toselli PA, Russell LD *et al.* (1999) Globozoospermia in mice lacking the casein kinase II catalytic subunit. *Nat Genet* 23, 118–121.

Yan W, Assadi AH, Wynshaw-Boris A *et al.* (2003) Previously uncharacterized roles of platelet-activating factor acetylhydrolase 1b complex in mouse spermatogenesis. *Proc Natl Acad Sci USA* 100, 7189–7194.

Yao R, Ito C, Natsume Y *et al.* (2002) Lack of acrosome formation in mice lacking a Golgi protein, GOPC. *Proc Natl Acad Sci USA* 99, 11211–11216.

Yoshinaga K, Tanii I and Toshimori K (1999) Molecular chaperone calmegin localization to the endoplasmic reticulum of meiotic and post-meiotic germ cells in the mouse testis. *Arch Histol Cytol* 62, 283–293.

Zhou Q, Shima JE, Nie R *et al.* (2005) Androgen-regulated transcripts in the neonatal mouse testis as determined through microarray analysis. *Biol Reprod* 72, 1010–1019.

Sperm maturation in the human epididymis

Trevor G. Cooper and Ching-Hei Yeung

Institute of Reproductive Medicine of the University, Münster, Germany

4.1 Introduction

The current success of assisted reproduction using testicular sperm extraction may give the impression that the human epididymis is not necessary for the development of the fertilising capacity of spermatozoa. However, as all assisted reproduction techniques bypass the epididymal processes refined over millions of years of evolution to permit internal fertilisation naturally (Jones, 2002), this argument is disingenuous (see Cooper, 1990). Certainly, the scarcity of intact human epididymides and the unavailability of biopsies (Schirren, 1982) has delayed research on this organ in comparison with that on the human testis, but organs from autopsies and accident victims and at operations for prostatic carcinoma, radical prostatectomy and organ transplantation have provided information. The human epididymis does not present clear-cut divisions into head (caput), body (corpus) and tail (cauda) as in other species (Fig. 4.1) and the structural complexity of the human epididymal caput (Yeung et al., 1991) and the uncertainty of which regions have been sampled in many studies leave the field less clear than it could be. Unlike the mouse, where the expression is confined to the proximal caput epididymidis (Sonnenberg-Riethmacher et al., 1996), the proto-oncogene c-ros is expressed along the length of the human epididymis (Légaré and Sullivan, 2004). Nevertheless, the accumulated data obtained from these studies and reviewed here reveal a pattern of sperm maturation not unlike that found in other animals that have been studied more systematically.

This chapter updates the information relating to the changes that occur to spermatozoa during maturation in the human epididymis that add to our knowledge about the mechanisms by which the epididymis influences the maturing spermatozoa. The application of molecular biology techniques to the human epididymis has provided evidence of many novel proteins over the last 15 years. From this literature it is evident that spermatozoa are subjected to an ever-changing environment in the

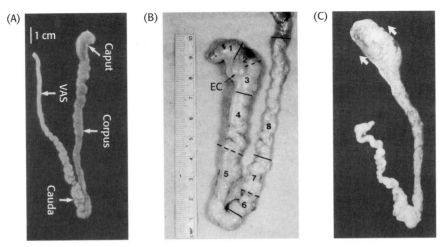

Figure 4.1   Photographs of the human epididymis from (A) TG Cooper and CH Yeung, unpublished;
(B) Turner (1997) and (C) Bedford (1991), with kind permission of Springer Science and
Business Media. Note the poor demarcation of caput, corpus and cauda, and the
distended caput in (C)

epididymis and come sequentially into contact with proteins that have the potential
to modify sperm–egg interactions. Recently, observations made on infertile transgenic mice have highlighted the importance of volume regulation in male fertility, a
property acquired by spermatozoa within the primate epididymis. This work has
suggested new functions for the high concentrations of low-molecular weight
organic compounds found in epididymal fluid.

4.2 Sperm maturation in the human epididymis

4.2.1 Sperm transit

Estimates of the time taken for sperm to migrate through the human epididymis
vary from a mean of 11 days (range 1–21) by thymidine labelling of spermatozoa
(Rowley *et al.*, 1970) to shorter values of 3–4 days (Amann and Howards, 1980;
Johnson and Varner, 1988) from measurement of extragonadal sperm reserves.
Faster transit (up to 2 days) was estimated for men with large daily sperm production (Johnson and Varner, 1988). Such rapid transit may be caused by the paucity
of spermatozoa, as human epididymal fluid is not viscous (Turner and Reich,
1985). Interestingly, rapid transit is also the norm for the chimpanzee (Smithwick
et al., 1996) in the very different situation of a large testis size and high sperm
production rate.

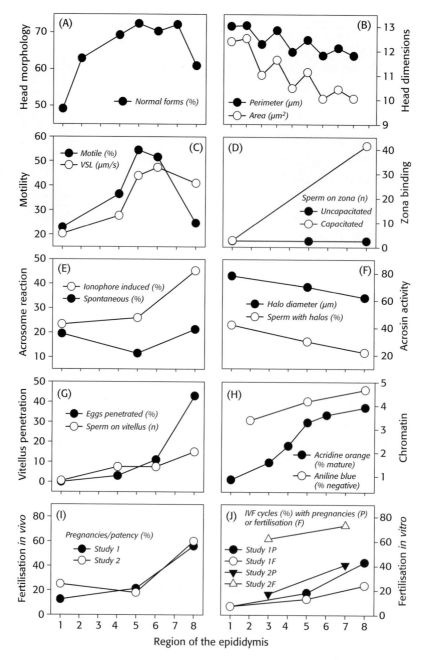

Figure 4.2   Maturation of spermatozoa in the human epididymis. Various functional parameters
(ordinate) are plotted for sperm obtained from different epididymal regions (abscissa):
(A) normal forms (Soler et al., 2000); (B) sperm head morphometry (Soler et al., 2000);
(C) motility and kinematics (Yeung et al., 1993); (D) sperm–zona binding (Delpech
et al., 1988; Moore et al., 1992); (E) acrosome reactions (Yeung et al., 1997a);

4.2.2 Morphology

4.2.2.1 Sperm heads

Subjecting human epididymal sperm to the same procedures as ejaculated sperm for morphological analysis (air-drying smears) results in artefactual swelling of the heads of many sperm from the caput region (Soler *et al.*, 2000; Yeung *et al.*, 1997a) but not those from the cauda epididymidis. This maturational change in the ability to resist air-drying was an unexpected demonstration of a maturational change that also affects primate spermatozoa (Gago *et al.*, 2000). Thus, the presence in human ejaculates of some spermatozoa with 'acorn-shaped' heads (Ludwig and Frick, 1987) may be indicating the appearance of immature spermatozoa in the ejaculate, as a consequence of abnormal epididymal function. Ignoring the obviously swollen types, the percentage of spermatozoa with normal heads still increases upon maturation (Fig. 4.2A), not as a result of removal of abnormal cells by the epididymal epithelium (Cooper *et al.*, 2002; Sutovsky *et al.*, 2001) but by the transformation into a more resistant cell type. Increased intramolecular disulphide bonding within sperm during transit through the epididymis (Bedford *et al.*, 1973) may permit maturing sperm to withstand the stresses associated with air drying.

The dimensions of the heads of the non-swollen sperm also changes upon maturation (Fig. 4.2B). This cell shrinkage may reflect dehydration caused by high intraluminal osmotic pressure, but little is known about this in man with values of 342 mmol/kg being reported for fluid obtained from the human vas deferens (Hinton *et al.*, 1981). As the osmolality of fluid entering the human epididymis is 280 mmol/kg (Table 4.1) this represents a 22% increase in osmolarity experienced by cells during their epididymal sojourn. An increase in compactness of nuclear contents may also explain the decrease in head size (see Fig. 4.2H).

4.2.2.2 Cytoplasmic droplets

A distinction needs to be made between the cytoplasmic droplets of morphologically normal cells and excess residual cytoplasm of abnormal cells (Cooper *et al.*, 2004). The air-drying procedure of seminal smears routinely employed for the morphological analysis of human spermatozoa has recently been shown to be inadequate for the preservation of normal cytoplasmic droplets on the majority of spermatozoa in fixed preparations (Cooper *et al.*, 2004). The human seems to be

Caption for fig 4.2 (*cont.*)   (F) acrosin content (Haidl *et al.*, 1994); (G) sperm–egg fusion (Moore *et al.*, 1983); (H) chromation condensation (Golan *et al.*, 1996; Haidl *et al.*, 1994); (I) fertilisation after epididymovasostomy (Fogdestam *et al.*, 1986; Schmidt *et al.*, 1976); (J) fertilisation *in vitro* (Patrizio *et al.*, 1994). Regions are 1: efferent ducts (testicular sperm in spermatocoeles); 2: proximal caput; 3: distal caput; 4: proximal corpus; 5: mid corpus; 6: distal corpus; 7: proximal cauda; 8: distal cauda

Table 4.1. Composition of fluid [1]entering and [2]leaving the human epididymis

Parameter	Units	[1]RTF	[3]Ref.	[2]CEP/VDF	[3]Ref.
Osmolality	mmol/kg	280	1	342	6
Protein	mg/ml	3.4	2,3	28.7	7
K^+	mM	5.9	2	111	6
Na^+	mM	148	2	30	6
Ca^{2+}	mM	2.1	2,3,4	1.5	8
Cl^-	mM	139	2	103	6
Phosphate	μM	27.3	2	24.4	6
Androgens	nM	66	2	0.28	9
Carnitine	mM	0	2	5.5	6,10
Inositol	mM	2	5	5.9	6
GPC	mM	0	2	0	6

[1]RTF: spermatocoele fluid; [2]CEP: cauda epididymidal fluid; [2]VDF: vas deferens fluid.
[3]References
1. TG Cooper, unpublished data + data cited in Cooper and Yeung, (2003)
2. Cooper *et al.* (1992)
3. Huggins and Johnson (1933)
4. Quinlivan (1968)
5. A Pruneda and TG Cooper, unpublished data
6. Hinton *et al.* (1981)
7. Turner and Reich (1985)
8. Morton *et al.* (1978)
9. Adamopoulos *et al.* (1979)
10. DE Brooks and SS Howards, cited in Brooks (1979).

peculiar in regard to the location of this droplet (at the neck and not the annulus as in other mammals) on mature spermatozoa in the ejaculate. One of the earliest electron micrographs showed a neck droplet on human epididymal spermatozoon (Ånberg, 1957) and well fixed seminal preparations display the same (Holstein and Roosen-Runge, 1981). Spermatozoa leaving the human testis present in fluid collected from epididymal spermatocoeles, which are in reality accumulations of testicular fluid (Cooper *et al.*, 1992), also bear droplets at the neck (Fig. 4.3). The failure of droplet migration along the midpiece in man may reflect a heat stress secondary to the wearing of clothes (JM Bedford, personal communication), since spermatozoa from the ascrotal shrew, with an inguinal testis and epididymis, display neck droplets after imposition of abdominal temperature *via* cryptorchidism (Bedford *et al.*, 1982). The failure of migration could conceivably reflect the low

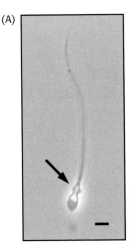

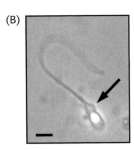

Figure 4.3   Photomicrograph of (A) a human testicular spermatozoon (obtained from an epididymal
spermatocoele) and (B) an ejaculated spermatozoon, both fixed in glutaraldehyde. Bars
5 μm. Note the location of the cytoplasmic droplet at the neck region both before and
after epididymal transit

sperm concentration within the epididymal lumen, which reduces the shear forces
incumbent upon more highly packed spermatozoa, since the migration of the droplet
along the midpiece can be induced by centrifugation of porcine and caprine testicular spermatozoa (Kato *et al.*, 1983, 1984).

4.2.2.3 Sperm tails

Haidl *et al.* (1993) have suggested that abnormal sperm tail morphology is related
to human epididymal dysfunction, but causal relationships were not discussed.

4.2.3 Motility

Within the human epididymis spermatozoa are held immotile, not by the viscosity
of the fluid (Turner and Reich, 1985) but presumably by low pH (Carr *et al.*, 1985),
and they are activated to motility upon release into female tract or physiological
fluids. Sperm obtained from epididymal spermatocoeles are weakly motile (Cooper
et al., 1992), as are those obtained in the caput epididymidis (Yeung *et al.*, 1993).
Belonoschkin (1943) examined the duration and intensity of motility *in vitro* of
sperm released from epididymides obtained from 21–44 year-old men within 1–5 h
of death. The duration was far higher for sperm from the cauda (18.7 h) than those
from the caput (4.6 h) or testis (2.1 h). These suggestions of a maturation in motility from observations on duration of motility have been extended to motility analysis at one time point for spermatozoa obtained from several regions of the human
epididymis from older men undergoing castration for prostatic carcinoma. The

percentage of motile sperm (assessed subjectively upon release into suitable medium) increases as they pass through the epididymis but in the old men examined, a decrease in motility of sperm was observed when recovered from the cauda (Fig. 4.2C). This is thought to reflect the ageing population of sperm stored there that had not been voided in these patients. Computer-aided sperm motion analysis reveals improved progressive swimming reflecting an increased velocity and linearity of the sperm tracks (Fig. 4.2C). The velocity of the sperm from the corpus are as fast as those of ejaculated (caudal) sperm from younger men, attesting to the normal functioning of the epididymis in these old patients. Initiation of motility may be a time-dependent phenomenon, rather than a result of epididymal secretions, since sperm recovered from the testis and caput are only motile after ductal occlusion (Jow *et al.*, 1993) and sperm obtained by testicular biopsy become motile upon *in vitro* incubation (Emiliani *et al.*, 2000). Whether this improvement occurs in the absence of epididymal secretions is not so clear since a proximal reflux of epididymal secretions could occur in situations where ductal occlusion prevents normal distal movement of spermatozoa through the lumen. The epididymal region where sperm motility normally develops is shifted proximally after vasectomy (Mooney *et al.*, 1972) or ductal occlusion (Mathieu *et al.*, 1992) and motile sperm are recovered in the testis only when the attached epididymis is occluded (Jow *et al.*, 1993).

4.2.4 Sperm–zona binding

The first results on the binding of human epididymal spermatozoa to the human zona pellucida did not detect differences in binding capacity between caput and cauda (Delpech *et al.*, 1988; Fournier-Delpech and Guérin, 1991) (Fig. 4.2D). This was most likely due to the non-physiological conditions employed (low temperature to reduce the velocity of the more mature cells in order to remove bias towards them by the greater number of sperm–egg collisions with more motile cells). When accepted capacitation conditions are used, a marked difference between the binding ability of caput sperm, which are unable to bind to the zona, and ejaculated spermatozoa (originating from the cauda epididymidis) which can, is evident (Fig. 4.2D). The co-culture with epididymal epithelium promotes the zona-binding ability of caput epididymidal spermatozoa (Moore *et al.*, 1992), implying the secretion from the epithelium of proteins taken up by spermatozoa under these conditions. The elution from spermatozoa by high salt treatment of proteins that can improve the zona-binding ability of other spermatozoa incubated with them, confirms that superficially orientated, electrostatically bound proteins are involved in zona binding (Jean *et al.*, 1995). Human epididymal proteins implicated in the binding of sperm to the zona pellucida are listed in Table 4.2. The protein for which most evidence is available is P34H, a glycosylphospatidylinositol (GPI)-anchored, membrane-intercolated protein.

Table 4.2. Human testicular and epididymal proteins suggested to be involved in human sperm–zona binding/penetration and motility

Name (pseudonym, orthologues, activity) [Reference]	MW/pI	Location in epithelium		Protein on epididymal CES	Location on sperm			Role in fertilisation
		mRNA	Protein		EJAC	CAP	AR	
Testis only								
PH-30 (fertilin) [Jury et al., 1997, 1998]	30	T						? (Pseudogene)
FA-1 antigen (fertilisation antigen 1) [Zhu and Naz, 1997]	18.2		T		Ac			1° zona binding
PH-20 (hyaluronidase) [Lin et al., 1993]	64	T			H	H	IAM	2° zona binding
Acrosin (proteinase) [Tesarik et al., 1988]			T		Ac	Ac	IAM	2° zona binding
FA-2 antigen (fertilisation antigen 2) [Naz et al., 1993]	95		T					Oocyte fusion
YWK-1 antigen [Yan et al., 1984]	84		T, ED > Cap	ED > Cap	M/PP			?
Epididymal region unstated								
p66 [Lasserre et al., 2003]	66		DCap > Cor/Cau		Ac > M/PP		Ac	Zona binding
DJ-1 (CAP1, SP22) [Yoshida et al., 2003]	24/5.7,5.8, 6.1,6.4		Ep		H/M			?
Prostaglandin D synthetase [Tokugawa et al., 1998]	27	T,Ep	Ep					Lipocalin
CD59 (protection membrane attack complex inhibitor) [Fenichel et al., 1994; Simpson and Holmes, 1994]	19,20	T,Ep	Ep		H/PP	H/PP	H/PP	Oocyte fusion immune suppression

Table 4.2. (cont.)

Name (pseudonym, orthologues, activity) [Reference]	MW/pI	Location in epithelium		Protein on epididymal CES	Location on sperm			Role in fertilisation
		mRNA	Protein		EJAC	CAP	AR	
2C6 antigen (human seminal plasma) [Isojima et al., 1990; Kameda et al., 1991]	15–25	Ep	Ep		H/PP			Zona binding oocyte fusion
HBD-1, HD-5, HNP1-3 [Com et al., 2003]					N			Immune suppression
All epididymal duct								
Trypsinogen (protease precursor) [Paju et al., 2000]		Cau	Cau					
3B2F7 antigen (HSP- gp, human seminal plasma glycoprotein) [Batova et al., 1990]	36		Cap,Cor,Cau	Cap,Cor,Cau				Zona binding
SOB2 (sperm–oocyte binding protein 2) [Lefevre et al. 1997]	17.5,18, 19/6.4	E	Cap,Cor,Cau	Cap,Cor,Cau	PAc/N			Oocyte fusion
ARP (hCRISP-1,2,3 (human cystein rich secretory protein), AEG- like protein (ARP)) [Cohen et al., 2001; Hayashi et al., 1996]	23,3/5.23	T,E	ED,Cap,Cor,Cau > Vas	Cap,Cor	PAc			Oocyte fusion
Proximal region only								
DEFB118 (β defensins; ESC42, epididymis specific clone 42) [Liu et al., 2001; Yamaguchi et al., 2002]	20		Ep		PAc/ N >M/PP			Immune suppression

Protein	MW / features	Tissue	Region		Sperm location		Function
HE6 (GPR64) [Obermann et al., 2003]	180,40 Ecto,endo		ED, Cap				Transporter?
Clusterin (SP-40,40, SGP2) [O'Bryan et al., 1994]	80		T, Cap		Ac/Eq/PP	X	Agglutination dead sperm
SOB1 (sperm–oocyte binding protein 1, FLB1, AKAP82) [Boué et al., 1995; Lefèvre et al., 1999]	94.7/5.7, 5.8,5.9	T	ED,Cap,Cor	Cor,Cau	PAc/N		Oocyte fusion
Eppin 1, 2, 3 (epididymal protease inhibitor) [Richardson et al., 2001; Yenugu et al., 2004c]	24,35	T,ED,Ep	ED,Cap,Cor		H/M/PP		Protease inhibitor microbicide
Cathepsin D [Raczek et al., 1995]	33,47,53		ED,Cor				Carbohydrase
Decreasing distally							
SPAM1 (PH-20) [Evans et al., 2003; Lin et al., 1993]		T,Cap,Cor	Cap,Cor	PH	H		Hyaluronidase
LCN6 (Lipocalin) [Hamil et al., 2003]			ED,Cap > Cor,Cau		PAc/PP		Fusion?
Cystatin 11 [Hamil et al., 2002]			Cap > Cau		PAc/PP		Microbicide
β- N-acetylglucosaminidase [Böstrom and Öckerman, 1971; Castéllon and Huidobro, 1999; Datti et al., 1993; Raczek et al., 1995]	29,54,63		ED > Cap > Cor,Cau				Carbohydrase
β-glucosidase [Castéllon and Huidobro, 1999]			ED > Ep > Vas				Carbohydrase
β-galactosidase [Böstrom and Öckerman, 1999]			ED > Ep > Vas				Carbohydrase

Table 4.2. (cont.)

Name (pseudonym, orthologues, activity) [Reference]	MW/pI	Location in epithelium		Protein on epididymal CES	Location on sperm			Role in fertilisation
		mRNA	Protein		EJAC	CAP	AR	
HE2 α2 β β2 (human epididymal protein 2) [Avellar et al., 2004; Hamil et al., 2000; Kirchhoff, 1998; Krull et al., 1993; Osterhoff et al., 1994; von Horsten et al., 2002:. Yenugu et al., 2003, 2004a, b;]	5.6–10.2/ 8.2–12.1	Cap > Cor > Cau		ED,Cap, Cor > Cau	PAc/N/Ac/Eq			Oocyte fusion microbicide
Galactosyl transferase (Ross et al., 1993)	45		Cap > Cor > Cau,Vas					Transferase
Maximum in corpus								
NW21 antigen [Poulton et al., 1996]	18		Cor	ES not TS	Y			
Fibronectin (integrin ligand) [Miranda and Tezón, 1992; Schaller et al., 1993]	220		T,Cap < Cor	Cap < Cor	Eq			Oocyte fusion
P34H (carbonyl reductase P26h P31m P25b) [Boué et al., 1994; Légaré et al., 1999; 2001]	34/6.0,6.2	Cap < Cor > Cau	Cap < Cor > Cau,Vas	Cap < Cor > Cau	Ac	X		1° zona binding
α fucosidase [Böstrom and Öckerman, 1971]			ED < Ep > Vas					Carbohydrase
α mannosidase [Böstrom and Öckerman, 1971; Castellon and Huidobro, 1999]			ED < Cap < Cor, Cau > Vas					Carbohydrase

β glucuronidase [Böstrom and Öckerman, 1971; Castellon and Huidobro, 1999]			ED < Cap < Cor, Cau > Vas				Carbohydrase
HE1 (human epididymal protein 1, EPI 1, ESP14.6, EPV20) [Kirchhoff et al., 1993; Krull et al., 1993; Larsen et al., 1997]	25–27	Cap,Cor > Cau < Vas	Cap < Cor > Cau < Vas	Cor			Sterol binding protein
HE3 a-β (human epididymal protein 3) [Kirchhoff et al., 1994]	14.9		Cap < Cor > Cau < Vas				?
HE5 (human epididymal protein 5, CD52, Campath1 antigen) [Hale et al., 1993; Kirchhoff et al., 1993; Yeung et al., 1997b]	20	Cap < Cor > Cau < Vas	Cap < Cor > Cau < Vas	Cap < Cor < Cau	H/PAc/PP		Motility? Storage?
SAGA-1 (sperm agglutination antigen 1, CD52, Campath1 antigen) [Diekman et al., 1997]	15–25		Ep				
Gp20 (glycoprotein 20, CD52, Campath1 antigen) [Focarelli et al., 1998, 1999a, b]	19–21/3–6		Ep	Ep	H	Eq	Oocyte fusion, capacitation
GZS-1 (CD52, Campath1 antigen) [Hutter et al., 1996]	20,25		Ep				Oocyte fusion immune suppression?

Table 4.2. (*cont.*)

Name (pseudonym, orthologues, activity) [Reference]	MW/pI	Location in epithelium		Protein on epididymal CES	Location on sperm			Role in fertilisation
		mRNA	Protein		EJAC	CAP	AR	
Increasing distally								
HSP70 (heat shock protein) [Légaré et al., 2004]	70	Cap,Cor,Cau	Cap,Cor,Cau					
hCAP-18 (human cationic antimicrobial protein, cathelecidin, SOB3) [Hammami Hamza et al., 2001; Malm et al., 2000]	18	T	Cap < Cor < Cau,Vas	Cap,Cor,Cau	N/PP			Microbicide
Sperm coating protein (SCP) [Sanjurjo et al., 1990; Tezón et al., 1985]	76,80		Cap < Cor < Cau	Cap < Cor < Cau	Ac			Oocyte fusion
α glucosidase [Castellon and Huidobro, 1999; Raczek et al., 1995; Yeung et al., 1990]			Cap < Cor < Cau	Cap < Cor < Cau				Storage?
Corpus and Cauda								
Serpin (serine protease inhibitor protein C inhibitor) [Elisen et al., 1998; Laurell et al., 1992; Moore et al., 1993]	57		T,Ep	Cau	Ac		Eq	Oocyte fusion zona binding
GP-83 (glycoprotein 83, lectin binding protein, ADAM7, protease) [Lin et al., 2001; Liu et al., 2000; Sun et al., 2000]	86/6.57	Cap < Cor < Cau	Cor,Cau	Cor,Cau	Ac	Eq	Eq	Protease

GP-39 (glycoprotein 39, lectin binding protein) [Liu et al., 2000]	39		Cor, Cau		Cor,Cau	Ac	Eq	Eq	Oocyte fusion

?: unknown; 1°: primary; 2°: secondary; Ac: acrosome; AR: acrosome reacted sperm; CAP: capacitated sperm; Cap: caput; Cau: cauda; Cor: corpus; D: distal; ED: efferent ducts; Ep: epididymis/al (region not stated); ES: epididymal sperm; EJAC: ejaculated sperm; Eq: equatorial region; H: head; IAM: inner acrosomal membrane; M: midpiece; N: neck; P: posterior; PAc: post-acrosomal; PP: principal piece; T: testis; TS: testicular sperm; Vas: vas deferens; X: not present; Y: present (region not stated); V: vas deferens.

Some confusion in this field is shown by the publication by Agerberth et al. (1995) who identified the hCAP-18 gene in the human testis. In fact, the authors used commercial filters that are preloaded with mRNA from various human organs. It is known from the presence of a purely epididymal secretion HE5 in the testis field of such arrays [C. Kirchhoff, personal communication] that such samples often contain mRNA from total scrotal contents and are not purely testicular RNA. In the case of hCAP-18/SOB3, antibodies do not detect the protein in the testis, making it likely to be a true epididymal secretion.

4.2.5 Acrosome reaction

The zona pellucida stimulates the spermatozoon to undergo the acrosome reaction (a fusion of the plasma membrane and the outer acrosomal membrane and eventual loss of the vesicles formed). In the absence of large numbers of human zonae, and the failure of recombinant human ZP3 to be of benefit, calcium ionophore has been used to mimic the increased intracellular calcium normally induced by the zona. The percentage of spontaneously acrosome-reacted human epididymal sperm is high but similar for sperm from all epididymal regions but upon challenge with ionophore, the response of cauda cells is greater than that of corpus cells and caput sperm do not respond at all (Fig. 4.2E). Clearly a change in the response of the cells to calcium influx occurs upon maturation that results in their being able to acrosome react. Epididymal sterol binding and lipid binding proteins (see Table 4.2) are capable of making membranes more fluid, which is a prerequisite for acrosomal vesiculation. In this regard it is interesting to note that human epididymal dysfunction has been associated with abnormally high sperm membrane rigidity (Wiese *et al.*, 1996).

4.2.6 Acrosin content

The proteolytic enzyme acrosin within the acrosome is liberated and the bound enzyme exposed on the inner acrosome membrane after the acrosome reaction. The amount of acrosin in the head has been measured from the area of a gelatin film that is digested by the enzyme released from sperm dried on the film (Fig. 4.2F). A smaller area of digestion is found around more mature sperm heads (Haidl *et al.*, 1994), but this may indicate a shift from soluble to bound acrosin rather than a loss of enzyme or reduction in activity. Bedford (2004) has emphasised the need for propulsive thrust in zona penetration rather than lytic enzymatic action.

4.2.7 Sperm oocyte binding and fusion

Capacitated and acrosome-reacted spermatozoa are able to bind to and eventually fuse with the vitelline membrane after their passage through the zona. Using the ethically acceptable, species-insensitive zona-free hamster oocyte as surrogate, capacitated human epididymal spermatozoa display an increasing ability to bind to and penetrate the vitellus (Fig. 4.2G). These results may partly be explained by the increased incidence of acrosome-reacted sperm in the mature population, but still a difference between the response of corpus and cauda sperm, both of which can acrosome react, is evident.

4.2.8 Chromatin condensation

The condensation of chromatin that occurs during epididymal maturation has been monitored indirectly by the exclusion of dyes that bind to nucleoproteins (aniline blue binds to the remaining histones) or deoxyribonucleic acid (DNA) itself (acridine orange fluoresces green with native, double stranded, DNA but red with single

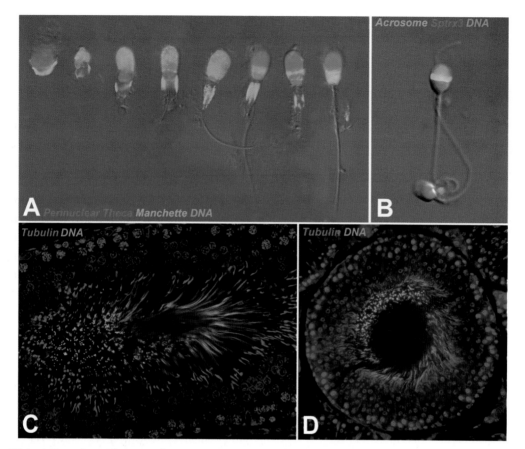

Plate 1 Snapshots of mammalian spermatogenesis and fertilization. (A) Biogenesis of sperm head Perinuclear theca (PT) and transient assembly of sperm caudal manchette as shown by immunofluorescence with antibodies against resident somatic cell type core histones of sperm PT (red; courtesy of Drs. R. Oko and P.R. Tovich, Queen's University, Kingston, ON, Canada; see Tovich *et al.*, 2004) and anti-tubulin antibody (green; E7-Developmental Studies Hybridoma Bank, DSHB, University of Iowa, Iowa City, IA), respectively. Note two possible routes of PT assembly through the deposition into subacrosomal layer and by the transport from cytoplasmic lobe along the manchette microtubules. (B) A morphologically normal spermatozoon (top) with an acrosome stained green with lectin Peanut lectin agglutinin-fluorescein isothiocynate (PNA-FITC) and a defective spermatozoon with superfluous retained cytoplasm labeled red with an antibody against spermatid specific thioredoxin Sptrx3 (courtesy of Dr. Antonio Miranda-Vizuete, CABD-CSIC, Universidad Pablo de Olavide, Sevilla, Spain; see Jimenez *et al.*, 2004). (C, D) Cross-sections of rat seminiferous tubule labeled with anti-tubulin antibody E7 (red; DSHB) (see page 14)

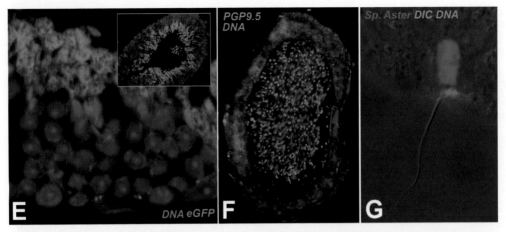

Caption for Plate 1 (*cont.*) (E) Testicular seminiferous tubule of a transgenic mouse expressing the enhanced green fluorescent protein (eGFP) under control of ubiquitin-C promoter. The accumulation of eGFP in the haploid spermatogenic cells near the lumen of the tubule reflects an increased need for substrate-specific, ubiquitin-dependent protein degradation during spermatid elongation. (F) After leaving testis, the caput epididymal spermatozoa of a mouse still carry the cytoplasmic droplet (CD), a remnant of germ cell cytoplasm eventually rejected by normal spermatozoa during epididymal passage or at ejaculation. Epididymal tubule section was labeled with antibody against CD's resident ubiquitin C-terminal hydrolase PGP9.5 (Biomol, Plymouth Meeting, PA). (G) A paternally contributed centriole organizes the zygotic centrosome, giving rise to sperm aster (red) responsible for the apposition of male and female pronuclei at an advanced stage of fertilization. This event of bovine fertilization *in vitro* was captured at the moment when the sperm tail Principal piece (PP) was not yet completely incorporated, remaining outside of the ooplasm at 7 hours and 30 minutes after insemination. Sperm aster microtubules (red) were labeled with anti-tubulin E7 (DSHB). Nuclear deoxyribonucleic acid (DNA) in all figures was labeled with DAPI (blue; Molecular Probes, Eugene, OR)

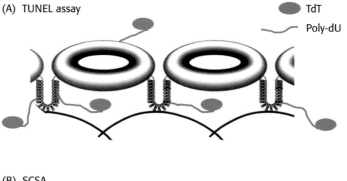

(A) TUNEL assay

TdT

Poly-dU

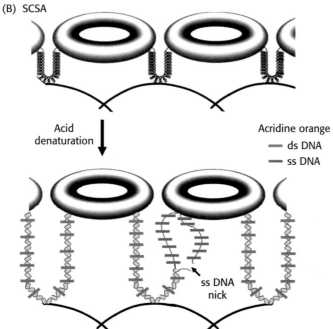

(B) SCSA

Acid
denaturation

Acridine orange
— ds DNA
— ss DNA

ss DNA
nick

Plate 2 *The TUNEL assay and SCSA considered with respect to the Donut-Loop model.* (A) The TUNEL assay uses the enzyme TdT to add uridine residues to 3′ OH ends of nicked and broken DNA. (B) The SCSA assay denatures DNA that has nicks, then uses acridine orange to detect ss and ds DNA (see Fig. 2.2)

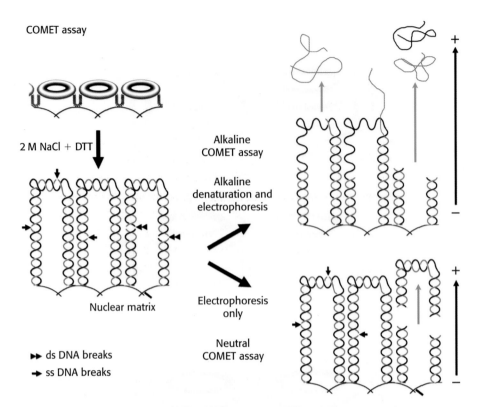

COMET assay

2 M NaCl + DTT

Nuclear matrix

Alkaline
COMET assay

Alkaline
denaturation and
electrophoresis

Electrophoresis
only

Neutral
COMET assay

▶▶ ds DNA breaks
➤ ss DNA breaks

Plate 3 *The neutral and alkaline COMET assays and the nuclear matrix.* Both COMET assays extract the histones and protamines with high salt, so that the Donut-Loop model is not relevant in this assay. The attachment sites of the DNA to the nuclear matrix, however, would remain intact in this assay. Note that DNA double-helices depicted in the extracted loop diagrams are not drawn to scale, but are shown as shorter segments for clarity (see Fig. 2.3)

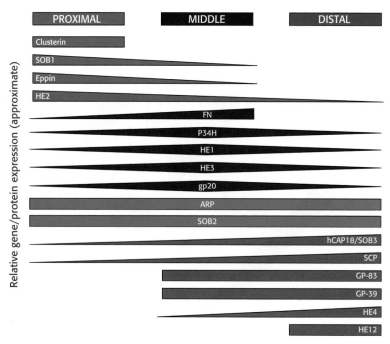

Plate 4 Schematic representation of the location (epididymal regions are approximate) of genes expressing secreted human epididymal proteins (for abbreviations see Table 4.2) (see Fig. 4.6)

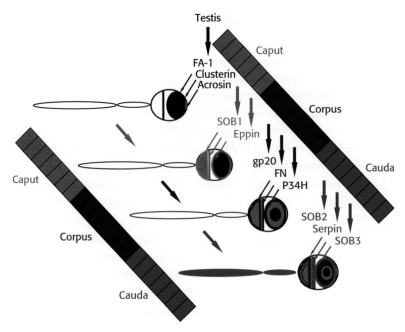

Plate 5 Schematic representation (not to scale) of the location of intrinsic (testicular) and extrinsic (secreted, epididymal) proteins on different membranes of the human sperm head with proposed functions in fertilisation (for abbreviations see Table 4.2) (see Fig. 4.7)

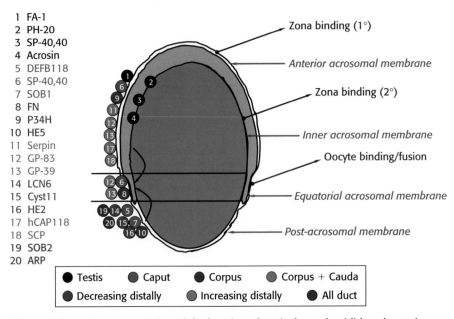

Plate 6 Schematic representation of the location of testicular and epididymal proteins on human epididymal sperm heads (for abbreviations see Table 4.2) (see Fig. 4.8)

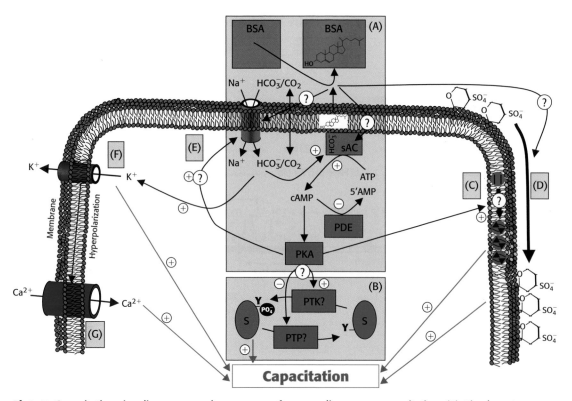

Plate 7 Capacitation signaling: proposed sequences of mammalian sperm capacitation. (A) Bicarbonate may enter sperm cells via a Na^+/HCO_3^- co-transporter or via diffusion as carbon dioxide. Intracellular bicarbonate switches on adenylyl cyclase (AC) and concomitant production of cyclic adenosine monophosphate (cAMP) activates protein kinase A (PKA). The role of cholesterol efflux in the activation of PKA is unclear. Cholesterol efflux may induce increased bicarbonate entry or may directly affect AC. (B) PKA induces tyr (Y) phosphorylation of several substrates (S) most likely via activation of protein tyr kinases (PTK) or inhibition of protein tyr phosphatases (PTP). PKA activation induces plasma membrane changes like in C and/or D. (C) Bilayer redistribution of aminophospholipids. (D) Lateral redistribution of seminolipid and cholesterol. The aminophospholipid scrambling is induced by PKA-dependent activation of a postulated scramblase. Most likely lateral redistribution of cholesterol is required before cholesterol depletion by bovine serum albumin (BSA). (E) The Na^+/HCO_3^- co-transporter could potentially be a substrate for PKA and may give rise to a sustained increase in HCO_3^- after its phosphorylation; thus having a positive feedback on cAMP synthesis. (F) Capacitation is also correlated with hyperpolarization of the sperm plasma membrane, which could be due to the opening of a potassium channel that senses alkalinization of the cytosol. (G) The consequent membrane hyperpolarization on turn may open voltage-dependent Ca^{2+} channels and induce the influx of Ca^{2+}. The increased tyr phosphorylation together with the ionic and lipidic changes in the membrane will induce downstream events involved in the process of capcitation (see Fig. 6.3). PDE: phosphodiesterase. (Adapted from Flesch and Gadella (2000) and Visconti and Kopf (1998) (see Fig. 6.1))

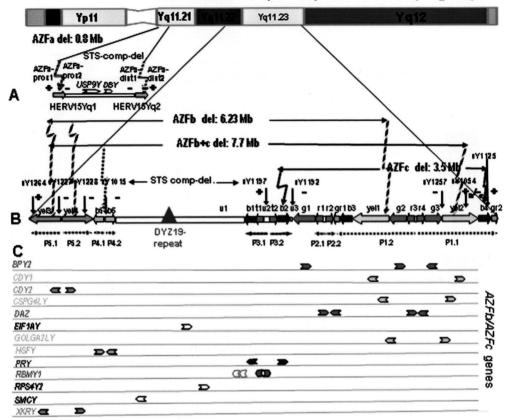

Plate 8 Schematic view on the AZF locus structure in Yq11 from men with haplogroup R*. (A) The AZF locus first marked by three distinct molecular deletion intervals (AZFa, AZFb, AZFc; Vogt et al., 1996) has now been sequenced. The AZFa deletion caused by recombination of two homologous HERV15 sequence blocks (HERV15Yq1/q2) is marked by a 0.8 Mb genomic DNA fragment in proximal Yq11. It contains the two *AZFa* genes, *USP9Y* and *DBY*. The AZFb deletion (extension 6.23 Mb) is largely overlapping with the AZFc deletion interval (extension 3.5 Mb) as indicated. Additionally a still larger AZFb deletion exists (coined AZFb+c del: 7.7 Mb; Repping et al., 2002), which however is not the sum of a complete AZFb + AZFc deletion interval. The indicated STS comp-del. markers can be used to diagnose complete AZFa, AZFb, AZFb+c, and AZFc deletions by a distinct deletion pattern. For example the sY1054 marker in distal AZFc is present in men with an AZFb+c deletion but absent in men with a complete AZFc deletion. (B) The approximate extension of the different palindromes formed by the AZFb/c amplicon structure is drawn below the amplicon blocks. Only the large P1 palindrome and the P3 palindrome include more than one amplicon type. (C) A schematic map of the location of all protein coding genes with a recognizable function (listed in Table 9.1A) are given for the AZFb and AZFc sequence interval. Their 5′–3′ polarity is indicated by the direction of the arrows marking the location of the different gene copies. Further pseudogene copies and the Testis-specific Transcript Y (*TTY*) genes (see Table 9.1B) mapping in the same sequence region (Skaletsky et al., 2003) are excluded to reduce the complexity of this map The colour code of the genes and associated arrow as indicates in which amplicon block the gene copies are located. Only the *EIF1AY*, *RPS4Y2*, and *SMCY* gene and two copies of the *RBMY1* gene family are located outside the amplicon blocks. One copy of the duplicated *CDY2* and *XKRY* gene is located proximal to the AZFb deletion interval (Repping et al., 2002). Please note that the ampliconic structure of the AZFb and AZFc sequence with its gene content as shown here is based on the GenBank Y chromosome sequence (http://www.ensembl.org/Homo_sapiens/mapview?chr=Y) and that this sequence belong to a Y chromosome of the R* lineage. Thus it can be different in men with another Y chromosomal haplogroup (for more details see Vogt, 2005b) (see Fig. 9.2)

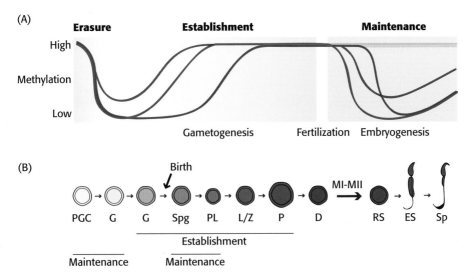

Plate 9 Methylation dynamics during germ cell and preimplantation embryo development. (A) Methylation dynamics of maternal (red) and paternal (blue) genomes. During gametogenesis, non-imprinted genes acquire their methylation similarly to imprinted genes, however, after fertilization, both the maternal and paternal genomes become demethylated while imprinted genes retain their methylation status, as shown by the paler red and blue lines. Some repeat sequences (dark gray) appear to escape complete demethylation during gametogenesis and retain a high proportion of their initial methylation marking during preimplantation development. Methylation levels are not to scale. (B) Progression of genomic methylation pattern acquisition during male germ cell development, as represented by the intensity of the blue shading. *De novo* and maintenance methylation events are indicated under the appropriate germ cell types. PGC: primordial germ cell; G: gonocyte; Spg: spermatogonia; PL: preleptotene; L/Z: leptotene/zygotene; P: pachytene; D: diplotene; RS: round spermatid; ES: elongating spermatid; Sp: sperm; MI–MII: meiosis I–II. Model based on mouse data and adapted from Lucifero *et al.* (2004b) (see Fig. 11.1)

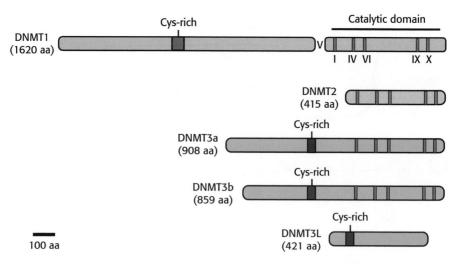

Plate 10 Organization of known mammalian DNMTs. Specific motifs are represented by boxes; five of the important amino acid motifs involved in catalysis are illustrated to demonstrate homology in the catalytic domain. Sizes in amino acids (aa) are those of the murine proteins (see Fig. 11.3)

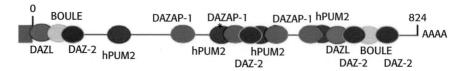

Plate 11 Screening of the *DAZR* 3′UTR (UnTranslated Region) for binding of multiple RNA-binding proteins. Diagrammed are results of binding assays with PUM2, BOULE, DAZL, DAZ2, DAZAP1 and DZIP1 proteins. The strongest reaction in the three-hybrid system was observed for sequences bound by PUM2 and DAZL. Binding by other proteins has not been investigated further. DAZAP1 was previously identified in the laboratory of Dr. Pauline Yen (Tsui *et al.*, 2000a) (see Fig. 12.7)

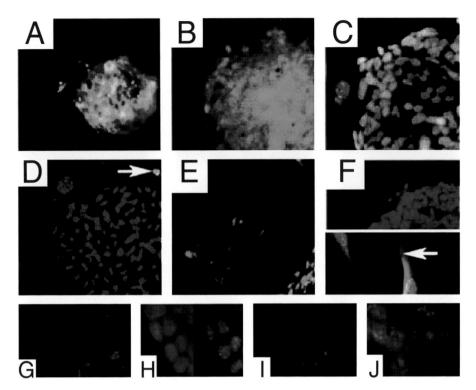

Plate 12 Protein expression in undifferentiated human (A–F) and mouse (G–J) ESCs. (A) SSEA3 (green) and TRA-1-81 (red) were used to assess status of hESC differentiation (orange indicates co-localization). Immunofluorescence: DAZL (B) and DAPI (C). Merged images of KDR and DAPI (D; white arrow shows positive cell); AFP (E) and NCAM1 (upper panel of F). NCAM1 was only detected in differentiated EBs (lower panel; F); white arrow shows cytoplasmic expression. mESC Immunofluorescence (G, I) Control preimmune for Dazl and Dzip; (H, J) specific antisera for Dazl and Dzip proteins. Immunofluorescence (lefthand) and DAPI (righthand panel) of G, I, H, J (see Fig. 12.12)

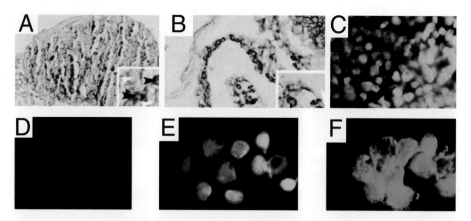

Plate 13 Immunohistochemistry and meiotic analysis of Day 14 EBs. See Clark *et al.*, for additional panels and controls. Day 14 EBs from HSF-6 and HSF-1 hESCs stained for VASA (A) and DAZL (B). Meiotic proteins (C–F). Undifferentiated hESCs stained with DAPI (C) and SCP3 antisera (D). Day 14 EBs stained for DAPI (E) and SCP3 (F) (see Fig. 12.13)

stranded DNA generated in DNA-denaturing acid conditions). With both methods a decrease in the accessibility of the dye upon maturation is interpreted as a maturational increase in the extent of chromatin condensation (Fig. 4.2H). Chromatin condensation reflects oxidation of sulphydryl groups of protamines (Bedford *et al.*, 1973) but nothing is known of any human enzymes involved in this process.

4.2.9 Fertilising ability *in vivo* and *in vitro*

The only *in vivo* studies on the fertilising capacity of sperm have been done on spermatozoa obtained from the epididymis of infertile men, for whom this offers hope of paternity. In these, epididymovasostomy is performed on azoospermic men with epididymal occlusion. The site of anastomosis of the vas to the epididymis is proximal to the site of occlusion so as to permit egress of the luminal spermatozoa. As this occurs at various sites in different individuals, different extents of the epididymis are bypassed. It has been observed that the more of the epididymis the sperm have passed through before entering the vas deferens, the higher the pregnancy rate (Fig. 4.2I).

Assisted reproduction techniques have also permitted pregnancies to be initiated by *in vitro* fertilisation (IVF) of sperm removed from different regions of an occluded epididymis. It has demonstrated that both fertilisation and pregnancy rates are higher, the longer the length of epididymis the spermatozoa have encountered (Fig. 4.2J). As expected, fertilisation *in vitro* occurs with the use of mature sperm retrieved from the vas deferens (Brindley *et al.*, 1986; Bustillo and Rajfer, 1986; Hirsch *et al.*, 1993).

The relationship between the length of the epididymal passage and fertilisation *in vitro* and *in vivo* supports the view that spermatozoa have a greater chance of interacting with relevant epididymal secretions before becoming competent at fertilisation. Occasional reports that pregnancies result from anastomosing the vas deferens to the efferent ducts (Silber, 1988; Weiske *et al.*, 1994), rete testis or a seminiferous tubule (Schoysman, 1993) may relate to a functional change in the vas deferens and its secretions consequent upon its abnormal exposure to testicular fluids, as demonstrated in rats and rabbits (Temple-Smith *et al.*, 1989, 1998). As all human observations are necessarily made on occluded epididymides, the effects of long-term ductal occlusion on normal epididymal function have to be contemplated. Reflux of epididymal secretions into this fluid may explain why testicular spermatozoa obtained from spermatocoeles can fertilise eggs *in vitro* (Hirsch *et al.*, 1996).

4.3 Sperm storage in the human epididymis

4.3.1 Sperm numbers

The small storage capacity of the human epididymis is demonstrated by the small size of the cauda region (see Fig. 4.1), the small reserves (about 3 days worth of testicular production: Bedford, 1990), which approximate those found after cauda bypass (Schoysman and Bedford, 1986), and the rapidity with which sperm reserves can be decreased or refilled after multiple ejaculation or abstention (see Cooper et al., 1993). After epididymal emptying by providing three ejaculates within 4 h, sperm numbers in the first of three subsequent ejaculates is increased from 50 millions after 1 day abstinence to over 300 millions after 10 days and is increased further with successive ejaculates (Fig. 4.4: from Cooper et al., 1993). Beyond this time ejaculate sperm numbers remain constant as the epididymis is filled and sperm enter the urine (Barratt and Cooke, 1988).

4.3.2 Sperm protection

Mammals have both adaptive (acquired) immunity, a function of T and B cells which are selected by nominal antigens and expand clonally, and innate (natural) immunity, which is triggered immediately in response to micro-organisms. Mechanisms of innate immunity include the generation of disinfectants (H_2O_2, NO), large antimicrobial proteins (lysozyme, cathepsins, lactoferrin, phospholipase A_2) and small antimicrobial peptides (cathelicidins (e.g. glycodelins) and defensins (α, β)) (Bourgeon et al., 2004; Com et al., 2003; Yang et al., 2002). A wide range of defensins have been identified in the human epididymis (Table 4.2). As defensins-α and -β are inhibited at high salt solutions, they would be more active in the low ionic strength

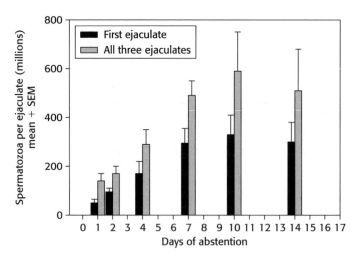

Figure 4.4   The increase in number of seminal spermatozoa obtained by multiple ejaculation after increasing periods of prior sexual abstinence (from Cooper et al., 1993). Note the increase from 50×10^6 in the first ejaculate after 1 day abstinence to 300×10^6 after 10 days abstinence. The total number of sperm in three ejaculates increases from about 150×10^6 to 600×10^6 over this time period

of epididymal fluid ($\mu = 0.122$ from data in Hinton *et al.*, 1981) and ideally situated to prevent the migration of invading micro-organisms into the male tract.

A variety of anti-oxidant enzymes are present in human seminal plasma but most are not of epididymal origin (Yeung *et al.*, 1998), although some anti-oxidant activity does originate there (Potts *et al.*, 1999).

4.4 Sperm volume regulation

The osmolality of spermatozoa in the cauda epididymidis must approximate that measured in the vas deferens (342 mmol/kg: Hinton *et al.*, 1981) but fluids in the female tract have been measured to be 276–302 mmol/kg (Edwards, 1974; Casslén and Nilsson, 1984; Menézo *et al.*, 1982; Rossato *et al.*, 1996). Thus within the female tract upon ejaculation spermatozoa should be considered to suffer a hypotonic challenge, especially as it is commonly held that seminal plasma is hyperosmotic (Rossato *et al.*, 2002). Recently, however, measurements of the sperm-rich, prostatic fraction of split ejaculates (Björndahl and Kvist, 2003) and unliquefied whole semen measured within 5 min of ejaculation (Cooper *et al.*, 2005) have revealed osmolalities in these fluids to be 294–304 mmol/kg, that is within the female range. This demonstrates that the osmotic challenge actually occurs within the male urethra during the ejaculatory process and that cell swelling would be anticipated within the female tract unless otherwise prevented.

4.4.1 Ejaculated spermatozoa

Human spermatozoa, as somatic cells, are able to regulate their volume when subjected to such hypotonic conditions as occur in the male and female tract. This is shown by swelling when ejaculated spermatozoa are provided with a physiological challenge by incubation in hypotonic medium together with inhibitors of channels employed by somatic cells for volume regulation. The broad-spectrum potassium channel blocker quinine is effective at preventing volume regulation and also renders sperm less able to migrate into and through surrogate mucus owing to a change to non-progressive motility; both quinine and the voltage-sensitive potassium channel blocker 4-aminopyridine induce volume increase with a simultaneous change to less progressive motility (Gu *et al.*, 2004; Yeung and Cooper, 2001; Yeung *et al.*, 2003). The ability of the potassium ionophores valinomycin and gramicidin to eliminate the quinine-induced change in size and kinematics suggests that K^+ ions are utilised in volume regulation (Yeung and Cooper, 2001) and the fact that raised extracellular K^+, by preventing intracellular K^+ efflux, is able to cause swelling under physiologically hypotonic conditions (Yeung *et al.*, 2003) suggests that this ion is an intracellular osmolyte that effluxes from spermatozoa with obliged water under hypotonic stress.

In the usual clinical situation, however, where semen is collected in a vessel and liquefied for 30 min at 37° (WHO, 1999), the osmolality of the fluid rises both during liquefaction (Cooper *et al.*, 2005) and after it (Abraham-Peskir *et al.*, 2002; Aitken *et al.*, 1996; Hofmann and Karlas, 1973; Velazquez *et al.*, 1977), so that the actual osmotic challenge to spermatozoa dispensed from the ejaculate to assisted reproductive technology (ART) medium is even greater than that normally encountered.

4.4.2 Epididymal spermatozoa

Spermatozoa acquire the ability to regulate their volume within the epididymis of mice (Yeung *et al.*, 1999, 2002) and monkeys (Yeung *et al.*, 2004). As no data are available on human epididymal spermatozoa, maturation in the cynomolgus monkey is presented. Epididymal spermatozoa from the caput, corpus and cauda were subjected to a physiological osmotic insult (290 mmol/kg) in the absence (control) or presence of the broad-spectrum cation channel inhibitor quinine. Cauda spermatozoa maintained their original volume except in the presence of quinine, when their volume increased over 20 min and remained that size. This indicates that the cells were regulating their volume in a quinine-sensitive manner under the physiologically hypotonic conditions, whereas caput spermatozoa never swelled in either the presence or absence of quinine (Fig. 4.5). The ability of spermatozoa to develop the capacity to regulate volume during epididymal transport is thought to reflect the epididymal provision of low molecular weight osmolytes (Cooper and Yeung, 2003) but this remains to be proved for humans.

4.5 Epididymal fluid

What little is known of the composition of human epididymal/vasal fluid is compared with that of fluid leaving the testis in Table 4.1. There is little change in calcium, chloride or phosphate and remarkably low concentrations of carnitine, GPC and inositol compared to those in rodents. The higher osmolality and protein concentration compared with testicular fluid and the high potassium and low sodium in epididymal fluid reflect the pattern seen in all mammals studied.

4.6 Epididymal proteins involved in sperm maturation

Several techniques have been applied to the study of epididymal proteins that may be involved in the maturation and storage of spermatozoa. The earlier work on proteins involved the raising of polyclonal or monoclonal antibodies against ejaculated spermatozoa; against proteins eluted from ejaculated sperm and against

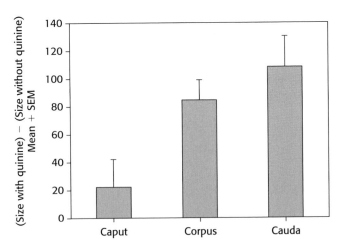

Figure 4.5   The size of monkey spermatozoa after incubation in physiologically hypotonic medium in the presence of the broad-spectrum cation channel blocker quinine (from Yeung *et al.*, 2004). As quinine prevents volume regulation in response to a physiologically hypotonic challenge, the regulatory response (cauda > corpus > caput) indicates a maturation of regulating ability during epididymal transit

seminal fluid proteins. More recently, molecular biology techniques such as cloning from gene-specific probes and differential library screening have been applied to the epididymis (see Kirchhoff, 1998) and revealed transcripts of genes that are expressed solely in the epididymis. Oligonucleotide sequence data and the consensus amino acid composition of these proteins have revealed surprising identities between proteins with different functions. The nucleotide sequence of one epididymal secretion involved in sperm–zona binding (P34H) identifies it as a member of the short-chain dehydrogenase/reductase family of proteins and it has carbonyl reductase activity. Another epididymal protein involved in sperm–zona binding (SOB3: Hammami-Hamza *et al.*, 2001) has the identical sequence as a human epididymal cationic anti-microbial protein (hCAP-18: Malm *et al.*, 2000). One major maturation antigen of the human epididymis (CD52) has been discovered by several groups and called variously H6-3C4 antigen (Kameda *et al.*, 1992), HE5 (Kirchhoff *et al.*, 1993), GZS-1 (Hutter *et al.*, 1996), SAGA-1 (Diekman *et al.*, 1997), S19 antigen (Mahony and Alexander, 1991) and gp20 (Focarelli *et al.*, 1999a, b, c) (see Diekman *et al.*, 2000). The uptake of CD52 by maturing spermarozoa (Yeung *et al.*, 1997b) and changes in antigen accessibility upon storage in the cauda and *in vitro* capacitation (Yeung *et al.*, 2000, 2001) suggest that it may be involved in sperm storage (Bedford, 2004).

Table 4.2 lists the proteins identified to date as secretions of the human epididymis that may be involved in the acquisition of fertilising capacity of epididymal spermatozoa. Their names, pseudonyms, molecular weight, pI, proven functions and suspected role in fertilisation are given. Where given, the site of expression of the gene and protein in the organ are presented, as well as the extent of expression, and the location in the epididymis where sperm are first coated by the secretion and the site of the sperm where the antigen is located.

4.6.1 Solely testicular proteins

Testicular proteins involved in sperm–egg contact are also listed for completeness. They are inherent components of sperm before they leave the testis and are thought to function in zona binding and fusion with the oocyte.

4.6.2 Testicular and epididymal proteins

Other proteins are expressed in both the testis and epididymis. The epididymal regions listed are those described in the papers cited, although as the human caput contains both a common epididymal duct and many efferent ducts (Yeung et al., 1991) the term 'caput' will include efferent ducts. Of those solely in the caput region, clusterin binds to lipids that are exposed on dead spermatozoa. Of efferent duct proteins also secreted more distally in the corpus epididymidis, one is a protease inhibitor/microbicide (Eppin) and three (SOB1, ARP and fibronectin) are involved in fusion with the oocyte. A role in egg fusion is deduced from the reduced number of sperm penetrating zona-free hamster oocytes after treatment of sperm with antibodies to the protein and showing that zona binding, motility and the acrosome reaction are not affected by the antibody. Steric hindrance by the antibody to an adjacent sperm site truly involved in binding is a concern and sometimes the smaller Fab Ig fragments are used. A location on the equatorial region of the acrosome (the site of sperm–egg contact) is usually consistent with a function in sperm–egg fusion. This is not always the case, however, and one sperm coating protein eluted by high ionic strength is located over the acrosomal region (Tezón et al., 1985) and yet its antibody prevents sperm–egg fusion not sperm–zona binding (Sanjurjo et al., 1990). This may be because the protein relocates to the equatorial segment during capacitation, which is the case for gp20/CD52 (from post-acrosomal to equatorial: Focarelli et al., 1998).

The location in the epididymis of several proteins also present in the testis (PDGS, a lipocalin) is not accurately given. In most cases it can be assumed, and in others it is clear from histological sections, that the corpus epididymidis was examined, however this does not necessarily imply that the protein is absent from other areas, since they may not have been examined or it may not be present (as in the case of BCAVD: He et al., 1995). Expression of serpin (involved in zona binding and oocyte fusion) and trypsinogen (a precursor for a proteolytic enzyme/zona binding protein) is found more distally in the cauda epididymidis as well.

4.6.3 Solely epididymal proteins

As found for the proteins above, some are expressed solely in the caput (or efferent ducts) and throughout the duct. HE6 (a suspected epithelial transporter) is solely located in the caput (Obermann *et al.*, 2003) but the reports of a caput expression of proteins C and S, proteases involved in immune suppression, may reflect the fact that only tissue from BCAVD patients was examined where no more distal tissue is present, so these proteins may also be present in more distal regions of normal epididymides.

Proteins involved in zona binding (3B2F antigen) and oocyte fusion (SOB2) are found throughout the epididymis but a regional gradation of expression/activity of other epididymal proteins is evident. The activities of the enzymes NAG, β-glucosidase and β-galactosidase are higher in the efferent ducts than the more distal regions of epididymis and vas deferens. The expression of HE2 (oocyte fusion/anti-microbial activity) and galactosyl transferase activity are also greater in the caput region.

On the other hand, α-fucosidase, α-mannosidase and β-glucuronidase are more active in the epididymis than efferent ducts or vas. The corpus epididymidis similarly displays higher expression than the caput or cauda of P34H (zona binding). For HE1 (a sterol binding protein) and the novel HE3, a biphasic expression is present with expression higher in the vas deferens than the cauda. Some epididymal proteins secreted into the lumen are taken up by spermatozoa locally and thus carried downstream to more distal regions. Indeed, for secretions P34H (Boué *et al.*, 1994) and HE5/CD52 (Yeung *et al.*, 1997b) there are higher amounts of protein on sperm from the cauda than corpus despite the lower gene expression in the cauda.

Nevertheless, proteins expressed along the entire duct but in higher amounts in the more distal regions would provide more secretion per sperm than others and may be involved in storage of sperm in the cauda. A sperm coating protein involved in egg fusion, the enzyme α-glucosidase and the anti-microbial hCAP-18 all provide such distal gradients of secretion. Other proteins are found solely in the corpus and cauda (the protease GP-83, GP-39, possibly involved in oocyte fusion), or cauda alone (HE4, HE12), the latter thought to be decapacitation factors that keep sperm quiescent until ejaculation.

Figure 4.6 (Color plate 4) shows schematically the general location and abundance of proteins secreted into the human epididymal lumen. Some are secreted proximally, some distally and some throughout the duct.

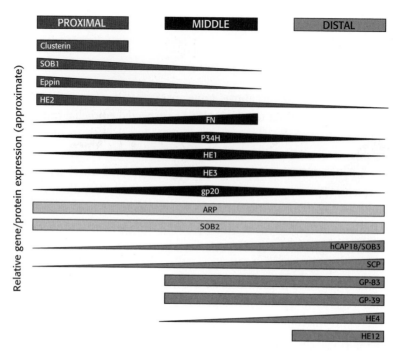

Figure 4.6   Schematic representation of the location (epididymal regions are approximate) of genes expressing secreted human epididymal proteins (for abbreviations see Table 4.2) (see Color plate 4)

4.6.4 Interaction of proteins with spermatozoa

Epididymal proteins held electrostatically to the sperm surface can be eluted with high ionic strength medium and include sperm coating protein (Sanjurjo *et al.*, 1990) and ARP (Krätzschmar *et al.*, 1996). The former was implicated in sperm–egg fusion because antibodies to it blocked penetration of human sperm into zona-free hamster eggs. By contrast, ARP was easily eluted from the sperm surface and was not considered to function in sperm–egg fusion in the way that the rodent equivalent (Protein D/E [AEG]) does in the rat (Rochwerger and Cuasnicú, 1992). Recent studies, however, have indicated that some ARP remains on the sperm equatorial region after high salt extraction and that antibodies against ARP block sperm–egg penetration (Cohen *et al.*, 2001). By analogy with the rat epididymis (about which most is known in this regard: Cooper, 1998) it is possible that the ionic strength within the human epididymal canal is low, because of high concentrations of uncharged organic solutes, and this would keep these proteins on the sperm (Cooper, 1998).

At least two epididymal secretions (CD52 and P34H) are held by glycerophoshoinositol anchors to the sperm membrane. These first serve to anchor

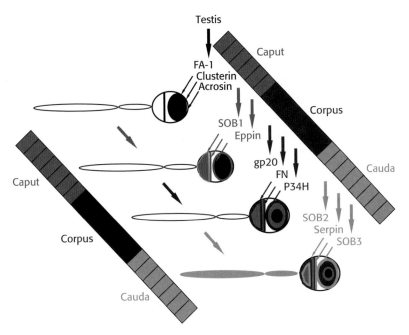

Figure 4.7   Schematic representation (not to scale) of the location of intrinsic (testicular) and extrinsic (secreted, epididymal) proteins on different membranes of the human sperm head with proposed functions in fertilisation (for abbreviations see Table 4.2) (see Color plate 5)

the secretory protein to the membrane of the epididymal cell that sheds vesicular 'epididymosomes' into the lumen. For both molecules, transfer to sperm is mediated by such vesicles (Frenette and Sullivan, 2001; Yeung *et al.*, 1997b). P34H protein remains on the sperm head until the acrosome reaction, when its role in zona binding is complete (Boué *et al.*, 1994).

Figure 4.7 (Color plate 5) summarises the sequence of sperm modification by secreted human epididymal proteins. FA-1 antigen, clusterin and acrosin are present in and on spermatozoa before they enter the epididymis; SOB2 and Eppin are caput secretions that bind to the equatorial and acrosomal regions, respectively; gp20, fibronectin (FN) and P34H are corpus secretions adhering to the post-acrosomal, equatorial and acrosomal regions, respectively, whereas SOB2, Serpin and SOB3 are caudal secretions similarly binding to the post-acrosomal, equatorial and acrosomal regions of the sperm cell.

The role of these proteins, irrespective of their origin, may be related to primary zona binding (acrosomal antigens) and oocyte binding/fusion (equatorial antigens). Some post-acrosomal and acrosomal antigens may migrate during capacitation to the equatorial region (Fig. 4.8, Color plate 6).

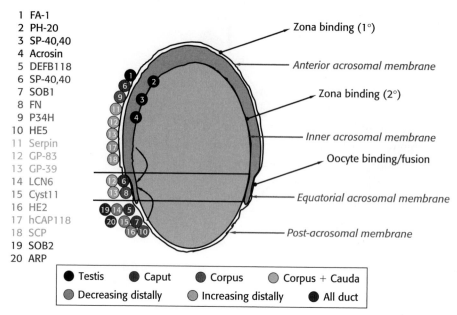

Figure 4.8   Schematic representation of the location of testicular and epididymal proteins on human epididymal sperm heads (for abbreviations see Table 4.2) (see Color plate 6)

4.7 Summary

As sperm move though the human epididymis they encounter a varied and varying environment with respect to the proteins they encounter. They acquire additional proteins, sometimes the same as those as testicular proteins but more often different, epididymis-specific proteins and come into contact with water soluble low molecular weight compound that may be important for volume regulation. In the proximal epididymis sperm are subjected to the action of certain enzymes and exposure to proteins involved in membrane modification and sperm–egg fusion. In the middle region another set of enzymes become active and proteins associated with sterol transport (HE1) predominate that could modify the membrane in such a way as to permit the uptake of GPI-anchored zona binding proteins. More distally sperm encounter increasing concentrations of glucosidase and protease, proteins involved in zona binding and oocyte fusion, the major maturation antigen CD52, anti-microbial activity and decapacitation factors, that help them to survive before ejaculation.

Adherence of the proteins to different domains (plasma membrane over the acrosome or equatorial acrosomal segment) may depend on the nature of the protein, the lipid composition of the particular membrane and the ionic and environment in which the sperm finds itself. The eventual location on a capacitated sperm (acrosomal membrane) or acrosome-reacted sperm (equatorial region) may dictate their role in, for example, zona-binding (P34H) or oocyte-binding (gp20). Both the proteins and the sperm membranes may be modified during epididymal transit by the range of enzyme activities to which sperm are subjected in different epididymal regions (e.g. glycosyltransferases, glycosidases and proteases) and which may add to or remove carbohydrates and peptides from the sperm surface. The activity of proteases is in turn modified by protease inhibitors liberated from the epithelium and attached to spermatozoa.

In addition to the secretion of macromolecules that bind to maturing spermatozoa, the secretion of low molecular weight ions and organic osmolytes are presumably taken up during epididymal transit endowing spermatozoa with the capacity to regulate volume when necessary and to keep sperm quiescent by keeping Na^+ low and K^+ high. The associated low ionic strength of the fluid would help to keep electrostatically bound proteins on the sperm surface and promote the activity of microbicidal proteins.

This knowledge could be used to develop diagnostic tests of male infertility or design post-testicular contraceptives for men.

Acknowledgments

Our work cited in this report was largely funded by the Deutsche Forschungsgemeinschaft and Ernst Schering Foundation/Rockefeller Foundation AMPPAI and Ernst Schering Foundation/CONRAD AMPPAII Research Networks.

REFERENCES

Abraham-Peskir JV, Chantler E, Uggerhoj E and Fedder J (2002) Response of midpiece vesicles on human sperm to osmotic stress. *Human Reprod,* 17, 375–382.

Adamopoulos DA, Lawrence DM, Vassilopoulos P, Kontogeorgos L, Ntounis A and Swyer GIM (1979) Testosterone concentration in different functional compartments of the male reproductive tract. *Arch Androl* 3, 13–18.

Agerberth B, Gunne H, Odeberg J, Kogner P, Boman HG and Gudmundsson GH (1995) FALL 39, a putative human peptide antibiotic, is cysteine-free and expressed in bone marrow and testis. *Proc Natl Acad Sci USA*, 92, 195–199.

Aitken RJ, Allan IW, Irvine DS and Macnamee M (1996) Studies on the development of diluents for the transportation and storage of human semen at ambient temperature. *Human Reprod* 11, 2186–2196.

Amann RP and Howards SS (1980) Daily spermatozoal production and epididymal spermatozoal reserves of the human male. *J Urol* 124, 211–215.

Ånberg Å (1957) The ultrastructure of the spermatozoon. An electronmicroscopic study of the spermatozoa from sperm samples and the epididymis including some observations of the spermatid. *Acta Obstet Gynecol Scand*, 36 (Suppl 2),1–133.

Avellar MC, Honda L, Hamil KG *et al.* (2004) Differential expression and antibacterial activity of epididymis protein 2 isoforms in the male reproductive tract of human and rhesus monkey (*Macaca mulatta*). *Biol Reprod* 71, 1453–1460.

Barratt CLR and Cooke ID (1988) Sperm loss in the urine of sexually rested men. *Int J Androl* 11, 201–207.

Batova I, Kameda K, Hasegawa A, Koyama K, Tsuji Y and Isojima S (1990) Monoclonal antibody recognising an apparent peptide epitope of human seminal plasma glycoprotein and exhibiting sperm immobilizing activity. *J Reprod Immunol* 17, 1–6.

Bedford JM (1990) Sperm dynamics in the epididymis. In: Gamete Physiology, eds RA Asch, JP Balmaceda and I Johnston. Norwell, MA, USA: Serono Symposia, pp. 53–67.

Bedford JM (1991) Effects of elevated temperature on the epididymis and testis: experimental studies. In: *Temperature and Environmental Effects on the Testis*, ed. AW Zorgniotti. New York: Plenum Press, pp. 19–32.

Bedford JM (2004) Enigmas of mammalian gamete form and function. *Biol Rev Camb Philos Soc* 79, 429–460.

Bedford JM, Calvin H and Cooper GW (1973) The maturation of spermatozoa in the human epididymis. *J Reprod Fertil Suppl* 18, 199–213.

Bedford JM, Berrios M and Dryden GL (1982) Biology of the scrotum. IV. Testis location and temperature sensitivity. *J Exp Zool* 224, 379–388.

Belonoschkin B (1943) Biologie der Spermatozoen im menschlichen Hoden und Nebenhoden. *Arch M Gynakoel* 174, 357–368.

Björndahl L and Kvist U (2003) Sequence of ejaculation affects the spermatozoon as a carrier and its message. *Reprod Biomed Online* 7, 440–448.

Böstrom K and Öckerman PA (1971) Glycosidases in human semen and male genital organs. *Scand J Urol Nephrol* 5, 117–122.

Boué F, Berubé B, De Lamirande E, Gagnon C and Sullivan R (1994) Human sperm-zona pellucida interaction in inhibited by an antiserum against a hamster sperm protein. *Biol Reprod* 51, 577–587.

Boué F, Duquenne C, Lassalle B, Lefevre A and Finaz C (1995) FLB1, a human protein of epididymal origin that is involved in the sperm–oocyte recognition process. *Biol Reprod* 52, 267–278.

Bourgeon F, Evrard B, Brillard-Bourdet M, Colleu D, Jegou B and Pineau C (2004) Involvement of semenogelin-derived peptides in the antibacterial activity of human seminal plasma. *Biol Reprod* 70, 768–774.

Brindley GS, Scott GI and Hendry WF (1986) Vas cannulation with implanted sperm reservoirs for obstructive azoospermia or ejaculatory failure. *Brit J Urol* 58, 721–723.

Brooks DE (1979) Biochemical environment of maturing spermatozoa. In: *The Spermatozoon*, eds DW Fawcett and JM Bedford. Baltimore, MD: Urban and Schwarzenberg, pp. 23–34.

Bustillo M and Rajfer J (1986) Pregnancy following insemination with sperm aspirated directly from vas deferens. *Fertil Steril* 46, 144–146.

Carr DW, Usselman MC and Acott, TS (1985) Effects of pH, lactate, and viscoelastic drag on sperm motility: a species comparison. *Biol Reprod* 33, 588–595.

Casslén B and Nilsson B (1984) Human uterine fluid, examined in undiluted samples for osmolarity and the concentrations of inorganic ions, albumin, glucose, and urea. *Am J Obstet Gynecol* 150, 877–881.

Castellón EA and Huidobro CC (1999) Androgen regulation of glycosidae secretion in epithelial cell cultures from human epididymis. *Human Reprod* 14, 1522–1527.

Cohen DJ, Ellerman DA, Busso D *et al.* (2001) Evidence that human epididymal protein ARP plays a role in gamete fusion through complementary sites on the surface of the human egg. *Biol Reprod* 65, 1000–1005.

Com E, Bourgeon F, Evrard B, Ganz T, Colleu D, Jegou B and Pineau C (2003) Expression of antimicrobial defensins in the male reproductive tract of rats, mice, and humans. *Biol Reprod* 68, 95–104.

Cooper TG (1990) In defense of a function for the human epididymis. *Fertil Steril* 90, 965–975.

Cooper TG (1998) Interaction of proteins with epididymal secretions. *J Reprod Fertil Suppl* 53, 119–136.

Cooper TG and Yeung CH (2003) Acquisition of volume regulatory response of sperm upon maturation in the epididymis and the role of the cytoplasmic droplet. *Microsc Res Techn* 61, 28–38.

Cooper TG, Raczek S, Yeung CH, Schwab E, Schulze H and Hertle L (1992) Composition of fluids obtained from human epididymal cysts. *Urol Res* 20, 275–280.

Cooper TG, Keck C, Oberdieck U and Nieschlag E (1993) Effects of multiple ejaculations after extended periods of sexual abstinence on total, motile and normal sperm numbers, as well as accessory gland secretions, from healthy normal and oligozoospermic men. *Human Reprod* 8, 1251–1258.

Cooper TG, Yeung CH, Jones R, Orgebin-Crist MC and Robaire B (2002) Rebuttal of a role for the epididymis in sperm quality control by phagocytosis of defective sperm. *J Cell Sci* 115, 5–7.

Cooper TG, Yeung CH, Fetic S, Sobhani A and Nieschlag E (2004) Cytoplasmic droplets are normal structures of human sperm but are not well preserved by routine procedures for assessing sperm morphology. *Human Reprod* 19, 2283–2288.

Cooper TG, Barfield JP and Yeung CH (2005) Changes in osmolality during liquefaction of human semen. *Int J Androl* 28, 58–60.

Datti A, Beccari T, Emiliani C, Stirling JL and Orlacchio A (1993) Blood testoterone levels are correlated with β-*N*-actylhexosaminidase activity in human caput epididymis. *Bichem Mol Biol Int* 30, 1013–1020.

Delpech S, Lecomte P and Lecomte C (1988) Étude *in vitro* chèz l'homme de la liason des spermatozoïdes épididymaires à la zone pellucida. *J Gynecol Obstet Biol Reprod* 17, 339–342.

Diekman AB, Westbrook-Case VA, Naaby-Hansen S, Klotz KL, Flickinger CJ and Herr JC (1997) Biochemical characterization of sperm agglutination antigen-1, a human sperm surface antigen implicated in gamete interactions. *Biol Reprod* 57, 1136–1144.

Diekman AB, Norton EJ, Westbrook VA, Klotz KL, Naaby-Hansen S and Herr JC (2000) Antisperm antibodies from infertile patients and their cognate sperm antigens: a review. Identity between SAGA-1, the H6-3C4 antigen, and CD52. *Am J Reprod Immunol* 43, 134–143.

Edwards RG (1974) Follicular fluid. *J Reprod Fertil* 37, 189–219.

Elisen MG, van Kooij RJ, Nolte MA, Marquart JA, Lock TM, Bouma BN and Meijers JC (1998) Protein C inhibitor may modulate human sperm-oocyte interactions. *Biol Reprod* 58, 670–677.

Emiliani S, Van den Bergh M, Vannin AS, Biramane J, Verdoodt M and Englert Y (2000) Increased sperm motility after in-vitro culture of testicular biopsies from obstructive azoospermic patients results in better post-thaw recovery rate. *Human Reprod* 15, 2371–2374.

Evans EA, Zhang H and Martin-DeLeon PA (2003) SPAM1 (PH-20) protein and mRNA expression in the epididymides of humans and macaques: utilizing laser microdissection/RT-PCR. *Reprod Biol Endocrinol* 1, 54.

Fenichel P, Cervoni F, Hofman P *et al.* (1994) Expression of the complement regulatory protein CD59 on human spermatozoa: characterization and role in gametic interaction. *Mol Reprod Dev* 38, 338–346.

Focarelli R, Giuffrida A, Capparelli S *et al.* (1998) Specific localization in the equatorial segment of gp20, a 20 kDa sialylglycoprotein of the capacitated human spermatozoon acquired during epididymal transit which is necessary to penetrate zona-free hamster eggs. *Mol Human Reprod* 4, 119–125.

Focarelli R, Francavilla S, Francavilla F, Giovampaola DC, Santucci A and Rosati F (1999a) gp20, a sialylglycoprotein of the human capacitated sperm surface is the homologue of the leukocyte CD52 antigen: analysis of the effect of anti-CD52 monoclonal antibody (CAMPATH-1) on capacitated sperm. *Mol Human Reprod* 5, 46–51.

Focarelli R, Giovampaola CD, Seraglia R, Brettoni C, Sabatini L, Pescaglini M and Rosati F (1999b) Biochemical and MALDI analysis of the human sperm antigen gp20, homologue of leukocyte CD52. *Biochem Biophys Res Commun* 258, 639–643.

Focarelli R, Giovampaola CD, Seraglia R *et al.* (1999c) Biochemical and MALDI analysis of the human sperm antigen gp20, homologue of leukocyte CD52. *Biochem Biophys Res Commun* 258, 639–643.

Fogdestam I, Fall M and Nilsson S (1986) Microsurgical epididymovasostomy in the treatment of occlusive azoospermia. *Fertil Steril* 46, 925–929.

Fournier-Delpech A and Guérin Y (1991) Interactions des spermatozoïdes avec le zone pellucide. *Contracept Fertil Steril* 19, 825–832.

Frenette G and Sullivan R (2001) Prostasome-like particles are involved in the transfer of P25g from the bovine epididymal fluid to the sperm surface. *Mol Reprod Develop* 59, 115–121.

Gago C, Soler C, Perez-Sanchez F, Yeung CH and Cooper TG (2000) Effect of cetrorelix on sperm morphology during migration through the epididymis in the cynomolgus macaque (*Macaca fascicularis*). *Am J Primatol* 51, 103–117.

Golan R, Cooper TG, Oschry Y, Oberpenning F, Schulze H, Shocat L and Lewin LM (1996) Changes in chromatin condensation of human spermatozoa during epididymal transit as determined by flow cytometry. *Human Reprod* 11, 1457–1462.

Gu Y, Kirkman-Brown JC, Korchev Y, Barratt CL and Publicover SJ (2004) Multi-state, 4-aminopyridine-sensitive ion channels in human spermatozoa. *Dev Biol* 274, 308–317.

Haidl G, Badura B, Hinsch K-D, Ghyczy M, Garei BJ and Schill W-B (1993) Disturbances of sperm flagella due to failure of epididymal maturation and their possible relationship to phospholipids. *Human Reprod* 8, 1070–1073.

Haidl G, Badura B and Schill W-B. (1994) Function of human epididymal spermatozoa. *J Androl* 15, 23ST–27ST.

Hale G, Rye PD, Warford A, Lauder I and Brito-Babapulle A (1993) The glycosylphosphatidyli-nositol-anchored lymphocyte antigen CDw52 is associated with the epididymal maturation of human spermatozoa. *J Reprod Immunol* 23, 189–205.

Hamil KG, Sivashanmugam P, Richardson RT *et al.* (2000) HE2beta and HE2gamma, new members of an epididymis-specific family of androgen-regulated proteins in the human. *Endocrinology* 141, 1245–1253.

Hamil KG, Liu Q, Sivashanmugam P *et al.* (2002) Cystatin 11: a new member of the cystatin type 2 family. *Endocrinology* 143, 2787–2796.

Hamil KG, Liu Q, Sivashanmugam P *et al.* (2003) LCN6, a novel human epididymal lipocalin. *Reprod Biol Endocrinol* 1, 112.

Hammami-Hamza S, Doussau M, Bernard J, Rogier E, Duquenn C, Richard Y, Lefèvre A and Finaz C (2001) Cloning and sequencing of SOB3, a human gene coding for a sperm protein homologous to an antimicrobial protein and potentially involved in zona pellucida binding. *Mol Human Reprod* 7, 625–632.

Hayashi M, Fujimoto S, Takano H *et al.* (1996) Characterization of a human glycoprotein with a potential role in sperm–egg fusion: cDNA cloning, immunohistochemical localization, and chromosomal assignment of the gene AEGL1. *Genomics* 32, 367–374.

He X, Shen L, Bjartel A, Malm J, Lilja H and Dahlbäck B (1995) The gene encoding vitamin K-dependent anticoagulant protein C is expressed in human male reproductive tissues. *J Histochem Cytochem* 43, 563–570.

Hinton BT, Pryor JP, Hirsch AV and Setchell BP (1981) The concentration of some inorganic ions and organic compounds in the luminal fluid of the human ductus deferens. *Int J Androl* 4, 457–461.

Hirsch AV, Mills C, Tan SL and Rainsbury P (1993) Pregnancy using spermatozoa aspirated from the vas deferens in a patient with ejaculatory failure due to spinal injury. *Human Reprod* 8, 89–90.

Hirsch AV, Dean NL, Mohan PJ, Shaker AG and Bekir JS (1996) Natural spermatocoeles in irre-versible obstructive azoospermia-reservoirs of viable spermatozoa for assisted conception. *Human Reprod* 11, 1919–1922.

Hofmann N and Karlas W (1973) Osmolality of the human seminal plasma. *Arch Dermatol Forsch* 246, 35–46.

Holstein AF and Roosen-Runge EC (1981) In: *Atlas of Human Spermatogenesis*, eds AF Holstein and EC Roosen-Runge. Berlin: Grosse Verlag.

Huggins CB and Johnson AA (1933) Chemical observations on fluids of the seminal tract. I. Inorganic phosphorus, calcium, non-protein nitrogen and glucose content of semen and of seminal vesicle, prostate and spermatocoele fluids in man. *Am J Physiol* 103, 574–581.

Hutter H, Hammer A, Blaschitz A *et al.* (1996) The monoclonal antibody GZS-1 detects a matur-ation-associated antigen of human spermatozoa that is also present on the surface of human mononuclear blood cells. *J Reprod Immunol* 30, 115–132.

Isojima S, Tsuji Y, Kameda K, Shigeta M and Hakamori SI (1990) Coating antigens of human sem-inal plasma involved in fertilization. In: *Gamete Interactions: Prospects for Immunocontraception*. New York: Wiley-Liss, pp. 155–174.

Jean M, Dacheux J-L, Dacheux F, Sagot P, Lopes P and Barriere P (1995) Increased zona-binding ability after incubation of spermatozoa with proteins extracted from spermatozoa of fertile men. *J Reprod Fertil* 105, 43–48.

Johnson L and Varner DD (1988) Effect of daily sperm production but not age on transit time of spermatozoa through the human epididymis. *Biol Reprod* 39, 812–817.

Jones RC (2002) Evolution of the vertebrate epididymis. In: *The Epididymis. From Molecules to Clinical Practice. A Comprehensive Survey of the Efferent Ducts, the Epididymis and the Vas Deferens*, eds B Robaire and BT Hinton. New York: Kluwer Academic/Plenum, pp. 11–33.

Jow WW, Steckel J, Schlegel PN, Magid MS and Goldstein M (1993) Motile sperm in human testis biopsy specimens. *J Androl* 14, 194–198.

Jury JA, Frayne J and Hall L (1997) The human fertilin α gene is non-functional: implications for its proposed role in fertilization. *Biochem J* 321, 577–581.

Jury JA, Frayne J and Hall L (1998) Sequence analysis of a variety of primate fertilin a genes: evidence for non-functional genes in the gorilla and man. *Mol Reprod Dev* 51, 92–97.

Kameda K, Takada Y, Hasegawa A, Tsuji Y, Koyama K and Isojima S (1991) Sperm immobilizing and fertilization – blocking monoclonal antibody 2C6 to human seminal plasma and characterization of the antigen epitope corresponding to the monoclonal antibody. *J Reprod Immunol* 20, 27–41.

Kameda K, Tsuji Y, Koyama K and Isojima S (1992) Comparative studies of the antigens recognized by sperm-immobilizing monoclonal antibodies. *Biol Reprod* 46, 349–357.

Kato S, Yasui T, Nano I and Kanda S (1984) Migration of cytoplasmic droplet in boar spermatozoa by centrifugation. *Jpn J Animal AI Res* 6, 15–18.

Kato S, Yasui T and Kanda S (1983) Migration of cytoplasmic droplet in goat testicular spermatozoa by centrifugation. *Jpn J Animal Reprod* 29, 214–216.

Kirchhoff C (1998) Molecular characterization of epididymal proteins. *Rev Reprod* 3, 86–95.

Kirchhoff C, Krull N, Pera I and Ivell R (1993) A major mRNA of the human epididymis principal cells, HE5, encodes the leucocyte differentiation CDw52 antigen peptide backbone. *Mol Reprod Dev* 34, 8–15.

Kirchhoff C, Pera L, Rust W and Ivell R (1994) Major human epididymis-specific gene product, HE3, is the first representative of a novel gene family. *Mol Reprod Dev* 37, 130–137.

Kirchhoff C, Osterhoff C and Young L (1996) Molecular cloning and characterization of HE1, a major secretory protein of the human epididymis. *Biol Reprod* 54, 847–856.

Krätzschmar J, Haendler B, Eberspaecher U, Roosterman D, Donner P and Schleuning W-D (1996) The human cysteine-rich secretory protein (CRISP) family. Primary structure and tissue distribution of CRISP-1, CRISP-2 and CRISP-3. *Eur J Biochem* 236, 827–836.

Krull N, Ivell R, Osterhoff C and Kirchhoff C (1993) Region-specific variation of gene expression in the human epididymis as revealed by in situ hybridization with tissue-specific cDNAs. *Mol Reprod Dev* 34, 16–24.

Lasserre A, Gonzalez-Echeverria F, Moules C, Tezón JG, Miranda PV and Vazquez-Levin MH (2003) Identification of human sperm proteins involved in the interaction with homologous zona pellucida. *Fertil Steril* 79 (Suppl 3), 1606–1615.

Larsen LB, Rovn P, Boisen A, Berglund L and Petersen TE (1997) Primary structure of EPV20, a secretory glycoprotein containing a previously uncharacterized type of domain. *Eur J Biochem* 243, 437–441.

Laurell M, Christensson A, Abrahamson P A, Stenflo J and Lilja H (1992) Protein C inhibitor in human body fluids. Seminal plasma is rich in inhibitor antigen deriving from cells throughout the male reproductive system. *J Clin Invest* 89, 1094–1101.

Lefevre A, Duquenne C, Rousseau-Merck MF, Rogier E and Finaz C (1999) Cloning and characterization of SOB1, a new testis-specific cDNA encoding a human sperm protein probably involved in oocyte recognition. *Biochem Biophys Res Commun* 259, 60–66.

Lefevre A, Ruis CM, Chokomian S, Duquenne C and Finaz C (1997) Characterization and isolation of SOB2, a human sperm protein with a potential role in oocyte membrane binding. *Mol Hum Reprod* 3, 507–516.

Légaré C, Thabet M, Olcard S and Sullivan R (2001) Effect of vasectomy on P34H messenger ribonucleic acid expression along the human excurrent duct: a reflection on the function of the human epididymis. *Biol Reprod* 64, 720–727.

Légaré C and Sullivan R (2004) Expression and localization of c-*ros* oncogene along the human excurrent duct. *Mol Human Reprod* 10, 697–703.

Légaré C, Gaudreault C, St-Jacques S and Sullivan R (1999) P34H sperm protein is preferentially expressed by the human corpus epididymidis. *Endocrinology* 140, 3318–3327.

Légaré C, Thabet M and Sullivan R (2004) Expression of heat shock protein 70 in normal and cryptorchid human excurrent duct. *Mol Human Reprod* 10, 187–202.

Lin Y, Kimmel LH, Myles DG and Primakoff P (1993) Molecular cloning of the human and monkey sperm surface protein PH-20. *Proc Natl Acad Sci USA* 90, 10071–10075.

Lin YC, Sun GH, Lee YM, Guo YW and Liu HW (2001) Cloning and characterization of a complementary DNA encoding a human epididymis-associated disintegrin and metalloprotease 7 protein. *Biol Reprod* 65, 944–950.

Liu HW, Lin YC, Chao CF, Chang SY and Sun GH (2000) GP-83 and GP-39, two glycoproteins secreted by human epididymis are conjugated to spermatozoa during maturation. *Mol Human Reprod* 6, 422–428.

Liu Q, Hamil KG, Sivashanmugam P *et al.* (2001) Primate epididymis-specific proteins: characterization of ESC42, a novel protein containing a trefoil-like motif in monkey and human. *Endocrinology* 142, 4529–4539.

Ludwig G and Frick J (1987) *Spermatology. Atlas and Manual.* Berlin: Springer-Verlag.

Mahony MC and Alexander NJ (1991) Sites of antisperm antibody action. *Human Reprod* 6, 1426–1430.

Malm J, Sorensen O, Persson T *et al.* (2000) The human cationic antimicrobial protein (hCAP-18) is expressed in the epithelium of human epididymis, is present in seminal plasma at high concentrations, and is attached to spermatozoa. *Infect Immun* 68, 4297–4302.

Mathieu C, Guerin J-F, Cognat M, Lejeune H, Pinatel M-C and Lornage J (1992) Motility and fertilizing capacity of epididymal human spermatozoa in normal and pathological cases. *Fertil Steril* 57, 871–876.

Menézo Y, Testart J, Thebault A, Frydman R and Khatchadourian C (1982) The preovulatory follicular fluid in the human: influence of hormonal pretreatment (clomiphene-hCG) on some biochemical and biophysical variables. *Int J Fertil* 27, 47–51.

Miranda PV and Tezón JG (1992) Characterization of fibronectin as a marker for human epididymal sperm maturation. *Mol Reprod Dev* 33, 443–450.

Mooney JK, Horan AH and Lattimer JK (1972) Motility of spermatozoa in the human epididymis. *J Urol* 108, 443–445.

Moore HDM, Hartmann TD and Pryor JP (1983) Development of the oocyte-penetrating capacity of spermatozoa in the human epididymis. *Int J Androl* 6, 310–318.

Moore HDM, Curry MR, Penfold LM and Pryor JP (1992) The culture of human epididymal epithelium and *in vitro* maturation of epididymal spermatozoa. *Fertil Steril* 58, 776–783.

Moore A, Penfold LM, Johnson JL and Latchman DS (1993) Human sperm–egg binding is inhibited by peptides corresponding to core region of an acrosomal serine protease inhibitor. *Mol Reprod Dev* 34, 280–291.

Morton BE, Sagadraca R and Fraser C (1978) Sperm motility within the mammalian epididymis: species variation and correlation with free calcium levels in epididymal plasma. *Fertil Steril* 29, 695–698.

Naz RQ, Morte C, Garcia-Framus V, Kaplan P and Martinez P (1993) Characterization of a sperm-specific monoclonal antibody and isolation of 95 kilodalton fertilization antigen-2 from human sperm. *Biol Reprod* 49, 1236–1244.

Obermann H, Samalecos A, Osterhoff C, Schroder B, Heller R and Kirchhoff C (2003) HE6, a two-subunit heptahelical receptor associated with apical membranes of efferent and epididymal duct epithelia. *Mol Reprod Dev* 64, 13–26.

O'Bryan MK, Mallidas C, Murphy BF and Baker HWG (1994) Immunohistological localization of clusterin in the male genital tract in humans and marmosets. *Biol Reprod* 50, 502–509.

Osterhoff C, Kirchhoff C, Krull N and Ivell R (1994) Molecular cloning and characteriztation of a novel human sperm antigen (HE2) specifically expressed in the proximal epididymis. *Biol Reprod* 50, 516–525.

Paju A, Bjartell A, Zhang WM, Nordling S, Borgstrom A, Hansson J and Stenman UH (2000) Expression and characterization of trypsinogen produced in the human male genital tract. *Am J Pathol* 157, 2011–2021.

Patrizio P, Ord T, Silber SJ and Asch RH (1994) Correlation between epididymal length and fertilization rate of men with congenital absence of the vas deferens. *Fertil Steril* 61, 265–268.

Potts RJ, Jefferies TM and Notarianni LJ (1999) Antioxidant capacity of the epididymis. *Human Reprod* 14, 2513–2516.

Poulton TA, Everard D, Baxby K and Parlsow JM (1996) Characterisation of a sperm coating auto-antigen reacting with anti-sperm antibodies of infertile males using monoclonal antibodies. *Br J Obstet Gynaecol* 103, 463–467.

Quinlivan WLG (1968) Analysis of proteins in human seminal plasma. *Arch Biochem Biophys* 127, 680–687.

Raczek S, Yeung CH, Hasilik A *et al.* (1995) Immunocytochemical localisation of some lysosomal hydrolases, their presence in luminal fluid and their directional secretion by human epididymal cells in culture. *Cell Tiss Res* 280, 415–426.

Richardson RT, Sivashanmugam P, Hall SH *et al.* (2001) Cloning and sequencing of human Eppin: a novel family of protease inhibitors expressed in the epididymis and testis. *Gene* 270, 93–102.

Rochwerger L and Cuasnicú PS (1992) Redistribution of a rat sperm epididymal glycoprotein after *in vitro* and *in vivo* capacitation. *Mol Reprod Dev* 31, 34–41.

Ross P, Vigneault N, Provencher S, Potier M and Roberts KD (1993) Partial characterization of galactosyltransferase in human seminal plasma and its distribution in the human epididymis. *J Reprod Fertil* 98, 129–137.

Rossato M, Di Virgillio F and Foresta C (1996) Involvement of osmo-sensitive calcium influx in human sperm activation. *Mol Human Reprod* 2, 903–909.

Rossato M, Balercia G, Lucarelli G, Foresta C and Mantero F (2002) Role of seminal osmolarity in the reduction of human sperm motility. *Int J Androl* 25, 230–235.

Rowley MJ, Teshima F and Heller CG (1970) Duration of transit of spermatozoa through the human male ductular system. *Fertil Steril* 21, 390–396.

Sanjurjo C, Dawidowsky AR, Cameo MS, González Echeverría F and Blaquier JA (1990) Participation of human epididymal sperm coating antigens in fertilization. *J Androl* 11, 476–483.

Schaller J, Glander HJ and Dethloff J (1993) Evidence of B1 integrins and fibronectin on spermatogenic cells in human testis. *Human Reprod* 8, 1873–1878.

Schirren C (1982) Gewebsentnahme aus dem Nebenhoden zu diagnostischen Zwecken? *Andrologia* 14, 461–462.

Schmidt SS, Schoysman R and Stewart BH (1976) Surgical approaches to male infertility. In: *Human Semen and Fertility Regulation in Men*, ed. ESE Hafez. St. Louis, MO, USA: C.V. Mosby Co., pp. 476–493.

Schoysman R (1993) Clinical situations challenging the established concept of epididymal physiology in the human. *Acta Eur Fertil* 24, 55–60.

Schoysman RJ and Bedford JM (1986) The role of the human epididymis in sperm maturation and sperm storage as reflected in the consequences of epididymovasostomy. *Fertil Steril* 46, 293–299.

Silber SJ (1988) Pregnancy caused by sperm from vasa efferentia. *Fertil Steril* 49, 373–375.

Simpson KL and Holmes CH (1994) Presence of the complement-regulatory protein membrane cofactor protein (MCP, CD46) as a membrane-associated product in seminal plasma. *J Reprod Fertil* 102, 419–424.

Smithwick EB, Gould KG and Young LG (1996) Estimate of epididymal transit time in the chimpanzee. *Tissue Cell* 28, 485–493.

Soler C, Pérez-Sánchez F, Schulze H, Bergmann M, Oberpenning F, Yeung C and Cooper TG (2000) Objective evaluation of the morphology of human epididymal sperm heads. *Int J Androl* 23, 77–84.

Sonnenberg-Riethmacher E, Walter B, Riethmacher D, Gödecke S and Birchmeier C. (1996) The c-*ros* tyrosine kinase receptor controls regionalization and differentiation of epithelial cells in the epididymis. *Genes Dev* 10, 1184–1193.

Sun GH, Lin YC, Guo YW, Chang SY and Liu HW (2000) Purification of GP-83, a glycoprotein secreted by the human epididymis and conjugated to mature spermatozoa. *Mol Human Reprod* 6, 429–434.

Sutovsky P, Moreno R, Ramalho-Santos J, Dominko T, Thompson WE and Schatten G (2001) A putative, ubiquitin-dependent mechanism for the recognition and elimination of defective spermatozoa in the mammalian epididymis. *J Cell Sci* 114, 1665–1675.

Temple-Smith PD, Southwick GJ, Herrera Castaneda E, Hamer J and McClatchey M (1989) Surgical manipulation of the epididymis: an experimental approach to sperm maturation. In: *Perspectives in Andrology*, ed. M Serio. New York NY, USA: Raven Press, pp. 281–290.

Temple-Smith PD, Zheng SS, Kadioglu T and Southwick GJ (1998) Development and use of surgical procedures to bypass selected regions of the mammalian epididymis: effects on sperm maturation. *J Reprod Fertil Suppl* 53, 183–195.

Tesarik J, Drahorad, J and Peknicova J (1988) Subcellular immunochemical localization of acrosin in human spermatozoa during the acrosome reaction and zona pellucida penetration. *Fertil Steril* 50, 133–141.

Tezón JG, Ramella E, Cameo MS, Vazquez MH and Blaquier JA (1985) Immunocytochemical localization of secretion antigens in the human epididymis and their association with spermatozoa. *Biol Reprod* 32, 591–597.

Tokugawa Y, Kunishige I, Kubota Y *et al.* (1998) Lipocalin-type prostaglandin S synthase in human male reproductive organs and seminal plasma. *Biol Reprod* 58, 600–607.

Turner TT (1997) The epididymis and accessory sex organs. In: *Infertility in the Male*, eds LI Lipshultz, SS Howards. St Louis: Mosby-Year Book Inc., pp. 138–151.

Turner TT and Reich GW (1985) Cauda epididymal sperm motility: a comparison among five species. *Biol Reprod* 32, 120–128.

Velazquez A, Pederon N, Delgado NM and Rosado A (1977) Osmolality and conductance of normal and abnormal human seminal plasma. *Int J Fertil* 22, 92–97.

von Horsten HH, Derr P and Kirchhoff C (2002) Novel antimicrobial peptide of human epididymal duct origin. *Biol Reprod* 67, 804–813.

Weiske W-H (1994) Pregnancy caused by sperm from the vasa efferentia. *Fertil Steril* 62, 642–643.

WHO (1999) *WHO Laboratory Manual for the Examination of Human Semen and Sperm Cervical Mucus Interaction.* Cambridge: Cambridge University Press.

Wiese K, Haidl G, Opper C and Schill W-B (1996) Erhöhte Membranrigidität bei Spermatozoen mit mangelnder Nebenhodenausreifung. *Fertilität* 12, 91–94.

Yamaguchi Y, Nagase T, Makita R *et al.* (2002) Identification of multiple novel epididymis-specific beta-defensin isoforms in humans and mice. *J Immunol* 169, 2516–2523.

Yan YC, Mitsudo SM, Wang LF and Koide SS (1984) Immunolocalization of a sperm membrane protein in human male reproductive organs. *Fertil Steril* 42, 614–617.

Yang D, Biragyn A, Kwak LW and Oppenheim JJ (2002) Mammalian defensins in immunity: more than just microbicidal. *Trend Immunol* 23, 291–296.

Yenugu S, Hamil KG, Birse CE, Ruben SM, French FS and Hall SH (2003) Antibacterial properties of the sperm-binding proteins and peptides of human epididymis 2 (HE2) family; salt sensitivity, structural dependence and their interaction with outer and cytoplasmic membranes of *Escherichia coli. Biochem J* 372, 73–83.

Yenugu S, Hamil KG, French FS and Hall SH (2004a) Antimicrobial actions of the human epididymis 2 (HE2) protein isoforms, HE2alpha, HE2beta1 and HE2beta2. *Reprod Biol Endocrinol* 2, 61.

Yenugu S, Hamil KG, Radhakrishnan Y, French FS and Hall SH (2004b) The androgen-regulated epididymal sperm-binding protein, human beta-defensin 118 (DEFB118) (formerly ESC42), is an antimicrobial beta-defensin. *Endocrinology* 145, 3165–3173.

Yenugu S, Richardson RT, Sivashanmugam P, Wang Z, O'Rand MG, French FS and Hall SH (2004c) Antimicrobial activity of human EPPIN, an androgen-regulated, sperm-bound protein with a whey acidic protein motif. *Biol Reprod* 71, 1484–1490.

Yeung CH and Cooper TG (2001) Effects of the ion-channel blocker quinine on human sperm volume, kinematics and mucus penetration, and the involvement of potassium channels. *Mol Human Reprod* 7, 819–828.

Yeung CH, Cooper TG and Senge T (1990) Histochemical localization and quantification of α-glucosidase in the epididymis of men and laboratory animals. *Biol Reprod* 42, 669–676.

Yeung CH, Cooper TG, Bergmann M and Schulze H (1991) Organization of tubules in the human caput epididymidis and the ultrastructure of their epithelia. *Am J Anat* 191, 261–279.

Yeung CH, Cooper TG, Oberpenning F, Schulze H and Nieschlag E (1993) Changes in movement characteristics of human spermatozoa along the length of the epididymis. *Biol Reprod* 49, 274–280.

Yeung CH, Perez-Sanchez F, Soler C, Poser D, Kliesch S and Cooper TG (1997a) Maturation of human spermatozoa (from selected epididymides of prostatic carcinoma patients) with respect to their morphology and ability to undergo the acrosome reaction. *Human Reprod Update* 3, 205–213.

Yeung C-H, Schröter S, Wagenfeld A *et al.* (1997b) Interaction of the human epididymal protein CD52 (HE5) with epididymal spermatozoa from men and cynomolgus monkeys. *Mol Reprod Dev* 48, 267–275.

Yeung CH, Cooper TG, DeGeyter M, DeGeyter C, Rolf C, Kamischke A and Nieschlag E (1998) Studies on the origin of redox enzymes in seminal plasma and their relationship with results of in-vitro fertilisation. *Mol Human Reprod* 4, 835–839.

Yeung CH, Sonnenberg-Riethmacher E, Cooper TG (1999) Infertile spermatozoa of c-*ros* tyrosine kinase receptor knockout mice show flagellar angulation and maturational defects in cell volume regulatory mechanisms. *Biol Reprod* 61, 1062–1069.

Yeung CH, Schröter S, Kirchhoff C and Cooper TG (2000) Maturational changes of the CD52-like epididymal glycoprotein on cynomolgus monkey sperm and their apparent reversal in capacitation conditions. *Mol Reprod Dev* 57, 280–289.

Yeung CH, Pérez-Sánchez F, Schröter S, Kirchhoff C and Cooper TG (2001) Changes of the major sperm maturation-associated epididymal protein HE5 (CD52) on human ejaculated spermatozoa during incubation. *Mol Human Reprod* 7, 617–624.

Yeung CH, Anapolski M, Cooper TG (2002) Measurement of volume changes in mouse spermatozoa using an electronic sizing analyzer and a flow cytometer: validation and application to an infertile mouse model. *J Androl* 23, 522–528.

Yeung CH, Anapolski M, Depenbusch M, Zitzman, M and Cooper TG (2003) Human sperm volume regulation. Response to physiological changes in osmolality, channel blockers and potential sperm osmolytes. *Human Reprod* 18, 1029–1036.

Yeung CH, Barfield JP, Anapolski M and Cooper TG (2004) Volume regulation of mature and immature spermatozoa in a primate model and possible ion channels involved. *Human Reprod* 19, 2587–2593.

Yoshida K, Sato Y, Yoshiike M, Nozawa S, Ariga H and Iwamoto T (2003) Immunocytochemical localization of DJ-1 in human male reproductive tissue. *Mol Reprod Dev* 66, 391–397.

Zhu X and Naz RK (1997) Fertilization antigen-1: cDNA cloning, testis-specific expression, and immunocontraceptive effects. *Proc Natl Acad Sci USA* 94, 4704–4709.

5

Controls of sperm motility

Claude Gagnon and Eve de Lamirande

Urology Research Laboratory, Royal Victoria Hospital and Faculty of Medicine, McGill University, Montréal, Canada

5.1 Introduction

Spermatozoa must be motile for their journey to the egg. In species that undergo external fertilization, such as sea urchins and fishes, the initiation of sperm motility occurs at spawning and movement is further regulated by factors released by oocytes. In mammals, the swimming ability is progressively acquired by spermatozoa during the epididymal transit even though motility is initiated only after dilution in seminal plasma. Factors from the female genital tract will later on trigger the hyperactivated motility that is needed for sperm penetration of the zona pellucida.

In this review, we will first examine the structure of the flagellum giving a special attention to the axonemal motility apparatus. Then, we will briefly discuss some of the factors that influence the initiation, maintenance and evolution of sperm motility.

5.2 Experimental approaches to study sperm movement

Before describing the flagellum, we will briefly mention some technical aspects of motility measurements and the most important experimental approaches or models that are used to evaluate the role, and mode of action, of specific structures in flagellar motility.

High speed videomicrography is an essential tool for the measurement of parameters such as the percentage of moving cells, the flagellar beat frequency (the number of complete beats per second; by stroboscopic illumination), the surface of flagellar beat envelope (surface covered by the flagellum over a complete beat) and the maximal wave amplitude (width of the beating envelope) (Brokaw and Kamiya, 1987; Cosson et al., 1999; Gingras et al., 1998). Most of the computer-aided semen analyzers (CASA) developed to study mammalian spermatozoa follow the movement of the head and not the flagellum. Therefore, the parameters evaluated, curvilinear and linear velocity, linearity of the trajectory, amplitude of the lateral head displacement, etc. are more related to cell trajectory (Burkman, 1991; Murad *et al.*, 1992).

One of the experimental approaches used to determine the importance of flagellar structures or external factors in sperm motility involves demembranation of the cells with a detergent (often Triton X-100) and reactivation of movement by the addition of adenosine triphosphate (ATP). This demembranated cell model bypasses the rather impermeable cell membrane and allows a direct access to the axoneme, the structure responsible for movement. The modeled flagella have similar motion patterns as intact flagella and the beat frequency depends on the concentration of ATP used. The demembranation–reactivation assay can be used for flagella of spermatozoa (sea urchin, fish, mammals) (de Lamirande and Gagnon, 1986, 1989, 1992a, b; Gingras *et al.*, 1996; Ho *et al.*, 2002) or of unicellular organisms such as *Chlamydomonas* reinhardtii and *Oxyrrhis marina* (Gagnon *et al.*, 1994, 1996; Gingras *et al.*, 1996, 1998). *Chlamydomonas* mutants lacking one of the axonemal components, and the potential reversal of these mutations, are also useful to determine the role of specific structures in motility (DiBella and King, 2001; Kamiya, 2002; Smith and Yang, 2004). We used monoclonal antibodies directed against targeted axonemal proteins to evaluate the role of these in the maintenance and type of motility (Gagnon *et al.*, 1994, 1996; Gingras *et al.*, 1996, 1998). This last approach has the major advantage of aiming at a specific protein/epitope in contrast to the previous methodology in which large ultrastructural defects are tested.

5.3 The flagellum

5.3.1 The axoneme

Flagellar motility results from undulatory waves propagating backwards to create forward propulsive thrust along the axis of the flagellum. The axoneme is the core structure responsible for motility and is common to most flagellated and ciliated cells from protozoans to man with relatively few modifications. This evolutionary stability indicates that axonemal components have sufficient diversity in structure and function to accommodate the different types of motility of flagella and cilia.

The axoneme (Fig. 5.1) is composed of nine peripheral microtubule doublets and two central microtubules that run the whole length of the flagellum (Inaba, 2003; Link, 2001; Turner, 2003). Dynein arms that project from microtubule A towards microtubule B of the adjacent doublet are major players in the active sliding of the microtubules. Neighboring microtubule doublets are also attached to each others by nexin links (Bozkurt and Wooley, 1993) and radial spokes point to the sheath surrounding the two singlet microtubules at the center of the axoneme (Smith and Yang, 2004).

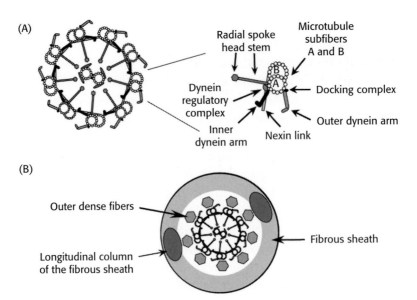

Figure 5.1   Schematic representation of the flagellum. (A) The axoneme. (B) In mammals, the axoneme is surrounded by outer dense fibers and fibrous sheath

Dynein is responsible for the conversion of chemical energy from ATP hydrolysis into mechanical energy for motility (Fig. 5.2). The two dynein arms have different functions. The outer dynein arms are spaced 24 nm apart along microtubule A and bound in an ATP-insensitive manner to tubulin by the dynein docking complex (three polypeptides) and their removal decreases the beat frequency by half (DiBella and King, 2001; Porter and Sale, 2000; Takada *et al.*, 2002). Inner dynein arms of three classes are equally distributed in each 96 nm segment of the axoneme (Porter and Sale, 2000). Dynein arms are complexes consisting of three classes of subunits. The heavy chains (α and β, $\cong 500$ kDa) have a central motor part with four ATP- and microtubule-binding sites. The 60–120 kDa intermediate chains are located at the base of the dynein molecules and play a role in the ATP-insensitive binding of the arms to microtubules. The light chains (8–20 kDa) are proteins of various functions, such as Ca^{++}-binding, thioredoxin-like, structure with a leucine-rich repeat or similar to mouse t-complex testis expressed Tctex1 or Tctex2 (DiBella and King, 2001; Inaba, 2002). The variety of structure and function of these chains indicate that many regulatory mechanisms are present and needed for the fine tuning of motility (DiBella and King, 2001; King *et al.*, 1991, 1995). Whereas outer dynein arms determine the maximal velocity of outer doublet microtubule sliding, inner dynein arms affect flagellar wave form, regulate beating symmetry or provide the additional force needed to maintain a high velocity in the presence of load (Brokaw and Kamiya, 1987). The dynein regulatory complex (seven polypeptides) is tightly bound to the microtubule lattice and could

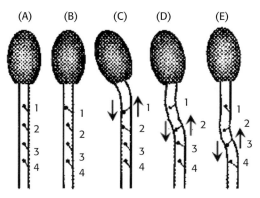

Figure 5.2   Schema of how microtubule slide under the action of dynein arms. For simplicity, only two outer microtubule doublets of the axoneme are drawn and each of the numbered arms is for a pair of inner and outer arms. No flagellar bend is seen when dynein arms are inactive (A). When the first dynein arm engages the adjacent microtubule (B) and generates a downward stroke (large arrow), the sliding force is translated into a bend in the axoneme (C) and the second dynein arm engages the adjacent microtubule doublet. The flagellar beat is then propagated with the first dynein arm relaxing, the second generating the downward stroke (D) and the third engaging into action (E). A similar sequence is continually repeated and occurs at the same time on the nine microtubule doublets in an asynchronous but coordinated fashion all along the flagellum and around the circumference allowing for swimming in three dimensions (From Turner, 2003; with permission.)

function as scaffold for enzymes that regulate and modify dynein activity or as a sensor for tension or strain within the axoneme to provide mechanical feedback to the dynein arms (Piperno, 1995; Porter and Sale, 2000).

Adjacent to the inner dynein arms and anchored on microtubules A, maybe through the dynein regulatory complex, are the radial spokes, T-shaped structures pointing to the central pair. *Chlamydomonas* mutants lacking radial spoke heads or stems are immotile (Porter and Sale, 2000; Smith and Yang, 2004). Some of the 23 polypeptides that form radial spokes are identified in *Chlamydomonas* and are A-kinase anchoring protein (AKAP; Feliciello *et al.*, 2001), kinesin-related protein, WD repeat protein, calmodulin, alanine/proline-rich protein, armadillo repeat protein and nucleoside diphosphate kinase (Inaba, 2003; Patel-King *et al.*, 2004; Smith and Yang, 2004). Because of their location, the radial spokes could provide a structural linkage between the central apparatus and dynein arms.

Isolated axonemes from mutants lacking central pair complex and radial spokes can be reactivated at low ATP concentration and undergo modest wave form conversion due to variations in Ca^{++} concentration. Therefore, the central pair complex and radial spokes are not essential for motility but the interaction of these structures could act as a mechanical and chemical signal transducer for controlling the size and the shape of the flagellar bend and for modifying motility in response to specific signals (Smith and Yang, 2004). The complex radial spokes–central pair regulates the velocity of microtubule sliding driven by dynein and coordinates the activity of inner and outer dynein arms at physiological levels of ATP (Porter and Sale, 2000). Data obtained with monoclonal antibodies that recognize radial spoke proteins indicate that these structures affect specific motility parameters, such as the movement in two or three dimensions and the flagellar beating envelope (Gingras *et al.*, 1998; White *et al.*, 2005).

Tubulin α and β, the main constituents of microtubules, are of paramount importance to flagellar structure and motility. These globular proteins of 50–55 kDa exist in a functional state as a heterodimer, one α- and one β-chain (Oakley, 2000). The longitudinal association of tubulins produce the protofilaments and the lateral association of 13 and 11 protofilaments builds microtubules A and B, respectively. Tubulin is often subjected to post-translational modifications, for example acetylation, palmitoylation, phosphorylation, polyglutamylation and polyglycation, that are important for axonemal motility (Gagnon *et al.*, 1996; Huitorel *et al.*, 1999, 2002; MacRae, 1997).

The outer doublet microtubules are bound by nexin links, possibly by association with dynein regulatory complexes (Wooley, 1997). One of the nexin link proteins corresponds to the p72 regulatory subunit of Ca^{++}-regulated nucleoside diphosphate kinase (Patel-King *et al.*, 2002).

5.3.2 Outer dense fibers, fibrous sheath and mitochondrial sheath

In spermatozoa from primitive species (such as sea urchins and fishes) and in flagellated unicellular organisms (such as *Chlamydomonas*), the flagellum consists of the 9 + 2 axoneme surrounded by the cell membrane. In animals with internal fertilization, the sperm axoneme is surrounded by outer dense fibers and the fibrous sheath (Fig. 5.1).

Each of the nine microtubule doublets is associated with an outer dense fiber, that has a characteristic size and shape (Fig. 5.1). These structures are composed of several cystein-, serine- and proline-rich intermediate filament-like proteins with a high degree of zinc-dependent disulfide cross-bridging (Oko and Clermont, 1990). Outer dense fibers could be involved in the maintenance of the passive elastic structure of the flagellum but their high and variable level of phosphoserine on proteins suggests some yet undetermined role in the regulation of flagellar motility (Inaba, 2003; Oko and Clermont, 1990).

The fibrous sheath is composed of three longitudinal columns attached to microtubule doublets 3 and 8 that run along the principal piece of spermatozoa (Oko and Clermont, 1990) (Fig. 5.1). This structural arrangement and the stabilization of proteins by disulfide bonds, suggest that the fibrous sheath influences the flexibility, the plane of flagellar motion and the shape of the flagellar beat (Eddy *et al.*, 2003). AKAPs represent more than 50% of the fibrous sheath mass in some species (Eddy *et al.*, 2003) and their tyrosine phosphorylation could be associated with fibrous sheath sliding (Carrera *et al.*, 1994; Mohri *et al.*, 1998; Si and Okuno, 1999). The Rho-binding protein, rhophilin, is located at the outer surface of the outer dense fibers and its binding protein, ropporin, is anchored at the inner surface of the fibrous sheath (Fujita *et al.*, 2000). Enzymes associated with the glycolytic pathway, such as glyceraldehyde 3-phosphate dehydrogenase-S (Miki *et al.*, 2004; Westhoff and Kamp, 1997), hexokinase HK1-S, glutathione S-transferase GSTM5 and an intermediate filament-like protein FS39, are also found in the fibrous sheath (Eddy *et al.*, 2003; Mohri *et al.*, 1998). The scaffolding of glycolytic enzymes and the presence of constituents of signal cascades on the fibrous sheath supports the importance of this structure for sperm motility.

Mammalian sperm mitochondria are condensed and elongated and they are tightly and helically disposed end to end around the outer dense fibers forming the mitochondrial sheath at the level of the sperm middle piece. These mitochondria have specific functional characteristics adapted for sperm motility such as resistance to hypotonic conditions and ability to use lactate as an oxidative substrate (Oko and Clermont, 1990).

5.3.3 Morphological abnormalities

Primary flagellar/ciliary dyskinesia is a syndrome characterized by a defect in axonemal structure or function that results in abnormal or absent flagellar/ciliary movement. In human spermatozoa, tail abnormalities range from coiled, short or bent tails (light microscopy level) (World Health Organization, 1999) and the percentages of cells with such defects are approximately 14% and 50% in fertile and infertile men, respectively (Kubo-Irie *et al.*, 2004). More defined structural alterations, such as missing or excess doublets or microtubules, outer dense fibers or central pair, double axonemes are observed by electron microscopy (Kubo-Irie *et al.*, 2004). Multiple molecular aberrations are also reported, such as the absence or reduced number of dynein arms (inner and/or outer), the absence of radial spokes, central pair or nexin links (Afzelius, 2004). Obviously, these disorders lead to infertility, chronic respiratory infections, etc.

5.4 Motility in marine species with external fertilization

5.4.1 Ionic factors

In sea urchin spermatozoa, the ionic changes that occur at the spawning of spermatozoa into sea water is a main determinant in the initiation of vigorous motility.

The lower CO_2 tension of sea water as compared to that of semen increases sperm intracellular pH (from $\cong 7.2$ to $\cong 7.5$) that results in dynein ATPase activation and consequently the initiation of motility. The adenosine diphosphate (ADP) produced then stimulates mitochondrial respiration. The lower K^+ content in sea water as compared to that of semen may also cause a hyperpolarization that could activate a voltage-dependent Na^+/K^+ exchanger and help to regulate intracellular pH (Morisawa et al., 1999; Neill and Vacquier, 2004).

Changes in the natural environment for spawning are also used by freshwater and seawater fishes as a trigger for motility initiation. In marine species, spermatozoa are quiescent when kept in medium isotonic to seminal plasma but become motile when diluted with a hypertonic solution. On the other hand, spermatozoa from freshwater fishes initiate motility when diluted in a medium hypotonic as compared to seminal plasma. Again, the decrease in external K^+ at spawning would stimulate K^+ efflux, via K^+ channels, cause hyperpolarization of sperm plasma membrane and subsequently activate adenylyl cyclase (Morisawa et al., 1999).

Conditions that cause hyperpolarization of the plasma membrane, such as addition of Ca^{++}, other divalent cations (Boitano and Okuno, 1991) or Ca^{++} ionophore A23187 (Oda and Morisawa, 1993) overcome the inhibitory effects of K^+ or isoosmolality and trigger sperm motility. Therefore, the increase in intracellular Ca^{++} is important for the control of axonemal movement and regulation of flagellar bending symmetry. The asymmetric waveform of demembranated sea urchin spermatozoa reactivated under low Ca^{++} concentration changes to increasing symmetry and then to quiescence, as Ca^{++} concentration is raised (Smith, 2002). Axonemes contain at least three Ca^{++}-binding proteins: (1) calmodulin, partly associated with radial spokes, which act as a key Ca^{++} sensor (Smith, 2002); (2) centrin/caltractin, present in the inner dynein arms; and (3) a light chain of the outer dynein arms that shares homology to centrin and calmodulin (Smith, 2002). In Chlamydomonas flagella, Ca^{++} regulates dynein activity through a mechanism involving the radial spokes, the central apparatus and signaling elements including axonemal calmodulin and a calmodulin-dependent kinase (Smith, 2002).

5.4.2 Protein phosphorylation

Pharmacological and physiological evidence indicate that protein phosphorylation is involved in the initiation and regulation of flagellar motility; the presence and anchoring of several kinases and phosphatases in the axoneme also suggest a tight control in the regulation of motility (Porter and Sale, 2000). The hyperpolarization of fish sperm plasma membrane that occurs at spawning stimulates adenylyl cyclase (Morisawa et al., 1999) and the resulting increase in cAMP activates protein kinase A (PKA). A portion of PKA activity is tightly bound to the axoneme, possibly by binding to AKAPs (Feliciello et al., 2001), such as those associated with the central pair apparatus (AKAP240) or with the radial spokes (AKAP97) in *Chlamydomonas* (Porter and Sale, 2000). PKA is also present in the detergent-soluble extracts of spermatozoa in many species including sea urchins, rainbow trout and mammals (Horowitz *et al.*, 1984; Ishuguro *et al.*, 1982; Yokota and Mabuchi, 1990).

Several axonemal proteins, of 45, 130 and 500 kDa in sea urchin (Bracho *et al.*, 1998), 21 kDa in salmons (Inaba *et al.*, 1999) and 21 and 26 kDa in Ciona (Nomura *et al.*, 2000) are phosphorylated by PKA when motility is initiated. In chum salmon spermatozoa, one of the seven proteins phosphorylated in relation to motility initiation is a 21 kDa light chain of the outer arm dynein (Inaba *et al.*, 1999). Dynein light chains from many fish and sea urchin species have a PKA-dependent phosphorylation motif and are homologous to t-complex testis expressed 2 (Tctex2). In salmonid fishes, proteasomes localized near the outer dynein arm may regulate the phosphorylation of the dynein light chain and the regulatory subunit of PKA (Inaba *et al.*, 1998). Furthermore, a tyrosine kinase is activated downstream of PKA and is responsible for the phosphorylation of a protein called movement-initiating phosphoprotein (Morisawa, 1994). Itoh *et al.* (2003) observed that the catalytic subunit of PKA in rainbow trout spermatozoa is anchored to the outer dynein arm of axonemes. The co-localization of PKA and its regulator, proteasomes and its substrate the dynein light chain, suggest the existence of an enzyme–substrate network that allows a rapid phosphorylation of the dynein light chain to support initiation of motility within 1 s of exposure to fresh water (Itoh *et al.*, 2003). Other enzymes are involved in flagellar motility, such as calmodulin, a calmodulin-dependent kinase II, casein kinase I, protein phosphatases, but only few of the protein targets of these enzymes are known (Inaba, 2002; Smith, 2002; Smith and Yang, 2004).

5.4.3 Chemotaxis

Chemotactic factors from the egg jelly cause spermatozoa to swim towards the eggs following the concentration gradient of these substances (Inaba, 2003; Morisawa *et al.*, 1999; Neill and Vacquier, 2004) (Fig. 5.3). Some of these factors are secreted by the eggs, such as speract and resact in sea urchins (Neill and Vacquier, 2004), L-tryptophan in abalone (Riffel *et al.*, 2002) and cholestane-3-ol in herring (Cosson, 1990). Others are synthesized by luminal epithelial cells and applied to eggs as they progress down the oviduct, such as the 21 kDa chemoattractant allurin in the frog Xenopus laevis (Xiang *et al.*, 2004). Chemoattractants are species specific and their binding to a plasma membrane receptor on sperm flagella triggers a complex cascade of events, including activation of guanylyl and adenylyl cyclases, opening of ion (K^+, Na^+/H^+, Ca^{++}) channels, hyperpolarization of the plasma membrane and protein phosphorylation (Morisawa *et al.*, 1999; Neill and Vacquier, 2004). The resulting activation of metabolism and modulation of flagellar waveform

(A)   (B)

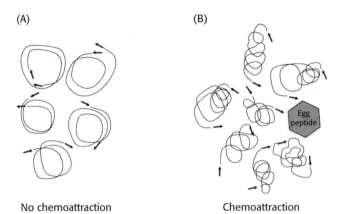

No chemoattraction   Chemoattraction

Figure 5.3   Schematic representation of the chemotactic response. Trajectories of sea urchin
              spermatozoa incubated in the (A) absence or (B) presence of egg peptide as
              chemoattractant

asymmetry direct sperm swimming towards the eggs (Inaba, 2003; Neill and
Vacquier, 2004).

5.5 Motility in mammalian species with external fertilization

5.5.1 Sources of ATP

The ability of mammalian spermatozoa to swim is acquired during their epididymal
transit but observed only upon dilution with seminal plasma at the time of ejaculation. Sugars from the seminal plasma, such as glucose and fructose, are the main
sources of ATP so that sperm motility is maintained for hours (Mukai and Okuno,
2004; Westhoff and Kamp, 1997). Even though oxidative phosphorylation from
mitochondrial respiration is more efficient than glycolysis for ATP production, the
latter energy-generating pathway is more important for sperm motility (Miki *et al.*,
2004; Mukai and Okuno, 2004). Glyceraldehyde 3-phosphate dehydrogenase-S,
a sperm-specific glycolytic enzyme, appears to be responsible for up to 90% of the
ATP generated in spermatozoa and its tight binding to the fibrous sheath supports its
importance in maintenance of motility (Miki *et al.*, 2004). In hamster spermatozoa,
a 58 kDa flagellar protein, localized more in mid piece and phosphorylated at motility initiation, appears to be the ATP synthase H^+ transporting F1 complex β subunit
and could be important for ATP production (Fujinoki *et al.*, 2003).

5.5.2 Bicarbonate, cAMP and PKA

The bicarbonate present in seminal plasma activates multiple sperm functions,
some of which are essential for the initiation of motility. At the biochemical level,

bicarbonate raises the intracellular pH, stimulates respiratory activity and facilitates opening of voltage-gated Ca^{++} channels, but also directly activates the sperm atypical adenylyl cyclase (Jaiswal and Conti, 2001; Wennemuth *et al.*, 2003). The resulting increases in cAMP and Ca^{++} stimulate sperm motility. The role of bicarbonate and cAMP in the induction of sperm motility is illustrated by experiments performed in mice. Mouse spermatozoa from the cauda epididymis are poorly motile upon dilution in a medium devoid of bicarbonate and, when demembranated, they do not reactivate motility unless cAMP is added with ATP (Si and Okuno, 1999). However, addition of bicarbonate to intact cauda spermatozoa induces a rapid increase in flagellar beat frequency and a decrease in flagellar beat asymmetry (Wennemuth *et al.*, 2003), and then cAMP is no longer needed for the demembranation–reactivation assay (Si and Okuno, 1999). The fact that pharmacological agents that raise intracellular cAMP, such as phosphodiesterase inhibitors, stimulate poorly motile spermatozoa after ejaculation suggests that a similar mechanism may exist in the human (Wennemuth *et al.*, 2003). The main action of cAMP is probably the stimulation of PKA activity since sperm motility is blocked by the PKA inhibitor H89 (Holt and Harrison, 2002) and enhanced by the protein phosphatase inhibitors calyculin and okadaic acid (Leclerc *et al.*, 1996; Wennemuth *et al.*, 2003).

The scaffolding of PKA to AKAPs is important for motility initiation since synthetic peptides that prevent the binding between the AKAP and the regulatory subunit of PKA block motility (Vijayaraghavan *et al.*, 1997a, b). During epididymal maturation in mice, the soluble precursor pro-AKAP82 becomes anchored to the sperm fibrous sheath, is phosphorylated and subsequently cleaved to produce the mature AKAP82 molecule (Yeung and Cooper, 2003). PKA regulatory subunits I and II are found on the fibrous sheath of mammalian spermatozoa (Vijayaragavan *et al.*, 1997a, b). In boar, bull and human spermatozoa, the catalytic subunit of PKA is found in detergent-resistant structures, on the fibrous sheath and outer dense fibers but not on microtubules, consistent with the proposed role of PKA in the sliding of the fibrous sheath on underlying outer dense fibers (Moos *et al.*, 1998).

The regulatory subunit II of PKA is one of the first substrates for PKA activity; this detergent-soluble 56 kDa phosphoprotein, axokinin, exists in flagella from sea urchin, dog and human spermatozoa and from *Chlamydomonas* (Tash *et al.*, 1986). In hamster spermatozoa, a 36 kDa protein is subjected to cAMP-dependent serine phosphorylation during motility initiation. This protein is localized in the fibrous sheath and has similarities with a pyruvate dehydrogenase EI component b subunit but lacks the N-terminal 30 amino acids (Fujinoki *et al.*, 2004). In intact boar spermatozoa, bicarbonate increases the PKA-dependent phosphorylation of 59, 64 and 96 kDa proteins within 80 s of contact; the 59 and 96 kDa proteins are both members of the outer dense fiber 2 family (Harrison, 2004).

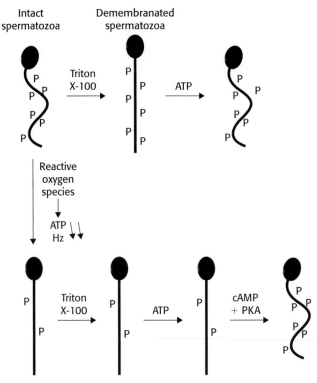

Figure 5.4   Use of demembranation–reactivation assay to study controls of sperm motility. Intact spermatozoa are immobilized after demembranation with a detergent but the motility is reactivated by ATP (upper panel) (P: phosphorylation site on protein). Intact spermatozoa immobilized by a treatment with ROS (ATP depletion and decreased protein phosphorylation) cannot be reactivated after demembranation and addition of ATP unless cAMP and PKA are also added

Exposure to reactive oxygen species (ROS) or rotenone cause ATP depletion and inhibit the motility of intact human spermatozoa (de Lamirande and Gagnon, 1992a, b). Under these circumstances demembranated spermatozoa cannot be reactivated unless cAMP + PKA or cAMP + PKA + sperm extract are added so that axonemes can be rephosphorylated (de Lamirande and Gagnon, 1992a, b) (Fig. 5.4). When motile spermatozoa are used for the demembranation–reactivation assay, both Triton-soluble (14.8 and 15.3 kDa) and insoluble (36 and 51 kDa) proteins are substrates for cAMP/PKA (Leclerc and Gagnon, 1996). When intact spermatozoa are first immobilized by ATP depleting treatment before the demembranation–reactivation assay, PKA phosphorylates proteins of 16.2, 46 and 93 kDa (Leclerc and Gagnon, 1996). Therefore, even though the need for PKA in the initiation of motility is recognized, the specific role of each of its phosphorylated substrates in sperm motility is still to be evaluated.

5.5.3 Other phosphorylation events associated with sperm motility

Sperm motility is increased by phorbol myristate acetate and blocked by sphingo-sine, staurosporine and H-7 suggesting the involvement of protein kinase C (PKC), which is localized in the equatorial segment and principal piece of the flagellum (Rotem *et al.*, 1990). Elements of the extracellular signal-regulated kinase (ERK) pathway are also present in mammalian spermatozoa (de Lamirande and Gagnon, 2002; Lu *et al.*, 1999; Naz *et al.*, 1992). The expression of ERK 1 and 2 varies during spermatogenesis in mice and these kinases could contribute to the acquisition of sperm motility (Lu *et al.*, 1999). In demembranated–reactivated fowl spermatozoa, the addition of ERK or p34cdc2 kinase substrate peptides inhibits motility, suggest-ing that these kinases mediate the phosphorylation of axonemal and/or accessory cytoskeletal proteins and are important for flagellar motility (Ashizawa *et al.*, 1997).

Ras, a small GTP-binding protein present on the sperm acrosomal cap (human; Naz *et al.*, 1992) and flagellum (hamster; NagDas *et al.*, 2002) could be involved in flagellar motility through interaction with some downstream effectors, the ERK pathway, PKC and phosphatidylinositol 3-kinase (PI3K) (NagDas *et al.*, 2002; Naz *et al.*, 1992). Another small GTP-binding protein, Rho, is found in bovine and murine sperm tails and its inactivation due to ADP-ribosylation by the C3 exoen-zyme blocks motility (Fujita *et al.*, 2000; Hinsch *et al.*, 1993). Rhophilin, a 71 kDa Rho-binding protein, is localized at the outer surface of the outer dense fibers and acts as an adaptor protein (Nakamura *et al.*, 1999). Finally, ropporin, a sperm-specific binding protein of rhophilin is localized exclusively on the sperm fibrous sheath and its N-terminal 40 amino acid sequence has a high homology to that of the regulatory subunit type II of PKA (Fujita *et al.*, 2000). Therefore, complexes of Rho, rophilin and ropporin, similar to those formed *in vitro*, may have a role *in vivo* in the regulation of sperm motility.

Protein phosphorylation is also regulated by phosphatases (Tash and Bracho, 1994). The motility of human ejaculated spermatozoa is improved by phosphatase inhibitors (okadaic acid, calyculin A) (Leclerc *et al.*, 1996). Similar compounds trigger motility in epididymal spermatozoa, suggesting that low protein kinase and high protein phosphatase activities control motility in these cells (Huang *et al.*, 2004). AKAPs could participate in this effect since they scaffold PKA, PKC and the protein phosphatase calcineurin (Feliciello *et al.*, 2001). Furthermore, the activity of protein phosphatase $1\gamma2$ decreases during epididymal maturation and motility acquisition. Protein phosphatase $1\gamma2$ is bound to protein 14-3-3, another scaffold for transduction elements involved in ERK activation (Huang *et al.*, 2004).

5.5.4 Other sperm enzymes or factors involved in motility

Demembranation–reactivation assays in the presence of protease inhibitors and substrates indicate that a trypsin-like protease of lysine/arginine ester bond specificity may be involved in human, rabbit, bull and rat sperm motility (de Lamirande and Gagnon, 1986). A similar role for protease activity in sperm motility has also been reported in chum salmon (chymotrypsin-like) (Inaba and Morisawa, 1992), carp and sea urchin (trypsin-like) (Cosson and Gagnon, 1988). On the other hand, substrates and inhibitors of transglutaminases also block the motility of demembranated–reactivated spermatozoa (de Lamirande and Gagnon, 1989). None of the agents affecting proteases and transglutaminases inhibit sperm dynein ATPase activity or affect flagellar beat frequency (de Lamirande and Gagnon, 1986, 1989; de Lamirande et al., 1990). However, aprotinin blocks the sliding of microtubules in carp and sea urchin spermatozoa (de Lamirande et al., 1990). It is hypothesized, in analogy to a theoretical model for the covalent interaction between actin and myosin in muscle (Loewy, 1968), that sperm motility is associated with the formation (through a transglutaminase) and the splitting (through a protease) of cross-links between two flagellar structures involved in microtubule sliding (de Lamirande and Gagnon, 1986, 1989; de Lamirande et al., 1990).

Spermatozoa possess protein-carboxyl methylase and protein-methyl esterase, that post-translationally and reversibly modify protein charge, structure and function (Gagnon et al., 1984, 1986). There is a positive correlation between the protein-carboxyl methylase activity in human spermatozoa and the percentage of motile cells (Gagnon et al., 1986). Furthermore, epididymal maturation in rats and bulls is associated with a 10- to 20-fold drop in protein-methyl esterase activity that parallels the progressive acquisition of sperm motility (Gagnon et al., 1984). These reports indicate the importance of the protein-carboxyl methylating–demethylating system in sperm motility (Gagnon et al., 1986).

Epididymal transit is associated with a decrease in the sulfhydryl : disulfide ratio of flagellar proteins (Huang et al., 1984) and sperm maturation induced by caput ligation causes an oxidation of sulfhydryl groups on sperm proteins rendering them similar to those of mature cauda spermatozoa (Seligman et al., 1992). Modification of sulfhydryl and disulfide groups affects the activity of many proteins, such as protein kinases, protein phosphatases and small GTP proteins (Forman et al., 2004; Mikkelsen and Wardman, 2003) that could be involved in initiation of motility. Removal of zinc (Zn^{++}) from spermatozoa during epididymal maturation by proteins such as the macrophage migration inhibitory factor (MIF) secreted by epithelial cells (Eickhoff et al., 2004), could be important for the acquisition of motility potential since flagellar zinc is negatively correlated with motility in human spermatozoa (Henkel et al., 2003). Most of the zinc binds to sulfhydryl groups of the outer dense fibers and removal of zinc allows the formation of disulfide bridges. This oxidation process may be associated with the increasing ability of spermatozoa to generate ROS during epididymal transit (Aitken et al., 2004).

5.5.5 Seminal plasma factors that affect sperm motility

Antioxidants, such as superoxide dismutase, catalase (low levels), vitamins C and E and small sulfhydryl-containing molecules (glutathione) (de Lamirande and Gagnon, 1999; Zini *et al.*, 1993), protect spermatozoa from oxidative stress and related loss of motility (de Lamirande and Gagnon, 1992a, b; de Lamirande and Gagnon, 1999; chapter by Aitken in this book). High levels of immunosuppressors, such as proteasomes, polyamines (spermine and spermidine) and transforming growth factor-β, are also present in seminal plasma and protect spermatozoa from a loss of motility during infection (Kelly, 1999).

Semenogelin (I and II) is the main protein of the semen coagulum in humans and represents upto 20% of seminal plasma proteins (Robert and Gagnon, 1999). After ejaculation, it is rapidly degraded by prostate specific antigen, a chymotrypsin-like protease (Robert and Gagnon, 1999). *In vitro*, sperm motility is inhibited by semenogelin and one of the degradation polypeptides, called the seminal plasma motility inhibitor, when added at levels similar to those found in semen (Robert and Gagnon, 1999). Semenogelin and its degradation peptides are associated with Triton-soluble and -insoluble sperm fractions and may have various biological effects, such as an inhibin-like activity, increase in sperm hyaluronidase activity, zinc shuttling and dynein ATPase inhibition (Robert and Gagnon, 1999).

5.5.6 Sperm hyperactivation

Capacitation, a maturation step that spermatozoa undergo during their transit through the female genital tract, involves multiple metabolic, biochemical, membrane and ionic changes (de Lamirande *et al.*, 1997; Yanagimachi, 1994; chapter by Visconti and Gadella in this book) and is temporally associated with the development of hyperactivated motility. The relatively linear and progressive swimming pattern of spermatozoa in seminal plasma is modified to motility patterns qualified as non-progressive, vigorous, whiplash type, frantic, high amplitude, etc. (Burkman, 1991; de Lamirande *et al.*, 1997; Ho and Suarez, 2001; Murad *et al.*, 1992; Yanagimachi, 1994) (Fig. 5.5). Even though sperm motility characteristics are species specific, common elements during hyperactivation are that the flagellar beating becomes less symmetrical and flagellar bends are more pronounced. The radius of curvature in flagellar bends appears to be larger in spermatozoa that have thicker outer dense fibers (Ho and Suarez, 2001). *In vitro*, in the mouse and the hamster, only hyperactivated spermatozoa can efficiently penetrate media of higher viscoelasticity or density, such as those of fluids from the female genital tract or zona pellucida (Ho and Suarez, 2001; Stauss *et al.*, 1995; Suarez and Dai, 1992). Observations of human spermatozoa co-cultured with epithelial cells from fallopian tubes (Pacey *et al.*, 1995) or mouse spermatozoa in oviducts of naturally mated mice (Demott and Suarez, 1992) indicate that hyperactivation helps spermatozoa to break free from the oviduct and progress along this tissue.

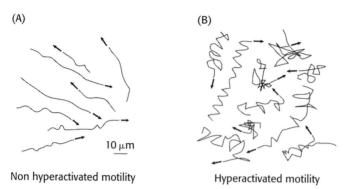

Figure 5.5 Human sperm hyperactivation. Motility patterns of (A) non hyperactivated or (B) hyperactivated spermatozoa. Tracks (2/3 second) were obtained using the CellSoft Research Module

Intracellular Ca^{++} is probably the most important factor in the regulation of sperm hyperactivation and is responsible for the increased flagellar asymmetry (Ho and Suarez, 2001). Intracellular Ca^{++} increases during hamster sperm hyperactivation and the local fluctuations in Ca^{++} concentration that occur throughout whole spermatozoa correlate best with the flagellar beat cycle detected in the proximal flagellar midpiece (Suarez et al., 1993). Furthermore, human spermatozoa submitted to a progesterone gradient to simulate the approach to the oocyte, show cyclical transitions in flagellar beating that parallel the induction of Ca^{++} oscillations (Harper et al., 2004). Ca^{++} acts on the axoneme since it increases the curvature of the principal flagellar bend and causes hyperactivated motility in demembranated–reactivated bull spermatozoa (Ho et al., 2002). The origin of the Ca^{++} needed for hyperactivation is still debated and could be from an influx from the extracellular medium and/or intracellular stores (Ho and Suarez, 2001; Harper et al., 2004). Sperm hyperactivation is complex and ionic changes represent only a part of the requirements. Hyperactivated spermatozoa demembranated and reactivated with cytosolic extracts from hyperactivated spermatozoa had higher velocity and lower linearity than control spermatozoa demembranated and reactivated in control cytosolic extracts indicating that sperm hyperactivation is accompanied by interdependent changes at cytosolic and axonemal levels (Murad et al., 1992).

Depending on the species and the level of maturity of spermatozoa, the requirement for bicarbonate in hyperactivation varies. Epididymal spermatozoa (mouse or hamster) require high bicarbonate concentrations (25 mM) for hyperactivation (Boatman and Robbin, 1991). However, ejaculated spermatozoa exposed to bicarbonate (25 mM) in seminal plasma (Okamura et al., 1985) require lower concentrations (2–3 mM) of this anion to initiate hyperactivation when using biological fluids used as inducers (de Lamirande and Gagnon, 1993a, b; de Lamirande *et al.*, 1993; Murad *et al.*, 1992). Bicarbonate activates adenylyl cyclase (Okamura *et al.*, 1985) but the cAMP produced is not sufficient for hyperactivation of whole spermatozoa (Mujica *et al.*, 1994) and not needed for that of demembranated–reactivated spermatozoa (Ho *et al.*, 2002). It is proposed that activation of cyclic nucleotide-gated channels with the resulting Ca^{++} entry may be one of the mechanisms by which cAMP is involved in sperm hyperactivation (Ho and Suarez, 2001). Bicarbonate could also increase intracellular pH and create the alkaline environment that seems to promote hyperactivation in intact human spermatozoa (Burkman, 1991). It is worth noticing that the pH of the fluids from the female genital tract is close to 8 during the preovulatory period (Nichol *et al.*, 1997), at the time spermatozoa are expected to need hyperactivated motility. A basic pH, 7.9–8.5, is also essential so that demembranated–reactivated bull spermatozoa acquire hyperactivated motility (Ho *et al.*, 2002). Therefore, the actions of bicarbonate appear to be multiple and affect different cellular systems.

Human sperm hyperactivation is prevented by the ROS scavengers, superoxide dismutase and catalase (de Lamirande and Gagnon, 1993a, b; de Lamirande *et al.*, 1997), inhibitors of nitric oxide synthase (Donnelly *et al.*, 1997; Herrero and Gagnon, 2001) and nicotinamide adenine dinucleotide phosphate (NADPH) oxidase (de Lamirande *et al.*, 1997). On the other hand, exogenous ROS promotes hyperactivation (de Lamirande and Gagnon, 1993a, b; de Lamirande *et al.*, 1997; Herrero and Gagnon, 2001). Spermatozoa themselves produce low and controlled amounts of extracellular ROS when incubated under conditions that support hyperactivation (de Lamirande and Gagnon, 1995; de Lamirande *et al.*, 1997). The sharp rise in oxygen tension from ≅5% to ≅20% in fluids from the female reproductive tract at ovulation time could promote the generation of ROS by spermatozoa (Maas *et al.*, 1976). The sperm enzyme that generates ROS is unknown but is suggested to be located at the sperm surface and to be an oxidase that shares few similarities with NADPH oxidases of other cell types (de Lamirande and Gagnon, 1995; de Lamirande *et al.*, 1997; Ford, 2004; Lassègue and Clempus, 2003; Leclerc *et al.*, 1996). The sulfhydryl/disulfide pair on sperm proteins could be some of the targets for ROS since they readily react with ROS and modifications are easily reversed (de Lamirande and Gagnon, 1998, 2003).

Sperm capacitation is associated with an increased tyrosine phosphorylation mainly of two proteins from the fibrous sheath (Aitken *et al.*, 1995; Carrera *et al.*, 1996; de Lamirande *et al.*, 1997; Leclerc *et al.*, 1996, 1997), but the requirement for this in hyperactivation is debated. Tyrosine phosphorylation occurs when hyperactivation is initiated and is increased with the triggering of the acrosome reaction (de Lamirande *et al.*,1998), a time at which spermatozoa need vigorous motility to swim through the zona pellucida. However, bull spermatozoa are hyperactivated by procaine or caffeine, much before tyrosine phosphorylation is increased;

furthermore, H89 and Rp-cAMPS (PKA inhibitors) prevent the cAMP/PKA-dependent tyrosine phosphorylation but not sperm hyperactivation (Marquez and Suarez, 2004). On the other hand, tyrosine phosphorylation of Triton-soluble, rather than Triton-insoluble, proteins could modulate human sperm hyperactivation (Bajpai and Doncel, 2003).

Spontaneous sperm hyperactivation in semen occurs in 16% of infertile men with normal semen analysis but only in 3% of normal men (de Lamirande and Gagnon, 1993c). Semenogelin could prevent premature hyperactivation and the related infertility since it blocks *in vitro* capacitation and hyperactivation at a concentration 200-fold lower than that found in seminal plasma, probably by interaction and inhibition of the sperm oxidase responsible for the superoxide production (de Lamirande *et al.*, 2001). Even though seminal plasma contains other substances, such as cholesterol (Cross, 1996; Purdy and Graham, 2004), zinc (Andrews *et al.*, 1994; de Lamirande *et al.*, 1997) and ROS scavengers (de Lamirande and Gagnon, 1993c), that are known factors that could prevent premature hyperactivation, this fluid also contains factors that can, at low concentrations, induce sperm hyperactivation (de Lamirande *et al.*, 1993c). Therefore, a fine balance between inhibitory and stimulatory factors is needed to prevent premature sperm hyperactivation in semen.

5.5.7 Sperm chemotaxis

Although sperm chemotaxis is well recognized in sea urchins and fishes, chemotaxis in mammals is still debated maybe because of differences in methods and substances tested (Eisenbach, 1999). Oviductal fluid (Oliveira *et al.*, 1999), follicular fluid (Eisenbach, 1999) and cumulus oophorus (Bronson and Hamada, 1977) attract spermatozoa, suggesting the possibility of sequential chemotaxis on the sperm journey to the egg. The active components of follicular fluid could be heat-stable peptides, heparin, epinephrine and atrial natriuretic peptide (Eisenbach, 1999) but not progesterone, which causes sperm hyperactivation but no chemotaxis (Jaiswal *et al.*, 1999). Only a small sperm population is responsive to chemoattraction and appears to consist mainly of capacitated cells (Cohen-Dayag *et al.*, 1995; Eisenbach, 1999).

Contrarily to what is observed in sea urchins, human and rabbit spermatozoa respond similarly to factors from human, rabbit or bovine eggs indicating that chemotaxis factors are common or very similar and that mammals do not rely on this mechanism to avoid interspecies fertilization (Sun *et al.*, 2003). In humans, the chemotactic response depends on the activation of several factors, such as the sperm olfactory receptor hOR17-4, the membrane-associated adenylyl cyclase and the G(olf) protein, all of which are located in the flagellum (Eisenbach, 1999; Spehr *et al.*, 2004).

5.6 Conclusion

Sperm motility is a complex phenomenon and its fine regulation by ionic, metabolic and enzymatic factors allows rapid and very specific changes in response to the environment so that fertilization occurs. The components of the axoneme, the motility apparatus in all flagella, are highly conserved. Some factors, such as cAMP and Ca^{++}, involved in motility initiation and alterations (chemotaxis and hyperactivation) appear common between species. Others, such as phosphorylation of proteins or chemoattractants, are more species specific. Motility disorders associated with missing or deficient flagellar components or with abnormal environment factors can cause infertility.

Acknowledgment

We thank Mr Daniel White for helpful comments in reviewing the chapter.

REFERENCES

Afzelius BA (2004) Cilia-related diseases. *J Pathol* 204, 470–477.

Aitken RJ, Paterson M, Fisher H, Buckingham DW and van Duin M (1995) Redox regulation of tyrosine phosphorylation in human spermatozoa and its role in the control of human sperm function. *J Cell Sci* 180, 2017–2025.

Aitken RJ, Ryan AL, Baker MA and McLaughlin EA (2004) Redox activity associated with the maturation and capacitation of mammalian spermatozoa. *Free Radic Biol Med* 36, 994–1010.

Andrews JC, Noland JP, Hammerstedt RH and Bavister BD (1994) Role of zinc in hamster sperm capacitation. *Biol Reprod* 51, 1238–1247.

Ashizawa A, Hashimoto K, Higashio M and Tsuzuki Y (1997) The addition of mitogen-activated protein kinase and p34cdc2 kinase substrate peptide inhibits the flagellar motility of demembranated fowl spermatozoa. *Biochem Biophys Res Commun* 240, 116–121.

Bajpai M and Doncel GF (2003) Involvement of tyrosine kinase and cAMP-dependent kinase cross-talk in the regulation of human sperm motility. *Reprod* 126, 183–195.

Boatman DE and Robbins RS (1991) Bicarbonate: carbon-dioxide regulation of sperm capacitation, hyperactivated motility, and acrosome reactions. *Biol Reprod* 44, 806–813.

Boitano S and Okuno CK (1991) Membrane hyperpolarization activates trout sperm without an increase in intracellular pH. *J Cell Sci* 98, 343–349.

Bozkurt HH and Wooley DM (1993) Morphology of nexin links in relation to interdoublet sliding in the sperm flagellum. *Cell Motil Cytoskeleton* 24, 109–118.

Bracho GE, Fritch JJ and Tash JS (1998) Identification of flagellar proteins that initiate the activation of sperm motility in vivo. *Biochem Biophys Res Comm* 242, 231–237.

Brokaw CJ and Kamiya R (1987) Bending patterns of *Chlamydomonas* flagella: IV. Mutants with defects in inner and outer dynein arms indicate differences in dynein arm function. *Cell Motil Cytoskeleton* 8, 68–75.

Bronson R and Hamada Y (1977) Gamete interactions *in vitro. Fertil Steril* 28, 570–576.

Burkman LJ (1991) Discrimination between non hyperactivated and classical hyperactivated motility patterns in human spermatozoa using computerized analysis. *Fertil Steril* 55, 363–371.

Carrera A, Gerton GL and Moss SB (1994) The major fibrous sheath polypeptide of mouse sperm: structural and functional similarities to the A-kinase anchoring proteins. *Dev Biol* 165, 272–284.

Carrera A, Moss J, Ning XP, Gerton GL, Tesarik J, Kopf GS and Moss SB (1996) Regulation of protein tyrosine phosphorylation in human sperm by a calcium/calmodulin dependent mechanism: identification of A kinase anchor proteins as major substrate for tyrosine phosphorylation. *Dev Biol* 180, 284–296.

Cohen-Dayag A, Tur-Kaspa I, Dor J, Mashiach S and Eisenbach M (1995) Sperm capacitation in humans is transient and correlates with chemotactic responsiveness to follicular factors. *Proc Natl Acad Sci USA*, 92, pp. 11039–11043.

Cosson J, Billiard R, Cibert C, Dréanno C and Suquet M (1999) Ionic factors regulating the motility of fish sperm. In: *The Male Gamete: From Basic Knowledge to Clinical Applications*, ed. C Gagnon. Vienna, IL: Cache River Press, pp. 161–186.

Cosson M-P (1990) Sperm chemotaxis. In: *Controls of Sperm Motility: #Biological and Clinical Aspects*, ed. C Gagnon. Boca Raton, FL: CRC Press, pp. 103–135.

Cosson M-P and Gagnon C (1988) Protease inhibitor and substrates block motility and microtubule sliding of sea urchin and carp spermatozoa. *Cell Motil Cytoskeleton* 10, 518–527.

Cross NL (1996) Human seminal plasma prevents sperm from becoming acrosomally responsive to the agonist progesterone: cholesterol is the major inhibitor. *Biol Reprod* 54, 138–145.

de Lamirande E and Gagnon C (1986) Effect of protease inhibitors and substrates on motility of mammalian spermatozoa. *J Cell Biol* 102, 1378–1383.

de Lamirande E and Gagnon C (1989) Effect of transglutaminase substrates and inhibitors on the motility of demembranated reactivated spermatozoa. *Gamete Res* 22, 179–192.

de Lamirande E and Gagnon C (1992a) Reactive oxygen species and human spermatozoa. I. Effects on the motility of intact spermatozoa and on sperm axonemes. *J Androl* 13, 368–378.

de Lamirande E and Gagnon C (1992b) Reactive oxygen species and human spermatozoa. II. Depletion of adenosine triphosphate plays an important role in the inhibition of sperm motility. *J Androl* 13, 379–386.

de Lamirande E and Gagnon C (1993a) A positive role for the superoxide anion in triggering hyperactivation and capacitation of human spermatozoa. *Int J Androl* 16, 21–25.

de Lamirande E and Gagnon C (1993b) Human sperm hyperactivation and capacitation as parts of an oxidative process. *Free Radic Biol Med* 14, 157–166.

de Lamirande E and Gagnon C (1993c) Human sperm hyperactivation in whole semen and its association with low superoxide scavenging capacity in seminal plasma. *Fertil Steril* 59, 1291–1295.

de Lamirande E and Gagnon C (1995) Capacitation associated production of superoxide anion by human spermatozoa. *Free Radic Biol Med* 18, 487–495.

de Lamirande E and Gagnon C (1998) Paradoxical effect of reagents for sulfhydryl and disulfide groups on human sperm capacitation and superoxide production. *Free Radic Biol Med* 25, 803–817.

de Lamirande E and Gagnon C (1999) The dark and bright sides of reactive oxygen species on sperm function. In: *The Male Gamete: From Basic Science to Clinical Applications*, ed. C Gagnon. Vienna, IL: Cache River Press, pp. 455–467.

de Lamirande E and Gagnon C (2002) The extracellular signal-regulated kinase (ERK) pathway is involved in human sperm function and modulated by the superoxide anion. *Mol Human Reprod* 8, 124–135.

de Lamirande E and Gagnon C (2003) Redox control of changes in protein sulfhydryl levels during human sperm capacitation. *Free Radic Biol Med* 35, 1271–1285.

de Lamirande E, Cosson M-P and Gagnon C (1990) Protease involvement in sperm motility. In: *Controls of Sperm Motility: Biological and Clinical Aspects*. ed. C Gagnon. Boca Raton, FL: CRC Press, pp. 241–254.

de Lamirande E, Eiley D and Gagnon C (1993) Inverse relationship between the induction of human sperm capacitation and spontaneous acrosome reaction by various biological fluids and the superoxide scavenging capacity of these fluids. *Int J Androl* 16, 258–266.

de Lamirande E, Leclerc P and Gagnon C (1997) Capacitation as a regulatory event that primes spermatozoa for the acrosome reaction and fertilization. *Mol Human Reprod* 3, 175–194.

de Lamirande E, Tsai C, Harakat A and Gagnon C (1998) Involvement of reactive oxygen species in human sperm acrosome reaction induced by A23187, lysophosphatidylcholine, and biological fluid ultrafiltrates. *J Androl* 19, 585–594.

de Lamirande E, Yoshida K, Yoshiike M, Iwamoto T and Gagnon C (2001) Semenogelin, the main protein of semem coagulum, inhibits human sperm capacitation by interfering with the superoxide anion generated during this process. *J Androl* 22, 672–679.

Demott RP and Suarez SS (1992) Hyperactivated sperm progress in the mouse oviduct. *Biol Reprod* 46, 779–785.

DiBella LM and King SM (2001) Dynein motors of the *Chlamydomonas* flagellum. *Int Rev Cytol* 210, 227–268.

Donnelly ET, Lewis SEM, Thompson W and Chakravarthy U (1997) Sperm nitric oxide and motility: the effect of nitric oxide synthase stimulation and inhibition. *Mol Human Reprod* 3, 755–762.

Eddy EM, Toshimori K and O'Brien D (2003) Fibrous sheath of mammalian spermatozoa. *Micros Res Tech* 61, 103–115.

Eickhoff RE, Baldauf C, Koyro H-W, Wennemuth G, Suga Y, Seitz J, Henkel R and Meinhardt A (2004) Influence of macrophage migration inhibitory factor (MIF) on the zinc content and redox state of protein-bound sulphydryl groups in rat sperm: indications for a new role in sperm maturation. *Mol Human Reprod* 10, 605–611.

Eisenbach M (1999) Mammalian sperm chemotaxis and its association with capacitation. *Dev Genet* 25, 87–94.

Feliciello A, Gottesman ME and Avvedimento EV (2001) The biological functions of A-kinase anchor proteins. *J Mol Biol* 308, 99–114.

Ford WCL (2004) Regulation of sperm function by reactive oxygen species. *Human Reprod Rev* 10, 387–399.

Forman HJ, Fukuto JM and Torres M (2004) Redox signaling: thiol chemistry defines which reactive oxygen and nitrogen species can act as second messengers. *Am J Physiol-Cell Physiol* 287, C246–C256.

Fujinoki M, Kawamura T, Toda T, Ohtake H, Shimizu N, Yamaoka S and Okuno M (2003) Identification of the 58-kDa phosphoprotein associated with motility initiation of hamster spermatozoa. *J Biochem* 134, 559–565.

Fujinoki M, Kawamura T, Toda T, Ohtake H, Ishimoda-Takagi T, Shimizu N, Yamaoka S and Okuno M (2004) Identification of 36 kDa phosphoprotein in fibrous sheath of hamster spermatozoa. *Comp Biochem Biophys Part B* 137, 509–520.

Fujita A, Nakamura K, Kato T, Watanabe N, Ishizaki T, Kimura K, Mizoguchi A and Narumiya S (2000) Ropporin, a sperm-specific binding protein of rophilin, that is localized in the fibrous sheath of sperm flagella. *J Cell Sci* 113, 103–112.

Gagnon C, Harbour D, de Lamirande E, Bardin CW and Dacheux J-L (1984) Sensitive assay detects protein methylesterase in spermatozoa: decrease in enzyme activity during epididymal maturation. *Biol Reprod* 30, 953–958.

Gagnon C, de Lamirande E and Sherins RJ (1986) Positive correlation between the level of protein-carboxyl methylase in spermatozoa and sperm motility. *Fertil Steril* 45, 847–853.

Gagnon C, White D, Huitorel P and Cosson J (1994) A monoclonal antibody against the dynein IC1 peptide of sea urchin spermatozoa inhibits the motility of sea urchin, dinoflagellate, and human flagellar axonemes. *Mol Biol Cell* 5, 1051–1063.

Gagnon C, White D, Cosson J *et al.* (1996) The polyglutamylated lateral chain of alpha-tubulin plays a key role in flagellar motility. *J Cell Sci* 109, 1545–1553.

Gingras D, White D, Garin J *et al.* (1996) Purification, cloning, and sequence analysis of a Mr = 30,000 protein from sea urchin axonemes that is important for sperm motility. Relationship of the protein to a dynein light chain. *J Biol Chem* 271, 12807–12813.

Gingras D, White D, Garin J *et al.* (1998) Molecular cloning and characterization of a radial spoke head protein of sea urchin sperm axonemes: involvement of the protein in the regulation of sperm motility. *Mol Biol Cell* 9, 513–522.

Harper CV, Barratt CLR and Publicover SJ (2004) Stimulation of human spermatozoa with progesterone gradients to simulate approach to the oocyte. Induction of $[Ca^{2+}]_i$ oscillations and cyclical transitions in flagellar beating. *J Biol Chem* 279, 46315–46325.

Harrison RAP (2004) Rapid PKA-catalysed phosphorylation of boar sperm proteins induced by the capacitating agent bicarbonate. *Mol Reprod Dev* 67, 337–352.

Henkel RR, Defosse K, Koyro HW, Weissmann N and Schill WB (2003) Estimate of oxygen consumption and intracellular zinc concentration of human spermatozoa in relation to motility. *Asian J Androl* 5, 3–8.

Herrero MB and Gagnon C (2001) Nitric oxide: a novel mediator of sperm function. *J Androl* 22, 349–356.

Hinsch KD, Habermann B, Just I, Hinsch EPfisterer, Schill WB and Aktories K (1993) ADP-ribosylation of Rho proteins inhibits sperm motility. *FEBS Lett* 334, 32–36.

Ho H-C and Suarez SS (2001) Hyperactivation of mammalian spermatozoa: function and regulation. *Reprod* 122, 519–526.

Ho H-C, Granish KA and Suarez SS (2002) Hyperactivated motility of bull sperm is triggered at the axoneme by Ca^{2+} and not cAMP. *Dev Biol* 250, 208–217.

Holt WV and Harrison RAP (2002) Bicarbonate stimulation of boar sperm motility via a protein kinase A-dependent pathway: between-cell and between-ejaculate differences are not due to deficiencies in protein kinase A activation. *J Androl* 23, 557–565.

Horowitz JA, Toeg H and Orr GA (1984) Characterization and localization of cAMP-dependent protein kinases in rat caudal epididymal sperm. *J Biol Chem* 259, 832–838.

Huang TTF, Kosower NS and Yanagimachi R (1984) Localization of thiols and disulfide groups in guinae pig spermatozoa during maturation and capacitation using bimane fluorescent labels. *Biol Reprod* 31, 797–809.

Huang Z, Myers K, Khatra B and Vijayaraghavan S (2004) Protein 14-3-3ζ binds to protein phosphatase PPIγ2 in bovine epididymal spermatozoa. *Biol Reprod* 71, 177–184.

Huitorel P, Audebert S, White D, Cosson J and Gagnon C (1999) Role of tubulin epitopes in the regulation of flagellar motility. In: *The Male Gamete: From Basic Knowledge to Clinical Applications*, ed. C Gagnon. Vienna, IL: Cache River Press, pp. 475–491.

Huitorel P, White D, Fouquet J-P, Kann M-L, Cosson J and Gagnon C (2002) Differential distribution of glutamylated tubulin isoforms along the sea urchin sperm axoneme. *Mol Reprod Dev* 62, 139–148.

Inaba K (2002) Dephosphorylation of Tctex2-related dynein light chain by type 2A protein phosphatase. *Biochem Biophys Res Comm* 297, 800–805.

Inaba K (2003) Molecular architecture of the sperm flagella: molecules for motility and signaling. *Zool Sci* 20, 1043–1056.

Inaba K and Morisawa M (1992) Chymotrypsin-like protease activity associated with demembranated sperm of chum salmon. *Biol Cell* 76, 329–333.

Inaba K, Morisawa S and Morisawa M (1998) Proteasomes regulate the motility of salmonid fish sperm through modulation of cAMP-dependent phosphorylation of an outer arm dynein light chain. *J Cell Sci* 111, 1105–1115.

Inaba K, Kagami O and Ogawa K (1992) Tctex2-related outer arm dynein light chain is phosphorylated at activation of sperm motility. *Biochem Biophys Res Comm* 256, 177–183.

Ishiguro K, Murofushi H and Sakai H (1982) Evidence that cAMP-dependent protein kinase and protein factor are involved in reactivation of Triton X-100 models of sea urchin and starfish spermatozoa. *J Cell Biol* 92, 777–782.

Itoh A, Inaba K, Ohtake H, Fujinoko M and Morisawa M (2003) Characterization of a cAMP-dependent protein kinase catalytic subunit from rainbow trout spermatozoa. *Biochem Biophys Res Commun* 305, 855–861.

Jaiswal BS and Conti M (2001) Identification and functional analysis of splice variants of the germ cell soluble adenylyl cyclase. *J Biol Chem* 276, 31698–31708.

Jaiswal BS, Tur-Kaspa, Dor J, Mashiach S and Eisenbach M (1999) Human sperm chemotaxis: is progesterone a chemoattractant? *Biol Reprod* 60, 1314–1319.

Kamiya R (2002) Functional diversity of axonemal dyneins as studied in *Chlamydomonas* mutants. *Int Rev Cytol* 219, 115–155.

Kelly RW (1999) Immunomodulators in human seminal plasma: a vital protection for spermatozoa in the presence of infection? *Int J Androl* 22, 2–12.

King SM, Wilkerson CG and Witman GB (1991) The Mr 78,000 intermediate chain of *Chlamydomonas* outer arm dynein interacts with alpha-tubulin. *J Cell Biol* 266, 8401–8407.

King SM, Patel-King RS, Wilerson CG and Witman GB (1995) The 78,000-Mr intermediate chain of *Chlamydomonas* outer arm dynein is a microtubule-binding protein. *J Cell Biol* 131, 399–409.

Kubo-Irie M, Matsumiya K, Iwamoto T and Kaneko S (2004) Morphological abnormalities in the spermatozoa of fertile and infertile men. *Mol Reprod Dev* 70, 70–81.

Lassègue B and Clempus RE (2003) Vascular NAD(P)H oxidases: specific features, expression, and regulation. *Am J Physiol Regul Integr Comp Physiol* 285, R277–R297.

Leclerc P and Gagnon C (1996) Phosphorylation of Triton X-100 soluble and insoluble protein substrates in a demembranated/reactivated human sperm model. *Mol Reprod Dev* 44, 200–211.

Leclerc P, de Lamirande E and Gagnon C (1996) Cyclic adenosine 3', 5' monophosphate-dependent regulation of protein tyrosine phosphorylation in relation to human sperm capacitation and motility. *Biol Reprod* 55, 684–692.

Leclerc P, de Lamirande E and Gagnon C (1997) Regulation of protein tyrosine phosphorylation and human sperm capacitation by reactive oxygen derivatives. *Free Radic Biol Med* 22, 643–656.

Link RW (2001) Cilia and Flagella. In: *Encyclopedia of Life Sciences*. London, UK: Nature Publishing Group, pp. 1–12.

Loewy AG (1968) A theory of covalent bonding in muscle contraction. *J Theor Biol* 20, 164–169.

Lu Q, Breitbart QY and Chen DY (1999) Expression and phosphorylation of mitogen-activated protein kinases during spermatogenesis and epididymal maturation in mice. *Arch Androl* 43, 55–66.

Maas DHA, Storey BT and Mastroianni L (1976) Oxygen tension in the oviduct of the Rhesus monkey (Macaca mulatta). *Fertil Steril* 27, 1312–1318.

MacRae TH (1997) Tubulin post-translational modifications-enzymes and their mechanisms of action. *Eur J Biochem* 244, 265–278.

Marquez B and Suarez SS (2004) Different signaling pathways in bovine sperm regulate capacitation and hyperactivation. *Biol Reprod* 70, 1626–1633.

Miki K, Qu W, Goulding EH, Willis WD *et al.* (2004) Glyceraldehyde 3-Phosphate dehydrogenase-S, a sperm-specific glycolytic enzyme, is required for sperm motility and male fertility. *Proc Natl Acad Sci USA*, 47, pp. 16501–16506.

Mikkelsen RB and Wardman P (2003) Biological chemistry of reactive oxygen and nitrogen and radiation-induced signal transduction mechanisms. *Oncogene* 22, 5734–5754.

Mohri C, Nakamura N, Welch JE, Gotoh H, Goulding EH, Fujioka M and Eddy EM (1998) Mouse spermatogenic cell-specific type 1 hexokinase (mHk1-s) transcripts are expressed by alternative splicing from the mHk1 gene and the HK1-S protein is localized mainly in the sperm tail. *Mol Reprod Dev* 49, 374–385.

Moos J, Peknicova J, Geussova G, Philimonenko V and Hozac P (1998) Association of protein kinase A type I with detergent-resistant structures of mammalian sperm cells. *Mol Reprod Dev* 50, 79–85.

Morisawa M (1994) Cell signaling mechanisms for sperm motility. *Zool Sci* 11, 647–662.

Morisawa M, Oda S, Yoshida M and Takai H (1999) Transmembrane signal transduction for the regulation of sperm motility in fishes and ascidians. In *The Male Gamete: From Basic Knowledge to Clinical Applications*, ed. C Gagnon, Vienna, IL: Cache River Press, pp. 149–160.

Mujica A, Neri-Bazan L, Tash J and Uribe S (1994) Mechanism for procaine-mediated hyperactivated motility in guinae pig spermatozoa. *Mol Reprod Dev* 38, 285–292.

Mukai C and Okuno M (2004) Glycolysis plays a major role for adenosine triphosphate supplementation in mouse sperm flagellar movement. *Biol Reprod* 71, 540–547.

Murad C, de Lamirande E and Gagnon C (1992) Hyperactivated motility is coupled with inter-dependent modifications at the axonemal and cytosolic levels in human spermatozoa. *J Androl* 13, 323–331.

NagDas SK, Winfrey VP and Olson GE (2002) Identification of Ras and its downstream signaling elements and their potential role in hamster sperm motility. *Biol Reprod* 67, 1058–1066.

Nakamura K, Fujita A, Murata T *et al.* (1999) Rhophilin, a small GTPase Rho-binding protein, is abundantly expressed in the mouse testis and localized in the principal piece of the sperm tail. *FEBS Lett* 445, 9–13.

Naz RK, Ahmad K and Kaplan P (1992) Expression and function of Ras proto-oncogene protein in human sperm cells. *J Cell Sci* 102, 487–494.

Neill AT and Vacquier VD (2004) Ligands and receptors mediating signal transduction in sea urchin spermatozoa. *Reprod* 127, 141–149.

Nichol R, Hunter RHF and Cooke GM (1997) Oviduct fluid pH in intach and unilaterally ovariectomized pigs. *Can J Physiol Pharmacol* 75, 1069–1074.

Nomura M, Inaba K and Morisawa M (2000) cAMP- and calmodulin-dependent phosphorylation of 21 and 26 kDa proteins in axoneme is a prerequisite for SAAF-induced motile activation in ascidian spermatozoa. *Dev Growth Differ* 42, 129–138.

Oakley BR (2000) An abundance of tubulins. *Cell Biol* 10, 537–542.

Oda S and Morisawa M (1993) Rise of intracellular Ca^{2+} and pH mediate the initiation of sperm motility by hyperosmolality in marine teleosts. *Cell Motil Cytoskeleton* 25, 171–178.

Okamura N, Tajima Y Soejima A, Masuda H and Sugita Y (1985) Sodium bicarbonate in seminal plasma stimulates the motility of mammalian spermatozoa through direct activation of adenylate cyclase. *J Biol Chem* 260, 9699–9705.

Oko R and Clermont Y (1990) Mammalian spermatozoa: structure and assembly of the tail. In *Controls of Sperm Motility: Biological and Clinical Aspects*, ed. C Gagnon. Boca Raton, FL: CRC Press, pp. 3–28.

Oliveira RG, Tomasi L, Rovasio RA and Giojalas LC (1999) Increased velocity and induction of chemotactic response in mouse spermatozoa by follicular fluids. *J Reprod Fertil* 115, 23–27.

Pacey AA, Davies N, Warren MA, Barratt CLR and Cooke ID (1995) Hyperactivation may assist human spermatozoa to detach from intimate association with the endosalpinx. *Human Reprod* 10, 2603–2609.

Patel-King RS, Benashski SE and King SM (2002) A bipartite Ca^{2+}-regulated nucleoside-diphosphate kinase system within the *Chlamydomonas* flagellum. The regulatory subunit p72. *J Biol Chem* 277, 34271–34279.

Patel-King RS, Gorgatyuk O, Takebe S and King SM (2004) Flagellar radial spokes contain a Ca^{2+}-stimulated nucleoside diphosphate kinase. *Mol Biol Cell* 15, 3891–3902.

Piperno G (1995) Regulation of dynein activity within *Chlamydomonas* flagella. *Cell Motil Cytoskeleton* 32, 103–106.

Porter ME and Sale WS (2000) The 9 + 2 axoneme anchors multiple inner arm dyneins and a network of kinases and phosphatases that control motility. *J Cell Biol* 151, F37–F42.

Purdy PH and Graham JK (2004) Effect of adding cholesterol to bull sperm membranes on sperm capacitation, the acrosome reaction, and fertility. *Biol Reprod* 71, 522–527.

Riffell JA, Krug PJ and Zimmer RK (2002) Fertilization in the sea: the chemical identity of an abalone sperm attractant. *J Exptl Biol* 205, 1439–1450.

Robert M and Gagnon C (1999) Semenogelin I: a coagulation forming multifunctional seminal vesicle protein. *Cell Mol Life Sci* 55, 944–960.

Rotem R, Paz GF, Homonnai ZT, Kalina M and Naor Z (1990) Protein kinase C is present in human sperm: possible involvement in flagellar motility. *Proc Natl Acad Sci USA*, 87, pp. 7305–7308.

Seligman J, Kosower NS and Shalgi R (1992) Effect of caput ligation on rat sperm and epididymis: protein thiols and fertilizing ability. *Biol Reprod* 46, 301–308.

Si Y and Okuno M (1999) Regulation of microtubule sliding by a 36-kDa phosphoprotein in hamster sperm flagella. *Mol Reprod Dev* 52, 328–334.

Smith E (2002) Regulation of flagellar dynein by calcium and role for an axonemal calmodulin and calmodulin-dependent kinase. *Mol Biol Cell* 13, 3303–3313.

Smith E and Yang P (2004) The radial spokes and central apparatus: mechano-chemical transducers that regulate flagellar motility. *Cell Motil Cytoskeleton* 57, 8–17.

Spehr M, Schwane K, Riffell JA, Babour J, Zimmer RK, Nauhaus EM and Hatt H (2004) Particulate adenylate cyclase plays a key role in human olfactory receptor-mediated chemotaxis. *J Biol Chem* 279, 40194–40203.

Stauss CR, Votta TJ and Suarez SS (1995) Sperm motility hyperactivation facilitates penetration of the hamster zona pellucida. *Biol Reprod* 53, 1280–1285.

Suarez SS and Dai X (1992) Hyperactivation enhanced mouse sperm capacity for penetrating viscoelastic media. *Biol Reprod* 46, 686–691.

Suarez SS, Varosi SM and Dai X (1993) Intracellular calcium increases with hyperactivation in intact, moving hamster sperm and oscillates with the flagellar beat cycle. *Proc Natl Acad Sci USA*, 90, pp. 4660–4664.

Sun F, Giojalas LC, Rovasio RA, Tur-Kaspa I, Sanchez R and Eisenbach M (2003) Lack of species-specificity in mammalian sperm chemotaxis. *Dev Biol* 255, 423–427.

Takada S, Wilkerson CG, Wakabayashi K-i, Kamiya R and Witman GB (2002) The outer dynein arm-docking complex: characterization of a subunit (Oda1) necessary for outer arm assembly. *Mol Biol Cell* 13, 1015–1029.

Tash JS and Bracho GE (1994) Regulation of sperm motility: emerging evidence for a major role for protein phosphatases. *J Androl* 15, 505–509.

Tash JS, Hidaka H and Mean AR (1986) Axokinin phosphorylation by cAMP-dependent protein kinase is sufficient for activation of sperm flagellar motility. *J Cell Biol* 103, 649–655.

Turner RM (2003) Tales from the tail: what do we really know about sperm motility? *J Androl* 24, 790–803.

Vijayaraghavan S, Goueli SA, Davey MP and Carr DW (1997a) Protein kinase A-anchoring inhibitor peptides arrest sperm motility. *J Biol Chem* 272, 4747–4752.

Vijayaraghavan S, Olson GE, NagDas S, Winfrey VP and Carr DW (1997b) Subcellular localization of the regulatory subunits of cyclic adenosine 3′, 5′-monophosphate-dependent protein kinase in bovine spermatozoa. *Biol Reprod* 57, 1517–1523.

Wennemuth G, Carlson AE, Harper AJ and Babcock DF (2003) Bicarbonate actions on flagellar and Ca^{2+}-channel responses: initial events in sperm activation. *Development* 130, 1317–1326.

Westhoff D and Kamp G (1997) Glyceraldehyde 3-phosphate dehydrogenase is bound to the fibrous sheath of mammalian spermatozoa. *J Cell Sci* 110, 1821–1829.

White D, Aghigh S, Magder I, Cosson J, Huitorel P and Gagnon C (2005) Two anti-radial spoke monoclonal antibodies inhibit *Chlamydomonas* axonemal motility by different mechanisms. *J Biol Chem* 280, 14803–14810.

Wooley DM (1997) Studies on the eel sperm flagellum. I. The structure of the inner dynein arm complex. *J Cell Sci* 110, 85–94.

World Health Organization (1999) *WHO Laboratory Manual for the Examination of Human Semen and Semen–Cervical Mucus Interaction*, 4th edn. Cambridge, UK: Cambridge University Press, pp. 1–107.

Xiang X, Burnett L, Rawls A, Bieber A and Chandler D (2004) The sperm chemoattractant 'allurin' is expressed and secreted from the xenopus oviduct in a hormone-regulated manner. *Dev Biol* 275, 343–355.

Yanagimachi R (1994) Mammalian fertilization. In: *The Physiology of Reproduction*, eds E Knobil and JD Neill, 2nd edn. New York, NY: Raven Press Ltd, pp. 189–317.

Yeung C-H and Cooper TG (2003) Developmental changes in signalling transduction factors in maturing sperm duling epididymal transit. *Cell Mol Biol* 49, 341–349.

Yokota E and Mabuchi I (1990) The cAMP-dependent protein kinase in sea urchin sperm tails: association of the enzyme with the flagellar axonemes. *J Biochem* 108, 1–3.

Zini A, de Lamirande E and Gagnon C (1993) Reactive oxygen species in semen of infertile patients: levels of superoxide dismutase- and catalase-like activities in seminal plasma and spermatozoa. *Int J Androl* 16, 183–188.

Regulation of capacitation

Bart M. Gadella[1,2] and Pablo E. Visconti[3]

Departments of [1]Biochemistry and Cell Biology
[2]Farm Animal Health, Faculty of Veterinary Medicine, Utrecht University, Yalelaan, Utrecht, The Netherlands
[3]Department of Veterinary and Animal Sciences, University of Massachusetts, Amherst, MA, USA

6.1 Introduction

Mammalian sperm are not able to fertilize eggs immediately after ejaculation. They acquire fertilization capacity after residing in the female tract for a finite period of time that varies depending on the species. In 1951, Chang (1951) and Austin (1951) independently demonstrated that such a period of time in the female tract is required for the sperm to acquire their fertilizing capacity. Both authors observed that freshly obtained rabbit sperm introduced into the Fallopian tubes shortly after ovulation were not able to penetrate the eggs; instead if sperm were introduced a few hours before ovulation, the majority of the eggs were later observed to be fertilized. This observation led them to conclude that freshly ejaculated sperm are incapable of penetrating the zona pellucida immediately, and that sperm must remain within the female tract for a period before they are able to penetrate the eggs. Following these original observations, many studies confirmed that the environment of the female tract induces a series of physiological changes in the sperm; these changes are collectively called 'capacitation'. Inherent to these first observations was that capacitation state became defined using fertilization as end-point. However, a variety of evidences suggest that the functional changes occurring in the sperm during capacitation are not one event, but a combination of concomitant processes; mainly, the sperm acquisition of the ability to undergo an agonist (e.g. zona pellucida, progesterone) induced acrosome reaction and the modification in the motility pattern known as hyperactivated motility (both enabling efficient zona drilling so that the sperm can reach the oolemma).

Although more than 50 years have passed since sperm capacitation was first reported and conditions for *in vitro* capacitation has been established in a variety of mammalian species, it is noteworthy that the molecular basis of this process is still today not well understood. Nevertheless, recent work is beginning to point to a unified model of how this event is controlled at the molecular level. To dissect the molecular mechanisms involved in sperm capacitation, most authors have used *in vitro* capacitation systems incubating the sperm in chemically defined buffers that mimic the glucose and electrolyte content of the oviduct and are enriched with serum albumin components. It is important though to keep in mind that capacitation occurs in the female tract and sooner or later, *in vitro* capacitation models will need to be validated *in vivo* taking into consideration the physiology of the female track that is under hormonal control. The purposes of this chapter are to consider some recent contributions towards our understanding of capacitation, to summarize open questions in this field, and to discuss future avenues of research. Reviews by Baldi *et al.* (2000), Cohen-Dayag and Eisenbach (1994), de Lamirande *et al.* (1997), Flesch and Gadella (2000), Florman and Babcock (1991), Harrison (1996), Visconti and Kopf (1998), Visconti *et al.* (1998), and Yanagimachi (1994) provide supplementary reading and complement the material of this chapter.

6.2 Heterogeneity in sperm populations and in sperm

Sperm are highly differentiated and polarized cells that can be divided into three main components: head, mid-piece, and flagellum. The head consists of the acrosome, the nucleus, some cytoskeletal structures, and cytoplasm. The flagellum contains a central axoneme surrounded by outer dense fibers; in addition, the anterior part of the flagellum (mid-piece) contains mitochondria and the posterior part of the tail (principal piece) contains a fibrous sheath surrounding the outer dense fibers (Eddy and O'Brien, 1994). Taking the sperm structures into account, when one attempts to understand the process of capacitation at the molecular level, events occurring in the sperm head (i.e. acrosome reaction) and in the tail (i.e. motility changes) must be considered. Therefore, one may postulate that components involved in the exocytotic and motility machinery of sperm are modified during capacitation. Some of these alterations may be initiated by changes in the lipid organization of the sperm plasma membrane; these modifications in the lipid order are likely to be essential to enhance the fusogenicity of the sperm membranes as a preparative step for the agonist (zona pellucida) induced acrosome reaction. In addition to this, capacitation may involve alterations in ion currents, changes in the phosphorylation status of certain proteins, changes in protein localization, and/or modification of protein–protein interactions. Experiments leading to the identification and characterization of the molecules involved will further increase our understanding of capacitation.

Regarding the signaling pathways associated with sperm capacitation, it is necessary to consider two main problems. First, several lines of evidence suggest that only a particular fraction of the sperm population undergoes capacitation. Second, as mentioned above, sperm are compartmentalized into several spatially separated structures; therefore, it is essential to analyze the topology of the molecular changes observed during capacitation. Due to difficulties in experimental conditions, most observations regarding the molecular basis of capacitation have been done in complete sperm suspensions containing sperm in different stages of capacitation as well as a subpopulation of deteriorated sperm cells. In addition, most of these experiments do not address localization of the observed molecular changes within the cell. To solve these problems related to sperm heterogeneity and compartmentalization, recent studies have used flow cytometric assessment of capacitated sperm (Gadella and Van Gestel, 2004; Harrison and Gadella, 2005), single cell analysis (Arnoult et al., 1999; Carlson et al., 2003; Fukami et al., 2003), and a combination of these methodologies; that is, microscopic visualization of signaling pathways after separation of the sperm subpopulations by flow cytometry (de Vries et al., 2003; Flesch et al., 2001a). In this respect, it is also necessary to distinguish among static and dynamic experimental approaches; the first referring to experiments such as immunolocalization of signaling molecules in fixed cells and the second to experimental approaches using imaging techniques of living sperm. Altogether, these experimental approaches will be essential to understand what is happening in the capacitating sperm cells and to discriminate certain features from degenerating sperm that can skew the conclusions of a particular experiment.

An additional problem derived from the division of the sperm in several structures is the distribution of energy among different compartments. Given that mitochondria are located in a specific region of the sperm, oxidative respiration and the consequent adenosine triphosphate (ATP) generation is restricted to the mid-piece of the flagellum. How then do other compartments such as the principal piece of the flagellum and the head of the sperm meet their energy needs? In sea urchin sperm, a phosphocreatine shuttle has been observed to transfer high-energy phosphate from the mitochondria to the principal piece (Tombes and Shapiro, 1985); however, this system is poorly developed or entirely absent in mammalian species (Kaldis et al., 1996). The findings of a unique hexokinase type 1 (HK1) in the head and in the entire flagellum (Visconti et al., 1996) as well as the discovery of glyceraldehyde-3-phosphate-dehydrogenase (GAPDH) in the fibrous sheath of several mammalian species (Bunch et al., 1998) suggest that glycolysis could be the source of energy for these extra-mitochondrial compartments. Moreover, GAPDH-S, the sperm-specific GAPDH is needed for motility and subsequently for fertilization as demonstrated by the analysis of knock-out mice for this enzyme (Miki et al., 2004). Supporting the importance of glycolysis in sperm motility, it has been shown that prior to capacitation, porcine and mouse sperm produce an important fraction of their ATP anaerobically, via the glycolytic pathway (Marin et al., 2003; Mukai and Okuno, 2004). Also, recent unpublished data from Sostaric and Gadella suggest that glycolysis is up regulated under incubation conditions that support hyperactive motility in bovine sperm. Altogether, these data suggest that glycolysis is important in the regulation of sperm motility and in the events leading to hyperactivation. It is necessary to stress the implications of these findings because the ATP and energy needs associated with capacitation are not restricted to the mid-piece of the sperm flagellum.

Finally, it is also important to take into consideration whether sperm capacitation is intrinsic to the sperm or whether there are first messengers from the female track involved in the induction of the capacitation response. It has been observed that certain factors isolated from the oviduct may support capacitation *in vivo* (Killian, 2004; McCauley *et al.*, 2003); however, the fact that sperm could be capacitated *in vitro* in a defined medium may argue against a female factor responsible for the induction of capacitation. If capacitation is intrinsic to the sperm, there are two main possibilities to analyze. First, sperm capacitation could be induced by a change in the environment, such as changes in HCO_3^- concentration or the presence of cholesterol acceptors *in vivo* and *in vitro*. Second, it is possible that in addition to these environmental changes, the sperm secretes a factor that is indeed responsible for capacitation. In this respect, incubation of sperm with the ether phospholipid 1-O-alkyl-2-acetyl-*sn*-glyceryl-3-phosphocholine, also known as platelet activating factor (PAF) in albumin-free media appears to increase the percentage of capacitated sperm based on the chlortetracycline (CTC) fluorescence assay (Huo and Yang, 2000). Recently, release of sperm PAF into the capacitation medium and binding to its receptor on the sperm membrane was shown to induce capacitation *in vitro* by an autocrine loop mechanism (Wu *et al.*, 2001). These different possibilities are open problems in the capacitation field.

6.3 Molecular basis of capacitation

To facilitate consideration of the complex cascade of molecular events that occur during capacitation, a discussion of this process may be divided into events that initiate capacitation and events that are a consequence of this process. Molecular events implicated in the initiation of capacitation include lipid rearrangements in the sperm plasma membrane, ion fluxes resulting in alteration of sperm membrane potential, and increased tyrosine (tyr) phosphorylation of proteins involved in induction of hyperactivation and the acrosome reaction. A working model for initiation of capacitation based on recent work is presented in Figure 6.1(see also Plate 7).

6.3.1 HCO_3^- and the cyclic adenosine monophosphate pathway in mammalian sperm

Multiple studies have shown that sperm capacitation is a HCO_3^--dependent process (Boatman and Robbins, 1991; Gadella and Harrison, 2000; Lee and Storey,

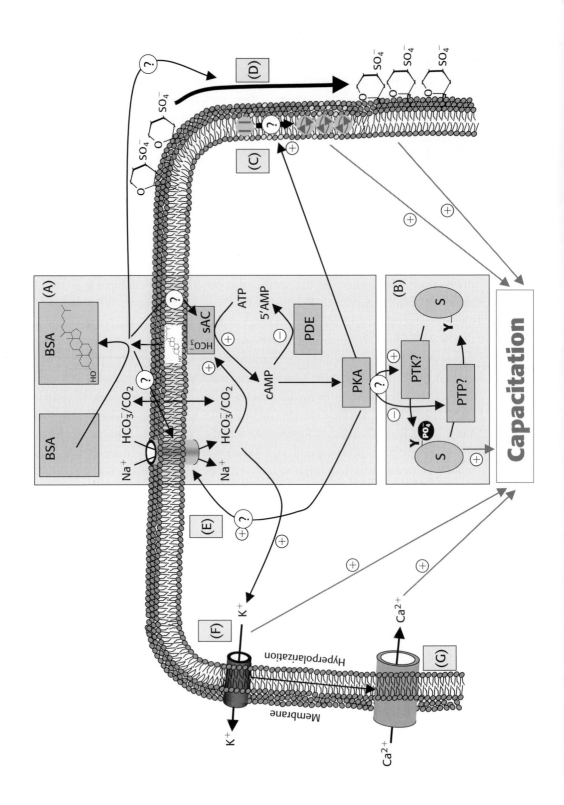

Figure 6.1   Capacitation signaling: proposed sequences of mammalian sperm capacitation. (A) Bicarbonate may enter sperm cells via a Na^+/HCO_3^- co-transporter or via diffusion as carbon dioxide. Intracellular bicarbonate switches on adenylyl cyclase (AC) and concomitant production of cyclic adenosine monophosphate (cAMP) activates protein kinase A (PKA). The role of cholesterol efflux in the activation of PKA is unclear. Cholesterol efflux may induce increased bicarbonate entry or may directly affect AC. (B) PKA induces tyr (Y) phosphorylation of several substrates (S) most likely via activation of protein tyr kinases (PTK) or inhibition of protein tyr phosphatases (PTP). PKA activation induces plasma membrane changes like in C and/or D. (C) Bilayer redistribution of aminophospholipids. (D) Lateral redistribution of seminolipid and cholesterol. The aminophospholipid scrambling is induced by PKA-dependent activation of a postulated scramblase. Most likely lateral redistribution of cholesterol is required before cholesterol depletion by bovine serum albumin (BSA). (E) The Na^+/HCO_3^- co-transporter could potentially be a substrate for PKA and may give rise to a sustained increase in HCO_3^- after its phosphorylation; thus having a positive feedback on cAMP synthesis. (F) Capacitation is also correlated with hyperpolarization of the sperm plasma membrane, which could be due to the opening of a potassium channel that senses alkalinization of the cytosol. (G) The consequent membrane hyperpolarization on turn may open voltage-dependent Ca^{2+} channels and induce the influx of Ca^{2+}. The increased tyr phosphorylation together with the ionic and lipidic changes in the membrane will induce downstream events involved in the process of capcitation (see Fig. 6.3). PDE: phosphodiesterase. (Adapted from Flesch and Gadella (2000) and Visconti and Kopf (1998).) (see Color plate 7)

1986; Neill and Olds-Clarke, 1987; Shi and Roldan, 1995; Visconti *et al.*, 1995a). Although little is known about the mechanisms of HCO_3^- transport in sperm, recent evidence strongly suggests that HCO_3^- transport in these cells is mediated by a member of the Na^+/HCO_3^- co-transporter family, as first described by Romero and Boron (1999). This conclusion is based on findings that HCO_3^- transport in sperm has the following properties (Demarco *et al.*, 2003):

(1) it is electrogenic,
(2) it is Na^+ dependent,
(3) it increases pHi,
(4) it is blocked by stilbenes, such as 4,4′-diisothiocyanostilbene-2,2′-disulfonic acid (DIDS).

The transmembrane movement of HCO_3^- has been associated with the increase in intracellular pH (pHi) observed during capacitation (Parrish *et al.*, 1989; Zeng *et al.*, 1996). The role of these changes in pHi is not well understood. A second target for HCO_3^- action is the regulation of cyclic adenosine monophosphate (cAMP) metabolism (Garbers *et al.*, 1982). In 1985, Okamura and collaborators (Okamura and Sugita, 1983) demonstrated that boar semen contained a low molecular weight factor able to induce pig sperm motility; this small factor was also able to stimulate adenylyl cyclase (AC), the enzyme responsible for cAMP synthesis. This factor was later purified to homogeneity and shown to be HCO_3^- (Okamura *et al.*, 1985). The finding that HCO_3^- can stimulate sperm AC was later confirmed in bovine and hamster spermatozoa (Garty *et al.*, 1988; Visconti *et al.*, 1990).

The increase in cAMP during capacitation and the stimulation of AC activity in sperm by increased levels of intracellular HCO_3^- implicate a role for this enzyme and the cAMP signaling pathway in capacitation. Two types of ACs are responsible for cAMP synthesis in eukaryotes; a very well studied family of isoforms, known as transmembrane adenylyl cyclases (tmACs), and a recently isolated soluble adenylyl cyclase (sAC) (Buck *et al.*, 1999). The sAC and tmACs are regulated by different pathways; sAC is insensitive to G-protein or forskolin regulation and is at least 10 times more active in the presence of Mn^{2+} than in the presence of Mg^{2+}. The identity of the AC activated in capacitating sperm has been the subject of multiple studies; although it is still controversial how many ACs are present in the sperm (Baxendale and Fraser, 2003), multiple evidences demonstrate that one of them is a post-translationally modified form of sAC. This conclusion is supported by the following facts:

(1) Similar to the sperm AC activity, the enzymatic activity of recombinant testicular sAC is stimulated by HCO_3^- anions (Chen *et al.*, 2000).
(2) Both the sperm AC as well as sAC is 20 times more active in the presence of Mn^{2+} when compared with the activity in the presence of Mg^{2+}.
(3) Antibodies against the catalytic domain of the testicular sAC recognized two sperm proteins corresponding to the deduced molecular masses of the processed

and unprocessed forms of the testicular enzyme (Chen *et al.*, 2000) suggesting that this cyclase remains associated with sperm after spermatogenesis.

(4) Antibodies against sAC can immunoprecipitate a fraction containing AC activity from mouse sperm (Chen *et al.*, 2000).

Interestingly, the sequence from the catalytic domain of this cyclase has sequence homology to cyanobacterial AC and the cyanobacterial cyclase is also HCO_3^- dependent (Chen *et al.*, 2000). Although the testis cyclase has been found in the soluble fraction, it is significant that cyclase activity identified in mammalian sperm remains associated with the particulate membrane fraction. Further research should clarify to which extent and how sAC becomes associated to sperm membranes as well as where this process occurs during spermatogenesis or later during epididymal maturation.

The HCO_3^--induced sAC activity results in increasing levels of cAMP in the cell (Harrison and Miller, 2000). One of the main targets for cAMP action is the cAMP-dependent protein kinase A (PKA), which is composed of two regulatory subunits and two catalytic subunits. Both regulatory subunits isoforms (I and II) are present in sperm (Vijayaraghavan *et al.*, 1997; Visconti *et al.*, 1997) but do not share the same sperm localization. PKA catalytic subunit has a unique N-terminal domain in the sperm and it is speculated that this domain is important for the localization of the catalytic subunit within the flagellum after PKA activation (San Agustin *et al.*, 1998). Once activated, PKA phosphorylates various target proteins which are presumed to initiate several signaling pathways (Harrison, 2004; Harrison and Miller, 2000). In pig sperm, the kinetics of the sperm sAC response to bicarbonate is extremely rapid. The cAMP rises to a maximum within 60 s (Harrison and Miller, 2000), and the increase in PKA-dependent protein phosphorylation begins within 90 s (Harrison, 2004). Functional changes are initiated equally as rapid. It is interesting that cAMP levels fall after their initial rise and then, after some 7 min, begin to rise again (although more slowly); PKA-catalyzed protein phosphorylation follows a similar time course. One possible explanation of this pulse response to bicarbonate with respect to cAMP levels could be the presence of a feedback mechanism in which the stimulated PKA phosphorylates the enzymes responsible for synthesis and degradation of cAMP, thereby modulating their activity (Hanoune and Defer, 2001; Mehats *et al.*, 2002). In this respect the following second rise in cAMP levels appears to surpass this feedback mechanism and has the kinetics of a sustained response to bicarbonate.

6.3.2 Changes that occur at the level of the plasma membrane (see Fig. 6.2)

It is accepted that some of the most important changes accompanying the capacitation process are at the level of the sperm plasma membrane. Capacitation-associated alterations in the sperm plasma membrane architecture can be rapid (Gadella and

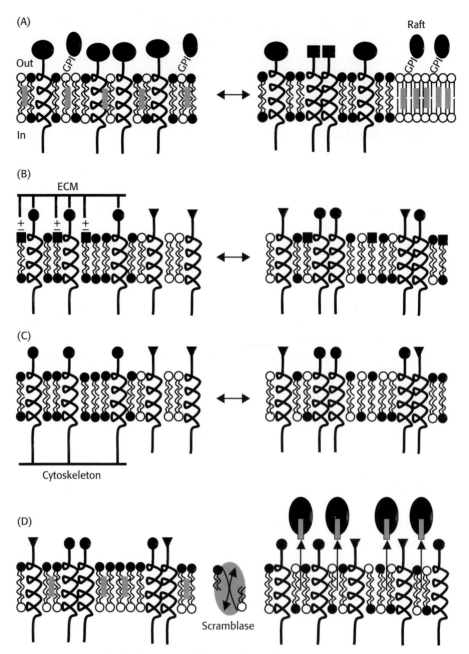

Figure 6.2   Current models for lateral membrane polarity dynamics upon sperm capacitation.
(A) Formation of lipid ordered microdomains in the membrane (lipid rafts) that exclude
freely diffusable transmembrane proteins and attracts GPI-anchored peripheral membrane
proteins. The raft area is presumably enriched in cholesterol and in saturated fatty acids
(for review see Rajendran and Simons (2005)). (B) The extracellular matrix (ECM)
surrounding the sperm in the female track is heterogeneous; therefore, the ECM may

Harrison, 2000, 2002; Harrison, 1996; Harrison and Miller, 2000) or slow (Flesch *et al.*, 2001b; Visconti *et al.*, 1999b). Interestingly, early changes in the sperm plasma membrane have been associated with the activation of the HCO_3^-/sAC/PKA pathway while the late effects are related with the presence of cholesterol acceptors in the *in vitro* incubation medium.

6.3.2.1 Early events (see Fig. 6.3)

For many years following the discovery of the bilayer structure of cell membrane lipids it was presumed that the component phospholipid species were distributed in a random fashion between the two lipid leaflets. However, some 30 years ago, it was discovered that the phospholipids are distributed asymmetrically, with sphingomyelin (SM) being essentially present only in the outer leaflet, phosphatidylcholine (PC) mostly in the outer leaflet, phosphatidylethanolamine (PE) mostly in the inner leaflet, and phosphatidylserine (PS) entirely confined to the inner leaflet (first reported by Verkleij *et al.* (1973)). More recent studies have shown that under normal conditions, this distribution is maintained by the combined activity of several phospholipid transferases: an aminophospholipid transferase ('flippase') that moves PS and PE from the outer to the inner leaflet; a non-specific phospholipid transferase ('floppase') that transfers phospholipids from the inner to the outer leaflet; and a bidirectional carrier ('scramblase') that moves all four phospholipids in both directions across the membrane bilayer. Although the phospholipid asymmetry is normally maintained throughout cell life, in certain circumstances the transverse asymmetry of the cell's plasma membrane collapses, with the result that PS and PE appear in the outer leaflet. Among other situations, such collapse (referred to as 'scrambling') is seen during activation of lymphocytes, during aging of red blood cells, and during apoptosis (see Balasubramanian and Schroit, 2003; Bevers *et al.*, 1998; Zachowski, 1993).

Although up to now most work on phospholipid asymmetry has been confined to mammalian somatic cells, recent investigations have shown that sperm plasma membrane phospholipids also show this characteristic, for example, ram (Pomorski *et al.*, 1995), bull (Nolan *et al.*, 1995), and boar (Gadella *et al.*, 1999). Furthermore, recent boar sperm studies have revealed that physiological levels of bicarbonate

Caption for fig. 6.2 (*cont.*)   assist in the creation of membrane domains via electrostatic interactions with glycolipids or with membrane proteins. Disruption of the ECM might allow mixing of lipids and proteins between the two lateral domains. (C) A similar scenario as described for B may be valid for the heterogeneous organization of the sperm cytoskeleton. (D) Processes A–C may be a result from an increase in disordered lipid packing in the sperm plasma membrane due to the bicarbonate induced phospholipids scrambling and related efflux of membrane cholesterol. (Adapted from Flesch and Gadella (2000))

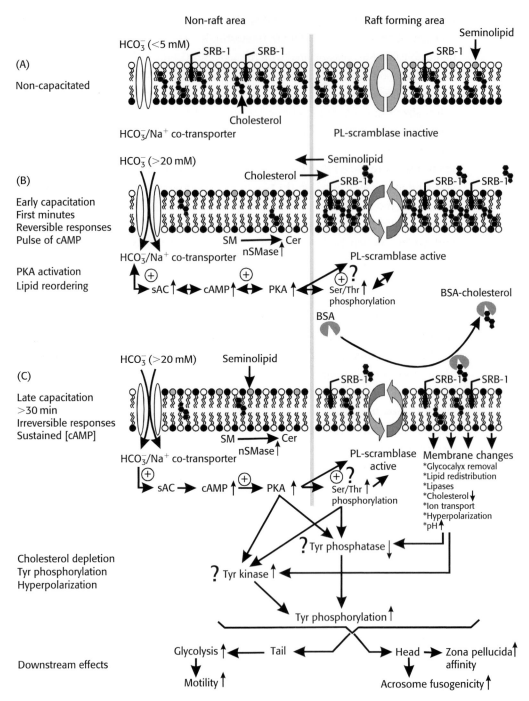

Figure 6.3   Early and sustained capacitation responses and relation to downstream events. (A) The non-capacitated sperm membrane (in low bicarbonate concentrations). Phospholipids are asymmetrically distributed over the membrane lipid bilayer, whereas sterols are diffuse

induce a collapse in the phospholipid asymmetry. The collapse is first seen as an increase in merocyanine stainability (Harrison *et al.*, 1996) and is subsequently detectable by direct staining of emergent surface PE and PS (Gadella and Harrison, 2002). The collapse is rapid, being first detectable after 2 min of incubation with 15 mM bicarbonate. Merocyanine stainability is maximal after 5 min, while the externalization of PE is maximal after 20 min. For a review about the relation of phospholipids asymmetry and merocyanine staining see Harrison and Gadella (2005). Analysis of phospholipid movements strongly suggests that the cause of the bicarbonate-induced collapse is an increase in the activity of a sperm scramblase (Gadella and Harrison, 2000). The resulting collapse ('scrambling') is reversible (at least in the short term (Harrison *et al.*, 1996)); it is mediated by PKA; and it is enhanced by protein phosphatase inhibitors (Gadella and Harrison, 2000; Harrison and Miller, 2000). Thus, one may deduce that the scramblase in spermatozoa is controlled directly or indirectly via a phosphorylation/dephosphorylation signaling pathway. In other cell types, the mechanisms of control of phospholipid asymmetry have not yet been elucidated, although it has been shown that scrambling can be induced in red blood cells through a rise in intracellular Ca^{2+}, which activates the scramblase and inhibits the flippase (Bevers *et al.*, 1998).

Three important points should be noted regarding HCO_3^--induced scrambling:

(1) It is not unique to boar spermatozoa but has also been detected in spermatozoa from human (de Vries *et al.*, 2003) and stallion (Rathi *et al.*, 2003); moreover, the investigations in humans have demonstrated that, as in boar, the phenomenon is driven via a PKA-dependent signaling pathway.

(2) While scrambling is a well-known characteristic of apoptosis (programmed cell death), HCO_3^--induced scrambling appears not to be related to this process in boar and human sperm. In fact, examples of non-apoptotic scrambling have been reported (Balasubramanian and Schroit, 2003).

Caption for fig. 6.3 (*cont.*)   distributed. The PKA signaling pathway is silent.
(B) Bicarbonate levels are high and enter the sperm cell by means of a Na^+/HCO_3^- co-transporter. The sAC/cAMP/PKA pathway is reversibly activated and induces ser/thr phosphorylation. Either directly or by indirect signaling pathways this lead to the activation of phospholipid scramblase causing a different lipid ordering (sperm raft aggregation and phospholipid scrambling). (C) Sustained bicarbonate influx possibly by PKA-dependent activation of the Na^+/HCO_3^- co-transporter (feed-forward principle, proposed in Fig. 6.1). The late responses become irreversible and the sustained membrane changes listed together with the rise in tyr phosphorylation of proteins will give rise to downstream events in the sperm tail (e.g. a rise in glycolysis and hyperactivated motility) and in the sperm head (e.g. increased zona affinity as well as acrosome fusogenicity which is zona dependent). SRB-1: Scavenger Receptor B type 1. (Adapted from Flesch *et al.* (2001a))

(3) HCO_3^--induced scrambling only takes place at physiological temperatures (Gadella and Van Gestel, 2004; Harrison and Gadella, 2005; Harrison et al., 1996).

6.3.2.2 Late events (see Fig. 6.3)

Serum albumin, a critical component of in vitro capacitation media, is believed to function as a sink for cholesterol by removing it from the sperm plasma membrane (Cross, 1996, 1998; Davis, 1981; Davis et al., 1979, 1980; Go and Wolf, 1985; Langlais and Roberts, 1985; Suzuki and Yanagimachi, 1989). Although serum albumin may have other roles during capacitation (Espinosa et al., 2000), its ability to facilitate cholesterol efflux is required for capacitation. For example, capacitation is inhibited by the addition of cholesterol and/or cholesterol analogs to the capacitation medium (Visconti et al., 1999b). Furthermore, to induce capacitation in vitro serum albumin can be substituted by cholesterol-binding compounds, such as high-density lipoproteins (HDL; Therien et al., 1997; Visconti et al., 1999b) and β-cyclodextrins (Choi and Toyoda, 1998; Cross, 1999; Osheroff et al., 1999; Visconti et al., 1999a).

As mentioned above, a very rapid lipid scrambling occurs as an early capacitation event. The major direct effect of scrambling observed so far is to enable and facilitate albumin-mediated cholesterol extraction (Flesch et al., 2001a; Gadella and Harrison, 2002). In pig sperm, albumin-mediated cholesterol depletion only occurs after the HCO_3^- induction of membrane lipid scrambling (Flesch et al., 2001a). The process may take place in two stages. In the absence of albumin, bicarbonate has the effect of altering the cholesterol distribution in the sperm head plasma membrane. Without HCO_3^- stimulation, cholesterol (measured using the cholesterol-binding antibiotic, filipin) is detected in both the post-acrosomal region and the acrosomal region; whereas in HCO_3^--stimulated cells, the post-acrosomal region is no longer labeled and the cholesterol is concentrated in the apical acrosomal region (Flesch et al., 2001a). In the presence of albumin, however, many of the HCO_3^--stimulated cells become largely devoid of filipin–cholesterol complexes in all regions of the head plasma membrane (de Vries et al., 2003; Flesch et al., 2001a; Gadella and Harrison, 2002; Visconti et al., 1999b). It was clear from these studies that the albumin-mediated cholesterol depletion was taking place in the same subpopulation that showed HCO_3^--induced lateral reorganization in the absence of albumin. These findings regarding the HCO_3^- dependence of cholesterol removal are very important with respect to establishing the initial sequence in capacitation. Results in pig sperm clearly show that the cholesterol loss is downstream of the HCO_3^-/cAMP pathway and follows the PKA-dependent collapse of phospholipid asymmetry. Nevertheless, it should be noticed that cholesterol efflux also modulates the cAMP pathway as was demonstrated in mouse sperm (Visconti et al., 1999b). A capacitation model should take into account cAMP involvement in both early and late capacitation-associated events. One possible hypothesis consistent with observations in several species is that initially, HCO_3^- transport increases cAMP levels and consequently PKA activity locally promoting scrambling but not other cAMP-dependent processes. Once scrambling occurs, cholesterol acceptors in the capacitation media, such as bovine serum albumin (BSA), are able to elicit cholesterol efflux. By some unknown mechanism this cholesterol exit has a feed-forward effect on HCO_3^- transport with the consequent activation of sAC and cAMP synthesis. This second more sustained increase of cAMP synthesis is likely to be responsible for late capacitation-associated processes, such as hyperactive motility and the increase in protein tyr phosphorylation.

Understanding how cholesterol efflux couples to the regulation of signal transduction pathways intrinsic to capacitation remains rudimentary at present. One possibility is that before capacitation, cholesterol concentrates in specialized sperm plasma membrane microdomains. It is now established that the lipids in a cell membrane display microheterogeneity due to the existence of dynamic complexes of cholesterol with sphingolipids (Brown and London, 2000; Simons and Ikonen, 1997, 2000; Simons and Vaz, 2004). These complexes, known as lipid rafts, sequester certain groups of membrane proteins; in addition, lipid rafts may also associate in a specific fashion with the cytoskeleton (Anderson and Jacobson, 2002; Kusumi *et al.*, 2004; Simons and Toomre, 2000).

Current concepts attribute important signaling properties to the existence of these rafts, acting as they do to bring protein assemblies together. Taking this into consideration, depletion or supplementation of cholesterol within the plasma membrane will have profound effects on the size and behavior of the raft complexes (for recent reviews, see Edidin, 2001; Mayorga *et al.*, 1994; Zajchowski and Robbins, 2002). In somatic cells, cholesterol removal is thought to disrupt lipid rafts, thus activating signaling events involving tyr kinases (TKs), G-proteins, and/or other molecules (Brown and London, 1998; Kabouridis *et al.*, 1997; Roy *et al.*, 1999). As the activation of similar signaling events during capacitation correlates to the removal of cholesterol from the plasma membrane, it can be hypothesized that in the sperm, cholesterol may likewise be concentrated in lipid rafts and that cholesterol efflux is related to changes in sperm lipid rafts. Supporting this hypothesis, in the last years, caveolin has been detected in the plasma membrane overlying the acrosomal region and the flagellum of mouse and guinea pig sperm (Travis *et al.*, 2000; Trevino *et al.*, 2001) suggesting the presence of a special type of lipid raft, called caveolae in these cells.

More recent studies have shown that a 2-h incubation in HCO_3^- and BSA-containing capacitation medium induces lateral redistribution of raft marker proteins such as the glycosyl phospatidyl inositol (GPI)-anchored cytoplasmic droplet (CD)59 and caveolin within the sperm head plasma membrane (Cross, 2004;

Shadan *et al.*, 2004). Although no particular sperm functional change has yet been ascribed to alterations of lipid raft structure and distribution, one may nevertheless expect that such changes, resulting from cholesterol removal, will have profound effects in subsequent signaling events. For example, it is now well established that cholesterol removal is necessary for the capacitation-associated increase in protein tyr phosphorylation observed in sperm (see below). It can be speculated that changes in lipid rafts play a role in this pathway (Edidin, 2001). In this respect, among human sperm incubated in the presence of HCO_3^-, only those with PE exposure in the apical head area showed extensive tyr phosphorylation in the tail (de Vries *et al.*, 2003) suggesting a tight connection between lipid changes and other capacitation-associated signaling events.

Capacitation has long been thought to involve the loss of coating proteins, leading to a different organization of the plasma membrane that some authors have described as membrane destabilization (references in Harrison (1996)). Such changes in the plasma membrane are clearly necessary to render the head plasma membrane fusogenic, not only with the underlying outer acrosomal membrane at the time of the acrosome reaction, but also with the oocyte plasma membrane at the time of sperm–egg fusion. Loss of coating proteins and membrane changes would expose surface receptors such as those through which the zona pellucida induces the acrosome reaction. Taking this into consideration, in addition to the lipid raft hypothesis, it is important to notice that removal of sterols decreases the cholesterol/phospholipid ratio as assessed by different criteria (Davis, 1981; Hoshi *et al.*, 1990; Tesarik and Flechon, 1986). This could further account for the membrane fluidity changes (Wolf and Cardullo, 1991; Wolf *et al.*, 1986) and redistribution of membrane proteins, observed with lectins (Cross and Overstreet, 1987) and antibodies (Rochwerger and Cuasnicu, 1992; Shalgi *et al.*, 1990) that occur during capacitation. One possible result of the HCO_3^--induced scrambling and subsequent loss of cholesterol could be to weaken the binding of surface proteins. Indeed, in both boar and ram sperm, HCO_3^- induces relatively slow alterations in the sperm surface coating (Ashworth *et al.*, 1995) visualized as a redistribution of seminolipid, a sperm-specific galacto-glycerolipid present in the outer lipid leaflet of the sperm plasma membrane (Gadella *et al.*, 1994, 1995). Other possible effects of changes in the sperm plasma membrane architecture are likely to be related to alterations in the steady-state intracellular ion concentrations with the resultant modification of the sperm resting plasma membrane potential. This topic is the focus of the following section.

6.3.3 Sperm plasma membrane potential

The role of ion flux in sperm function has been shown in multiple species (Darszon *et al.*, 2001). It is well established that ions play a role in the regulation of the acrosome reaction in sperm of both vertebrate and invertebrates. Other roles for ion transport in different aspects of sperm physiology have also been demonstrated. As examples, movement of ions has been associated with sperm motility (Gatti *et al.*, 1990; Morisawa and Suzuki, 1980), regulation of intracellular messengers (Visconti *et al.*, 1995b; Ward and Kopf, 1993), and mammalian sperm capacitation (Arnoult *et al.*, 1999; Zeng *et al.*, 1995). In all these cases, the *in vitro* influence of the external ion composition and the effect of channel blockers suggest that ion channels actively participate in the regulation of sperm function. During their transport through the male and female reproductive tracts, sperm are exposed to significant changes in their surrounding milieu. For example, the epididymal fluid is an environment that contains high K^+, low Na^+, and very low HCO_3^- concentrations (Brooks, 1983; Setchell *et al.*, 1994). After ejaculation, there is a drastic change in the ion concentrations, first in the seminal fluid and then in the female tract, K^+ is significantly reduced and the Na^+ and HCO_3^- concentrations are significantly increased (Brooks, 1983; Setchell *et al.*, 1994; Yanagimachi, 1994). As a consequence of these shifts in extracellular ion concentrations, there are changes in the intracellular concentrations of these ions that lead to alterations in the membrane potential of the sperm plasma membrane (Demarco *et al.*, 2003; Munoz-Garay *et al.*, 2001).

Mammalian sperm capacitation is accompanied by the hyperpolarization of the sperm plasma membrane (Zeng *et al.*, 1995). Hyperpolarization is observed as an increase in the intracellular negative charges when compared with the extracellular environment. What is the functional role of sperm plasma membrane hyperpolarization during capacitation? Florman and collaborators have speculated that since capacitation prepares the sperm for the acrosome reaction, capacitation-associated hyperpolarization may regulate the ability of sperm to generate transient intracellular Ca^{2+} elevations during acrosome reaction induced by physiological agonists (e.g. zona pellucida). In this respect, low voltage-activated (LVA) Ca^{2+} T channels currents have been measured in spermatogenic cells (Arnoult *et al.*, 1996; Lievano *et al.*, 1996); these channels may also be present in mature sperm. One unique property of LVA Ca^{2+} channels is that they are inactive at membrane potentials equivalent to those of sperm before capacitation (Arnoult *et al.*, 1996; Lievano *et al.*, 1996). Thus, if LVA Ca^{2+} T channels are involved in the regulation of the acrosome reaction, the sperm plasma membrane potential should hyperpolarize before they become able to undergo the acrosome reaction (Arnoult *et al.*, 1999; Florman *et al.*, 1998). Interestingly, individual sperm studies (Arnoult *et al.*, 1999) demonstrated that after 1 h capacitation, sperm can be divided into two different populations. Approximately 50% of the sperm remain at a membrane potential close to the uncapacitated population while the rest hyperpolarize to $-80\,mV$, a potential that can remove inactivation from LVA Ca^{2+} channels. Arnoult *et al.* (1999) demonstrated that only the hyperpolarized population was able to undergo the acrosome reaction when exposed to solubilized zona pellucidae.

Under normal conditions, sperm maintain an internal ion concentration markedly different from that in the extracellular medium. *In vitro*, the difference between intracellular and extracellular ion concentrations is determined by the relative permeability of the sperm plasma membrane to the ions that constitute the capacitation media. The ion composition of capacitation media mimics that of oviductal fluid (Yanagimachi, 1994). These media are high in Na^+ (about 130 mM) and Cl^- (about 100 mM), but low in K^+ (about 5.9 mM). Capacitation media also contain Ca^{2+} (about 2.7 mM) and HCO_3^- (10–25 mM). In contrast, intracellular fluids of sperm have a low concentration of Na^+ (about 14 mM) and high concentration of K^+ (about 90–120 mM) (Babcock, 1983; Zeng *et al.*, 1995). The free intracellular Ca^{2+} concentration of non-capacitated sperm is approximately 0.1 µM or less, but during the acrosome reaction it may increase to approximately 10 µM (Arnoult *et al.*, 1999; Bailey and Storey, 1994). To date, the intracellular concentrations of Cl^- and HCO_3^- in sperm have not been determined.

How are the changes in the sperm plasma membrane potential regulated? It can be hypothesized that the capacitation-associated hyperpolarization is the result of changes in the activity of ion-selective channels that control the extent of ion flow. Consistent with this hypothesis, different components of the capacitation media play important roles in the regulation of the sperm plasma membrane potential during capacitation. In mouse sperm, it has been shown that in the absence of BSA or HCO_3^- (Demarco *et al.*, 2003), the changes in membrane potential do not occur. These data suggest that HCO_3^- in the capacitation medium as well as cholesterol efflux may have a direct as well as an indirect function in controlling events leading to the hyperpolarization of the sperm plasma membrane. Additionally, it appears that membrane hyperpolarization may be partially due to an enhanced K^+ permeability as a result of a decrease in inhibitory modulation of K^+ channels (Zeng *et al.*, 1995). Recently, Muñoz-Garay *et al.* (2001) demonstrated with patch clamp techniques that inward rectifying K^+ channels are expressed in mouse spermatogenic cells and proposed that these channels may be responsible for the capacitation-associated membrane hyperpolarization. Consistent with this hypothesis, Ba^{2+} blocks these K^+ channels with an IC50 similar to that shown to inhibit the zona pellucida-induced acrosome reaction, one of the landmarks of capacitation. How the HCO_3^-, BSA, and different ion permeabilities integrate to regulate the changes in the sperm plasma membrane potential is not known and warrants further investigation.

6.3.4 Phosphorylation events during capacitation

Post-translational protein modifications through serine/threonine (ser/thr) or tyr phosphorylation by protein kinases and/or dephosphorylation of these residues by phosphoprotein phosphatases play a role in many cellular processes including transduction of extracellular signals, intracellular transport, and cell cycle progression

(Manning *et al.*, 2002). With the exception of PKA, kinase(s) involved in the regulation of sperm function are not well defined. Similarly, very little is known about the proteins undergoing phosphorylation during capacitation. Capacitation-associated changes in protein tyr phosphorylation have been demonstrated in multiple species including the mouse (Visconti *et al.*, 1995a), bovine (Galantino-Homer *et al.*, 1997), human (Leclerc *et al.*, 1996; Osheroff *et al.*, 1999), pig (Kalab *et al.*, 1998), and hamster (Devi *et al.*, 1999; Visconti *et al.*, 1999c). In addition, it has been demonstrated that the capacitation-associated increase in protein tyr phosphorylation is downstream of a cAMP/PKA pathway in mouse sperm (Visconti *et al.*, 1995b) and other species (Galantino-Homer *et al.*, 1997; Kalab *et al.*, 1998; Leclerc *et al.*, 1996; Osheroff *et al.*, 1999). This pathway appears to be tightly controlled by components in the capacitation medium; for example, in the absence of BSA, Ca^{2+}, or HCO_3^- neither capacitation nor the increase in tyr phosphorylation is observed. Furthermore, concentrations of these compounds needed for tyr phosphorylation are correlated with those required for capacitation (Visconti *et al.*, 1995a). As discussed in previous sections, HCO_3^- modulates the sustained cAMP pathway in sperm; therefore, its role in the regulation of tyr phosphorylation is likely to be associated with this sustained up regulation of the cAMP pathway in sperm. Two recent publications illustrate this point; first, sperm from mice that lack sAC do not display changes in their tyr phosphorylation pattern after incubation in a capacitation-supporting media (Esposito *et al.*, 2004); second, sperm from knock-out mice lacking C2α, the testis-specific PKA catalytic subunit, are not able to move actively and are unable to undergo the increase in tyr phosphorylation observed in wild type mouse (Nolan *et al.*, 2004). These knock-out mice confirm results obtained using cAMP agonists and antagonists on the capacitation-associated increase in tyr phosphorylation.

There are two important points to have in mind when analyzing the PKA pathway in sperm capacitation. First, as mentioned above, the HCO_3^-/cAMP pathway is involved in rapid and slow events related with capacitation. The rapid effect of HCO_3^- and PKA activation on lipid scrambling and phosphorylation of certain protein substrates (Harrison, 2004) is on a different time scale to its effect on protein tyr phosphorylation. The former occurs within 5 min of incubation in capacitation media while the later is detectable only after a longer incubation that varies dependent on the species, being around 45 min in mouse (Visconti *et al.*, 1995a) and more than 60 min in boar sperm (Harrison, unpublished observations). Second, PKA is a ser/thr kinase that is not able to directly phosphorylate proteins on tyr residues; thus, an intermediate TK must be involved in capacitation. Three possible mechanisms of interaction between PKA and protein tyr phosphorylation are as follows:

(1) Direct or indirect stimulation of a TK by PKA (a ser/thr kinase).
(2) Direct or indirect inhibition of a tyr phosphatase.

(3) Direct or indirect phosphorylation of proteins by PKA on ser or thr residues that prime these proteins for subsequent phosphorylation by a TK.

We discriminate between direct effects (e.g. when the enzymes involved in the signaling cross-talk are directly phosphorylated by PKA) and indirect effects (e.g. when PKA phosphorylation affect other intermediary pathways, such as other kinases, membrane reorganization, and/or ionic fluxes). These inter-related possibilities are currently being explored. It is predicted that identification of specific enzymes and substrates involved in the PKA/tyr phosphorylation signaling cross-talk pathways will improve our knowledge of sperm capacitation.

Recently, several groups have made efforts to identify the protein substrates that undergo tyr phosphorylation during capacitation. In this respect, the use of two-dimensional polyacrylamide gel electrophoresis (2-D PAGE) followed by mass spectrometry (MS/MS) provides a comprehensive approach to the analysis of proteins involved in cell signaling (Alms *et al.*, 1999; Blomberg, 1997; Lewis *et al.*, 2000; Soskic *et al.*, 1999). Specifically, changes in tyr phosphorylation can be monitored using 2-D PAGE (Gorg *et al.*, 1988; O'Farrell, 1975) followed by Western blot analysis with anti-phosphotyrosine antibodies. Proteins that undergo changes in tyr phosphorylation during cellular processes can then be isolated from a duplicated gel stained with silver and sequenced by tandem mass spectrometry MS/MS. This approach has been used to identify sperm proteins that undergo tyr phosphorylation during capacitation (Asquith *et al.*, 2004; Ficarro *et al.*, 2003; Mitra and Shivaji, 2004). When analyzing these works it is important to keep in mind that although identification of tyr phosphorylation substrates using 2-D PAGE strongly suggests that a given protein is phosphorylated on tyrosine residues, a full demonstration requires the use of independent methods (e.g. cross-reaction in immunoprecipitation experiments, direct sequencing, mutagenesis analysis). Similar approaches have been attempted with antibodies directed to consensus phosphorylation sequences. Noteworthy, recent studies used antibodies against consensus PKA phosphorylated sequences. These antibodies recognized a series of proteins after treatment with HCO_3^-, among them is oviduct fluid (ODF), a protein from the sperm outer dense fibers (Harrison, 2004).

Identification of phosphorylation substrates using 2-D PAGE is a powerful approach. However, although in some cases it is possible to get the exact site of phosphorylation of a candidate protein, more often the phosphorylation site remains elusive due to the presence of more abundant not phosphorylated peptides. Recently, direct sequencing of phosphopeptides by MS/MS has been attempted in human sperm (Ficarro *et al.*, 2003). In this work, the authors used Fe^{3+}-immobilized metal affinity chromatography (IMAC) prior to MS/MS to enrich sperm digests for peptides containing phosphorylated amino acids. To increase the selectivity of the IMAC column for phosphopeptides, acidic residues (i.e. glutamic and aspartic acid) were converted to methyl esters to block their binding to iron before IMAC was employed. Using this methodology, 5 sites of tyr, 56 sites of ser, and 2 sites of thr phosphorylation were characterized in capacitated human sperm (Ficarro *et al.*, 2003). Similar to other high-throughput methodologies, such as microarrays, the advantage of a global MS/MS approach to identify phosphopeptides is that this methodology is unbiased and is able to generate large amount of data in a relatively short time. On the minus side, these high-throughput techniques are often regarded as a descriptive analysis of a particular problem. More information can be achieved when these techniques are used to analyze functional changes occurring in a biological process. In the case of sperm capacitation, this goal could be achieved by comparison of the ratio of any particular phosphopeptide present in digests of proteins from capacitated and non-capacitated sperm cells. For this, the two populations should be labeled differentially. If the analysis is based in mass spectrometry, differential labeling could be achieved by the use of a different isotope of hydrogen for each sample. Ficarro *et al.* (2003) have used this method to compare human sperm before and after capacitation and were able to show a capacitation dependent increase in serine phosphorylation of A-kinase anchoring protein 3 (AKAP 3). Although this work has only identified one phosphopeptide, the methodology described here could potentially unveil other phosphorylation reactions in the near future.

Protein kinases play a pivotal role in intracellular signal transduction systems. Considering the importance of phosphorylation in the regulation of cellular mechanisms, it is not surprising that several protein kinases have been shown to be involved in spermatogenesis (Sassone-Corsi, 1997). However, it is not known whether kinases expressed in the testis are present or not in the mature sperm. As mentioned above the best-characterized kinase in sperm is PKA (Visconti *et al.*, 2002). Few other kinases have been described in mature mammalian sperm using antibodies; some of them are protein kinase C (PKC) (Rotem *et al.*, 1990), glycogen synthase kinase 3 (GSK 3) (Vijayaraghavan *et al.*, 2000), casein kinase II (Chaudhry *et al.*, 1991a, b), mitogen-activated protein kinase (MAP kinase) (Luconi *et al.*, 1998), and at least one member of the testis-specific serine kinase (Tssk) family (Hao *et al.*, 2004).

While these results show the presence of these kinases in the sperm, their role in sperm function is not yet understood. Even less is known about the identity of TKs in sperm. Although proteins with TK activity have been purified from boar (Berruti, 1994) and hamster sperm (Uma Devi *et al.*, 2000), the identity of the kinase responsible for this activity is still not known. There is some evidence on the presence of TK c-yes (Leclerc and Goupil, 2002) and also of a TK receptor in human sperm zona receptor kinase (ZRK) (Burks *et al.*, 1995); however, these reports have not been confirmed. Recently, Leclerc and collaborators have found janus kinase 1 (JAK 1) in human sperm and have shown that cytokines are able to stimulate this kinase (Laflamme *et al.*, 2005). This result could potentially open new avenues of investigation on first messenger involvement in the regulation of capacitation. Protein kinases are also important from the pharmacological point of view. These enzymes have become major targets for the development of novel drugs. Progress in the field of small molecule library generation using combinatorial chemistry methods coupled to high-throughput screening has accelerated the search for ideal cell-permeable inhibitors. In addition, structural-based design using crystallographic methods has improved the ability to characterize ligand–protein interaction sites that can be exploited for ligand design. Development of novel kinase inhibitors should be based on the combination of these technologies. In this respect, a sperm-specific kinase with an important role in capacitation will offer new opportunities towards an alternative approach for contraception.

6.3.5 Ca^{2+} and capacitation

Numerous studies have demonstrated that capacitation is Ca^{2+} dependent. The initiation and/or regulation of capacitation Ca^{2+} occurs via different targets, some of which are involved with cAMP metabolism. Since Ca^{2+} calmodulin can activate both the synthesis of cAMP by AC (Gross et al., 1987), as well as degradation by cAMP cyclic nucleotide phosphodiesterase (Wasco and Orr, 1984), it is not surprising that Ca^{2+} has both positive and negative actions on capacitation and related signaling events. In this respect, the effect of Ca^{2+} on the capacitation-associated increase in tyr phosphorylation is controversial. In the mouse, there is evidence supporting a positive (Visconti et al., 1995a, b) as well as a negative effect of Ca^{2+} in this pathway (Baker et al., 2004). In human sperm, Ca^{2+} has been demonstrated to inhibit protein tyr phosphorylation during the first 2 h of in vitro capacitation (Carrera et al., 1996; Luconi et al., 1996).

6.4 Hyperactivated motility

Hyperactivated motility refers to the changes in the pattern of flagellar beat that is observed in mammalian sperm as a result of capacitation. These changes in swimming behavior were reported first in the hamster and in the guinea pig by Yanagimachi (1970, 1972); followed by observations in the mouse (Fraser, 1977), dog (Mahi and Yanagimachi, 1976), and rabbit (Overstreet and Cooper, 1978). Since these initial reports, hyperactivation has been observed in sperm during in vitro capacitation and in sperm flushed from the oviduct near the time of fertilization. It is believed that hyperactivation enables sperm to penetrate mucoid oviductal secretions and the intercellular matrix in the cumulus oophorus, and also has a role after the acrosome reaction to help the penetration of the zona pellucida. As hyperactivation is believed to be necessary for fertilization to occur, this process is usually considered as part of the capacitation process. Hyperactivation is most likely related to signaling events occurring in the flagellum of the sperm. Although in general the studies on capacitation have not addressed the localization of the signaling pathways under investigation, it can be postulated that several of the changes reported to be associated with capacitation might correspond to signaling pathways linked to hyperactivated motility. Signaling and ionic events involved in motility and probably in the induction of hyperactivated motility are recently becoming clearer from normozoospermic knock-out mice whose sperm fail to develop normal and/or hyperactivated motility. Two of these knock outs are the aforementioned null mutant mouse for sAC (Esposito *et al.*, 2004) and the one for the sperm-specific PKA catalytic subunit (Nolan *et al.*, 2004). These mutant mice are both infertile due to lack of sperm motility and deficiency in HCO_3^--induced capacitation responses.

In the case of the sAC knock out, these defects were restored by addition of membrane permeable cAMP analogs to the sperm incubation medium. Another immotile infertile phenotype was obtained by silencing the two genes coding for sodium–hydrogen exchangers (NHE1 and NHE5) (Wang *et al.*, 2003). In these mice, addition of cAMP agonists is able to restore motility and fertility through direct activation of PKA. Another interesting phenotype is found in null mutants of a novel testis-specific family of cationic channels, CatSper 1 (Ren *et al.*, 2001) and CatSper 2 (Quill *et al.*, 2003). Sperm from the respective knock out of each of these genes also showed defects in hyperactivation despite normal tyr phosphorylation response (Carlson *et al.*, 2003). Interestingly, these mice present defects in the cAMP-induced increase in flagellar Ca^{2+} first described by Wiesner *et al.* (1998). Therefore, hyperactivated sperm motility appears to involve ionic changes upstream and downstream of the HCO_3^--stimulated cAMP/PKA pathway.

Other interesting knock-out studies strongly suggest that glycolytic enzymes in the tail are crucial for motility; null mutant mice for the sperm's fibrous sheath-specific glycolytic enzyme GAPDH-S are immotile (Miki *et al.*, 2004). In this respect, freshly ejaculated sperm cells produce >90% of their ATP by anaerobic metabolism and blocking of aerobic ATP production did not result in either a reduction of ATP levels or in decreasing sperm motility (Marin *et al.*, 2003; Mukai and Okuno, 2004). It is therefore likely that hyperactivated motility is a result of a further speeding up of glycolysis as the ATP production rate should equal the enhanced ATP consumption rate required for the hyperactive motility state.

6.5 Preparation for the acrosome reaction

In addition to the changes in motility pattern, capacitation is usually defined as a necessary process for the agonist-induced acrosome reaction. In this context, questions that are necessary to keep in mind when analyzing the capacitation process are: Why cannot acrosomal exocytosis occur before capacitation? Which molecular changes are necessary to allow an agonist, such as the *zona pellucida* to induce the acrosome reaction? As a first approach, to understand the link between capacitation and the acrosome reaction, an increased knowledge of the mechanisms that regulate this exocytotic event in sperm is necessary. Exocytosis is a tightly regulated, complex process that involves fusion of a subcellular vesicle, for example, acrosome, with its target membrane, for example, overlying plasma membrane, and the subsequent release of vesicle contents. Recent evidence suggests that membrane fusion is governed by a few conserved protein families regardless of whether membrane fusion occurs between intracellular organelles or between trafficking vesicles and the plasma membrane. Proteins involved in fusion events include a family of proteins commonly referred to as SNARE proteins (soluble N-ethylmaleimide-sensitive attachment protein receptors; Jahn and Sudhof, 1999). Sperm homologues of SNARE proteins as well as SNARE-associated proteins, such as Rab 3A and NSF (N-ethylmaleimide-sensitive factor), have been detected in sea urchin (Schulz *et al.*, 1997, 1998) and mammalian sperm (Michaut *et al.*, 2000; Ramalho-Santos *et al.*, 2000; Yunes *et al.*, 2000). These observations support the idea that the sperm acrosome reaction might be regulated in similar ways as exocytotic processes in somatic cells. It is also clear that the induction of the acrosome reaction requires calcium influxes and that the opening of these channels are linked to the activation of G-protein coupled receptors (Florman *et al.*, 1989; Ward *et al.*, 1992). Altogether this emerging knowledge on the regulation of the acrosome reaction brings up the following hypothesis about how capacitation might be linked to the acrosome reaction:

(1) a receptor(s) molecule changes its conformation during capacitation allowing recognition by specific agonists, such as the zona pellucida and/or progesterone;
(2) molecular changes occurring during capacitation couple downstream signaling molecules to the receptor;
(3) proteins directly related to exocytosis, such as the aforementioned SNAREs become docked and primed for membrane fusion during capacitation;
(4) changes in the plasma membrane lipid composition and architecture that increase the fusogenic nature of the plasma membrane;
(5) capacitation-associated changes in the sperm plasma membrane potential resulting in modifications of ion channel properties;
(6) a combination of all these possibilities.

Although it is still not understood which of these possibilities is correct, they can give a mark of reference to the study of capacitation.

6.6 Some precautions when working on sperm capacitation

Sperm capacitation is a lengthy process in which early changes take place as rapidly as 1 min whereas full capacitation is accomplished within hours (depending on the mammalian species of interest). Therefore, one cannot design a single *in vitro* capacitation assay, and the existing assays discriminate non-responding from responding cells at different time intervals of capacitation (Flesch *et al.*, 2001a). As it is generally considered that capacitation destabilizes sperm cells, it is important to avoid artificial destabilization of the sperm plasma membrane. In this respect, when measuring capacitation, one important parameter to consider is the temperature at which the sperm are capacitated. For example, in pig sperm, capacitation *in vitro* is usually performed at 38°C, the physiological temperature, in a tube that is placed under a 5% CO_2 humidified atmosphere, instead in mouse and human capacitation is performed at 37°C (Marin-Briggiler *et al.*, 2002; Visconti *et al.*, 1995a). Under these conditions, sperm can be kept alive for hours without notable cell decay. On the other hand, cooling of the sperm only slightly to 30°C results in cell deterioration and false acrosome reactions (Gadella and Harrison, 2000); in fact these membrane alterations resemble the ones observed after freeze thawing of sperm cells. Consequently the latter phenomenon has been described as cryocapacitation (Green and Watson, 2001); however, the validity of this concept has not been tested and is subject of debate (Cornelius, 1995; Pommer *et al.*, 2003). Similarly, it is important to be careful when cholesterol acceptors, such as β-cyclodextrins, are used. These compounds could potentially disrupt membranes in the bicarbonate responsive cells (by virtue of lipid modifications) resulting in detection of an increased percentage of the spontaneous acrosome reactions (Visconti *et al.*, 1999a) and will not shed new light on the mechanisms involved in capacitation and the physiologically induced acrosome reaction.

A battery of assays have been used to measure capacitation, these can be classified as follows:
(1) Assays that observed the physiological state of the sperm, such as the ability of the sperm to fertilize an egg *in vitro*, the onset of the spontaneous acrosome reaction, and the percentage of cells undergoing an agonist-induced acrosome reaction.
(2) Assays that used changes in fluorescent patterns, such as the changes observed when the sperm are stained with the antibiotic CTC.
(3) Assays that use correlates of capacitation, such as the aforementioned phospholipid scrambling or the increase in tyr phosphorylation.
(4) Assays that consider the percentage of hyperactivated sperm.
(5) Assays that used pharmacological agents to induce the acrosome reaction, such as phorbol esters, lysophospholipids, or Ca^{2+} ionophore.

All these assays present advantages and disadvantages. For example, although only capacitated sperm are able to fertilize an egg, a failure in fertilization could be due to multiple factors such as an impediment in the ability to acrosome react. Another example is the use of CTC; this probe binds in a calcium-dependent manner to the surface of sperm and this intrinsic molecular property makes CTC questionable for discriminating the calcium-dependent and -independent pathways leading to capacitation (de Vries *et al.*, 2003; Rathi *et al.*, 2001). Finally, it is important to consider that pharmacological agents (like calcium ionophores and lysophospholipids) could potentially bypass the capacitation process (Yanagimachi, 1994). Due to restrictions in the length of this chapter these methods will not be analyzed in detail (for an overview of current multiparametric flow cytometric evaluation of sperm properties for review see Gillan *et al.* (2005)); however, it is important when analyzing a particular set of results to recognize the limitation of each of these methodologies.

6.7 Discussion and summary

In this chapter, we have attempted to review some of the advances in the sperm capacitation field in the last years. Although the molecular basis of this phenomenon is still not well understood, the use of novel technologies such as flow cytometry, single cell analysis and tandem mass spectrometry in combination with the examination of knock-out mice with phenotypes involving capacitation will result in considerable advances in our understanding of this process. As a final note, it should be highlighted that most of our knowledge of sperm capacitation is coming from *in vitro* experiments. While these observations are important, it should be taking into account for future studies the ability of the female tract to control the speed of capacitation and to deliver freshly capacitated sperm to all of the ovulated eggs. Comparison between *in vivo* and *in vitro* capacitation will be necessary to fully understand the capacitation process and warrant continued investigation in this field.

Acknowledgments

P.V. was supported by the National Institutes of Health, Grant HD38082 and HD44044. B.G. was supported by grants of the Royal Dutch Academy of Sciences and Arts (KNAW), the European Union Human Capability and Mobility Program (EU HCM), and the Dutch Research Council for Medical Sciences (NWO MW).

REFERENCES

Alms GR, Sanz P, Carlson M and Haystead TA (1999) Reg1p targets protein phosphatase 1 to dephosphorylate hexokinase II in *Saccharomyces cerevisiae*: characterizing the effects of a phosphatase subunit on the yeast proteome. *Embo J* 18, 4157–4168.

Anderson RG and Jacobson K (2002) A role for lipid shells in targeting proteins to caveolae, rafts, and other lipid domains. *Science* 296, 1821–1825.

Arnoult C, Cardullo RA, Lemos JR and Florman HM (1996) Activation of mouse sperm T-type Ca2+ channels by adhesion to the egg zona pellucida. *Proc Natl Acad Sci USA* 93, 13004–13009.

Arnoult C, Kazam IG, Visconti PE, Kopf GS, Villaz M and Florman HM (1999) Control of the low voltage-activated calcium channel of mouse sperm by egg ZP3 and by membrane hyperpolarization during capacitation. *Proc Natl Acad Sci USA* 96, 6757–6762.

Ashworth PJ, Harrison RA, Miller NG, Plummer JM and Watson PF (1995) Flow cytometric detection of bicarbonate-induced changes in lectin binding in boar and ram sperm populations. *Mol Reprod Dev* 40, 164–176.

Asquith KL, Baleato RM, McLaughlin EA, Nixon B and Aitken RJ (2004) Tyrosine phosphorylation activates surface chaperones facilitating sperm-zona recognition. *J Cell Sci* 117, 3645–3657.

Austin CR (1951) Observations on the penetration of the sperm in the mammalian egg. *Aust J Sci Res* (B)4, 581–596.

Babcock DF (1983) Examination of the intracellular ionic environment and of ionophore action by null point measurements employing the fluorescein chromophore. *J Biol Chem* 258, 6380–6389.

Bailey JL and Storey BT (1994) Calcium influx into mouse spermatozoa activated by solubilized mouse zona pellucida, monitored with the calcium fluorescent indicator, fluo-3. Inhibition of the influx by three inhibitors of the zona pellucida induced acrosome reaction: tyrphostin A48, pertussis toxin, and 3-quinuclidinyl benzilate. *Mol Reprod Dev* 39, 297–308.

Baker MA, Hetherington L, Ecroyd H, Roman SD and Aitken RJ (2004) Analysis of the mechanism by which calcium negatively regulates the tyrosine phosphorylation cascade associated with sperm capacitation. *J Cell Sci* 117, 211–222.

Balasubramanian K and Schroit AJ (2003) Aminophospholipid asymmetry: a matter of life and death. *Annu Rev Physiol* 65, 701–734.

Baldi E, Luconi M, Bonaccorsi L, Muratori M and Forti G (2000) Intracellular events and signaling pathways involved in sperm acquisition of fertilizing capacity and acrosome reaction. *Front Biosci* 5, E110–E123.

Baxendale RW and Fraser LR (2003) Evidence for multiple distinctly localized adenylyl cyclase isoforms in mammalian spermatozoa. *Mol Reprod Dev* 66, 181–189.

Berruti G (1994) Biochemical characterization of the boar sperm 42 kilodalton protein tyrosine kinase: its potential for tyrosine as well as serine phosphorylation towards microtubule-associated protein 2 and histone H 2B. *Mol Reprod Dev* 38, 386–392.

Bevers EM, Comfurius P, Dekkers DW, Harmsma M and Zwaal RF (1998) Transmembrane phospholipid distribution in blood cells: control mechanisms and pathophysiological significance. *Biol Chem* 379, 973–986.

Blomberg A (1997) Osmoresponsive proteins and functional assessment strategies in *Saccharomyces cerevisiae*. *Electrophoresis* 18, 1429–1440.

Boatman DE and Robbins RS (1991) Bicarbonate: carbon-dioxide regulation of sperm capacitation, hyperactivated motility, and acrosome reactions. *Biol Reprod* 44, 806–813.

Brooks DE (1983) Epididymal functions and their hormonal regulation. *Aust J Biol Sci* 36, 205–221.

Brown DA and London E (1998) Functions of lipid rafts in biological membranes. *Annu Rev Cell Dev Biol* 14, 111–136.

Brown DA and London E (2000) Structure and function of sphingolipid- and cholesterol-rich membrane rafts. *J Biol Chem* 275, 17221–17224.

Buck J, Sinclair ML, Schapal L, Cann MJ and Levin LR (1999) Cytosolic adenylyl cyclase defines a unique signaling molecule in mammals. *Proc Natl Acad Sci USA* 96, 79–84.

Bunch DO, Welch JE, Magyar PL, Eddy EM and O'Brien DA (1998) Glyceraldehyde 3-phosphate dehydrogenase-S protein distribution during mouse spermatogenesis. *Biol Reprod* 58, 834–841.

Burks DJ, Carballada R, Moore HD and Saling PM (1995) Interaction of a tyrosine kinase from human sperm with the zona pellucida at fertilization. *Science* 269, 83–86.

Carlson AE, Westenbroek RE, Quill T, Ren D, Clapham DE, Hille B, Garbers DL and Babcock DF (2003) CatSper1 required for evoked Ca2+ entry and control of flagellar function in sperm. *Proc Natl Acad Sci USA* 100, 14864–14868.

Carrera A, Moos J, Ning XP, Gerton GL, Tesarik J, Kopf GS and Moss SB (1996) Regulation of protein tyrosine phosphorylation in human sperm by a calcium/calmodulin-dependent mechanism: identification of a kinase anchor proteins as major substrates for tyrosine phosphorylation. *Dev Biol* 180, 284–296.

Chang MC (1951) Fertilizing capacity of spermatozoa deposited into the fallopian tubes. *Nature* 168, 697–698.

Chaudhry PS, Nanez R and Casillas ER (1991a) Purification and characterization of polyamine-stimulated protein kinase (casein kinase II) from bovine spermatozoa. *Arch Biochem Biophys* 288, 337–342.

Chaudhry PS, Newcomer PA and Casillas ER (1991b) Casein kinase I in bovine sperm: purification and characterization. *Biochem Biophys Res Commun* 179, 592–598.

Chen Y, Cann MJ, Litvin TN, Iourgenko V, Sinclair ML, Levin LR and Buck J (2000) Soluble adenylyl cyclase as an evolutionarily conserved bicarbonate sensor. *Science* 289, 625–628.

Choi YH and Toyoda Y (1998) Cyclodextrin removes cholesterol from mouse sperm and induces capacitation in a protein-free medium. *Biol Reprod* 59, 1328–1333.

Cohen-Dayag A and Eisenbach M (1994) Potential assays for sperm capacitation in mammals. *Am J Physiol* 267, C1167–C1176.

Cornelius F (1995) Phosphorylation/dephosphorylation of reconstituted shark Na+, K(+)-ATPase: one phosphorylation site per alpha beta protomer. *Biochim Biophys Acta* 1235, 197–204.

Cross NL (1996) Effect of cholesterol and other sterols on human sperm acrosomal responsiveness. *Mol Reprod Dev* 45, 212–217.

Cross NL (1998) Role of cholesterol in sperm capacitation. *Biol Reprod* 59, 7–11.

Cross NL (1999) Effect of methyl-beta-cyclodextrin on the acrosomal responsiveness of human sperm. *Mol Reprod Dev* 53, 92–98.

Cross NL (2004) Reorganization of lipid rafts during capacitation of human sperm. *Biol Reprod* 71, 1367–1373.

Cross NL and Overstreet JW (1987) Glycoconjugates of the human sperm surface: distribution and alterations that accompany capacitation *in vitro*. *Gamete Res* 16, 23–35.

Darszon A, Beltran C, Felix R, Nishigaki T and Trevino CL (2001) Ion transport in sperm signaling. *Dev Biol* 240, 1–14.

Davis BK (1981) Timing of fertilization in mammals: sperm cholesterol/phospholipid ratio as a determinant of the capacitation interval. *Proc Natl Acad Sci USA* 78, 7560–7564.

Davis BK, Byrne R and Hungund B (1979) Studies on the mechanism of capacitation. II. Evidence for lipid transfer between plasma membrane of rat sperm and serum albumin during capacitation *in vitro*. *Biochim Biophys Acta* 558, 257–266.

Davis BK, Byrne R and Bedigian K (1980) Studies on the mechanism of capacitation: albumin-mediated changes in plasma membrane lipids during *in vitro* incubation of rat sperm cells. *Proc Natl Acad Sci USA* 77, 1546–1550.

de Lamirande E, Leclerc P and Gagnon C (1997) Capacitation as a regulatory event that primes spermatozoa for the acrosome reaction and fertilization. *Mol Human Reprod* 3, 175–194.

Demarco IA, Espinosa F, Edwards J, Sosnik J, De La Vega-Beltran JL, Hockensmith JW, Kopf GS, Darszon A and Visconti PE (2003) Involvement of a Na+/HCO-3 cotransporter in mouse sperm capacitation. *J Biol Chem* 278, 7001–7009.

Devi KU, Jha K and Shivaji S (1999) Plasma membrane-associated protein tyrosine phosphatase activity in hamster spermatozoa. *Mol Reprod Dev* 53, 42–50.

de Vries KJ, Wiedmer T, Sims PJ and Gadella BM (2003) Caspase-independent exposure of aminophospholipids and tyrosine phosphorylation in bicarbonate responsive human sperm cells. *Biol Reprod* 68, 2122–2134.

Eddy EM and O'Brien DA (1994) The spermatozoon. In: *The Physiology of Reproduction*, Vol. 1, eds E Knobil and JD Neill, New York: Raven Press, pp. 29–77.

Edidin M (2001) Membrane cholesterol, protein phosphorylation, and lipid rafts. *Sci STKE* 2001, PE1.

Espinosa F, Lopez-Gonzalez I, Munoz-Garay C, Felix R, De la Vega-Beltran JL, Kopf GS, Visconti PE and Darszon A (2000) Dual regulation of the T-type Ca(2+) current by serum albumin and beta-estradiol in mammalian spermatogenic cells. *FEBS Lett* 475, 251–526.

Esposito G, Jaiswal BS, Xie F *et al.* (2004) Mice deficient for soluble adenylyl cyclase are infertile because of a severe sperm-motility defect. *Proc Natl Acad Sci USA* 101, 2993–2998.

Ficarro S, Chertihin O, Westbrook VA *et al.* (2003) Phosphoproteome analysis of human sperm. Evidence of tyrosine phosphorylation of AKAP 3 and valosin containing protein/P97 during capacitation. *J Biol Chem* 278, 11579–11589.

Flesch FM and Gadella BM (2000) Dynamics of the mammalian sperm plasma membrane in the process of fertilization. *Biochim Biophys Acta* 1469, 197–235.

Flesch FM, Brouwers JF, Nievelstein PF, Verkleij AJ, van Golde LM, Colenbrander B and Gadella BM (2001a). Bicarbonate stimulated phospholipid scrambling induces cholesterol redistribution and enables cholesterol depletion in the sperm plasma membrane. *J Cell Sci* 114, 3543–3555.

Flesch FM, Wijnand E, van de Lest CH, Colenbrander B, van Golde LM and Gadella BM (2001b). Capacitation dependent activation of tyrosine phosphorylation generates two sperm head plasma membrane proteins with high primary binding affinity for the zona pellucida. *Mol Reprod Dev* 60, 107–115.

Florman HM and Babcock DF (1991) Progress towards understanding the molecular basis of capacitation. In: *Chemistry of Fertilization*. CRC: Uniscience, pp. 105–132.

Florman HM, Tombes RM, First NL and Babcock DF (1989) An adhesion-associated agonist from the zona pellucida activates G protein-promoted elevations of internal Ca2+ and pH that mediate mammalian sperm acrosomal exocytosis. *Dev Biol* 135, 133–146.

Florman HM, Arnoult C, Kazam IG, Li C and O'Toole CM (1998) A perspective on the control of mammalian fertilization by egg-activated ion channels in sperm: a tale of two channels. *Biol Reprod* 59, 12–16.

Fraser LR (1977) Differing requirements for capacitation *in vitro* of mouse spermatozoa from two strains. *J Reprod Fertil* 49, 83–87.

Fukami K, Yoshida M, Inoue T, Kurokawa M, Fissore RA, Yoshida N, Mikoshiba K and Takenawa T (2003) Phospholipase Cdelta4 is required for Ca2+ mobilization essential for acrosome reaction in sperm. *J Cell Biol* 161, 79–88.

Gadella BM and Harrison RA (2000) The capacitating agent bicarbonate induces protein kinase A-dependent changes in phospholipid transbilayer behavior in the sperm plasma membrane. *Development* 127, 2407–2420.

Gadella BM and Harrison RA (2002) Capacitation induces cyclic adenosine 3′,5′-monophosphate-dependent, but apoptosis-unrelated, exposure of aminophospholipids at the apical head plasma membrane of boar sperm cells. *Biol Reprod* 67, 340–350.

Gadella BM and Van Gestel RA (2004) Bicarbonate and its role in mammalian sperm function. *Anim Reprod Sci* 82–83, 307–319.

Gadella BM, Gadella Jr TW, Colenbrander B, van Golde LM and Lopes-Cardozo M (1994) Visualization and quantification of glycolipid polarity dynamics in the plasma membrane of the mammalian spermatozoon. *J Cell Sci* 107, 2151–2163.

Gadella BM, Lopes-Cardozo M, van Golde LM, Colenbrander B and Gadella Jr TW (1995) Glycolipid migration from the apical to the equatorial subdomains of the sperm head plasma membrane precedes the acrosome reaction. Evidence for a primary capacitation event in boar spermatozoa. *J Cell Sci* 108, 935–946.

Gadella BM, Miller NG, Colenbrander B, van Golde LM and Harrison RA (1999) Flow cytometric detection of transbilayer movement of fluorescent phospholipid analogues across the boar sperm plasma membrane: elimination of labeling artifacts. *Mol Reprod Dev* 53, 108–125.

Galantino-Homer HL, Visconti PE and Kopf GS (1997) Regulation of protein tyrosine phosphorylation during bovine sperm capacitation by a cyclic adenosine 3′5′-monophosphate-dependent pathway. *Biol Reprod* 56, 707–719.

Garbers DL, Tubb DJ and Hyne RV (1982) A requirement of bicarbonate for Ca2+-induced elevations of cyclic AMP in guinea pig spermatozoa. *J Biol Chem* 257, 8980–8984.

Garty NB, Galiani D, Aharonheim A, Ho YK, Phillips DM, Dekel N and Salomon Y (1988) G-proteins in mammalian gametes: an immunocytochemical study. *J Cell Sci* 91, 21–31.

Gatti JL, Billard R and Christen R (1990) Ionic regulation of the plasma membrane potential of rainbow trout (*Salmo gairdneri*) spermatozoa: role in the initiation of sperm motility. *J Cell Physiol* 143, 546–554.

Gillan L, Evans G and Maxwell WM (2005) Flow cytometric evaluation of sperm parameters in relation to fertility potential. *Theriogenology* 63, 445–457.

Go KJ and Wolf DP (1985) Albumin-mediated changes in sperm sterol content during capacitation. *Biol Reprod* 32, 145–153.

Gorg A, Postel W and Gunther S (1988) The current state of two-dimensional electrophoresis with immobilized pH gradients. *Electrophoresis* 9, 531–546.

Green CE and Watson PF (2001) Comparison of the capacitation-like state of cooled boar spermatozoa with true capacitation. *Reproduction* 122, 889–898.

Gross MK, Toscano DG and Toscano Jr WA (1987) Calmodulin-mediated adenylate cyclase from mammalian sperm. *J Biol Chem* 262, 8672–8676.

Hanoune J and Defer N (2001) Regulation and role of adenylyl cyclase isoforms. *Annu Rev Pharmacol Toxicol* 41, 145–174.

Hao Z, Jha KN, Kim YH *et al.* (2004). Expression analysis of the human testis-specific serine/threonine kinase (TSSK) homologues. A TSSK member is present in the equatorial segment of human sperm. *Mol Human Reprod* 10, 433–444.

Harrison RA (1996) Capacitation mechanisms, and the role of capacitation as seen in eutherian mammals. *Reprod Fertil Dev* 8, 581–594.

Harrison RA (2004) Rapid PKA-catalysed phosphorylation of boar sperm proteins induced by the capacitating agent bicarbonate. *Mol Reprod Dev* 67, 337–352.

Harrison RA and Gadella BM (2005) Bicarbonate-induced membrane processing in sperm capacitation. *Theriogenology* 63, 342–351.

Harrison RA and Miller NG (2000) cAMP-dependent protein kinase control of plasma membrane lipid architecture in boar sperm. *Mol Reprod Dev* 55, 220–228.

Harrison RA, Ashworth PJ and Miller NG (1996) Bicarbonate/CO2, an effector of capacitation, induces a rapid and reversible change in the lipid architecture of boar sperm plasma membranes. *Mol Reprod Dev* 45, 378–391.

Hoshi K, Aita T, Yanagida K, Yoshimatsu N and Sato A (1990) Variation in the cholesterol/phospholipid ratio in human spermatozoa and its relationship with capacitation. *Human Reprod* 5, 71–74.

Huo LJ and Yang ZM (2000) Effects of platelet activating factor on capacitation and acrosome reaction in mouse spermatozoa. *Mol Reprod Dev* 56, 436–440.

Jahn R and Sudhof TC (1999) Membrane fusion and exocytosis. *Ann Rev Biochem* 68, 863–911.

Kabouridis PS, Magee AI and Ley C (1997) S-acylation of LCK protein tyrosine kinase is essential for its signalling function in T lymphocytes. *Embo J* 16, 4983–4998.

Kalab P, Peknicova J, Geussova G and Moos J (1998) Regulation of protein tyrosine phosphorylation in boar sperm through a cAMP-dependent pathway. *Mol Reprod Dev* 51, 304–314.

Kaldis P, Stolz M, Wyss M, Zanolla E, Rothen-Rutishauser B, Vorherr T and Wallimann T (1996) Identification of two distinctly localized mitochondrial creatine kinase isoenzymes in spermatozoa. *J Cell Sci* 109, 2079–2088.

Killian GJ (2004) Evidence for the role of oviduct secretions in sperm function, fertilization and embryo development. *Anim Reprod Sci* 82–83, 141–153.

Kusumi A, Koyama-Honda I and Suzuki K (2004) Molecular dynamics and interactions for creation of stimulation-induced stabilized rafts from small unstable steady-state rafts. *Traffic* 5, 213–220.

Laflamme J, Akoum A and Leclerc P (2005) Induction of human sperm capacitation and protein tyrosine phosphorylation by endometrial cells and interleukin-6. *Mol Human Reprod* 11, 141–150.

Langlais J and Roberts JD (1985) A molecular membrane model of sperm capacitation and the acrosome reaction of mammalian spermatozoa. *Gamete Res* 12, 183–224.

Leclerc P and Goupil S (2002) Regulation of the human sperm tyrosine kinase c-yes. Activation by cyclic adenosine 3′,5′-monophosphate and inhibition by Ca(2+). *Biol Reprod* 67, 301–307.

Leclerc P, de Lamirande E and Gagnon C (1996) Cyclic adenosine 3′,5′-monophosphate-dependent regulation of protein tyrosine phosphorylation in relation to human sperm capacitation and motility. *Biol Reprod* 55, 684–692.

Lee MA and Storey BT (1986) Bicarbonate is essential for fertilization of mouse eggs: mouse sperm require it to undergo the acrosome reaction. *Biol Reprod* 34, 349–356.

Lewis TS, Hunt JB, Aveline LD *et al.* (2000) Identification of novel MAP kinase pathway signaling targets by functional proteomics and mass spectrometry. *Mol Cell* 6, 1343–1354.

Lievano A, Santi CM, Serrano CJ, Trevino CL, Bellve AR, Hernandez-Cruz A and Darszon A (1996) T-type Ca2+ channels and alpha1E expression in spermatogenic cells, and their possible relevance to the sperm acrosome reaction. *FEBS Lett* 388, 150–154.

Luconi M, Krausz C, Forti G and Baldi E (1996) Extracellular calcium negatively modulates tyrosine phosphorylation and tyrosine kinase activity during capacitation of human spermatozoa. *Biol Reprod* 55, 207–216.

Luconi M, Barni T, Vannelli *et al.* (1998) Extracellular signal-regulated kinases modulate capacitation of human spermatozoa. *Biol Reprod* 58, 1476–1489.

Mahi CA and Yanagimachi R (1976) Maturation and sperm penetration of canine ovarian oocytes *in vitro*. *J Exp Zool* 196, 189–196.

Manning G, Plowman GD, Hunter T and Sudarsanam S (2002) Evolution of protein kinase signaling from yeast to man. *Trend Biochem Sci* 27, 514–520.

Marin-Briggiler CI, Tezon JG, Miranda PV and Vazquez-Levine MH (2002) Effect of incubating human sperm at room temperature on capacitation-related events. *Fertil Steril* 77, 252–259.

Marin S, Chiang K, Bassilian S *et al.* (2003) Metabolic strategy of boar spermatozoa revealed by a metabolomic characterization. *FEBS Lett* 554, 342–346.

Mayorga LS, Beron W, Sarrouf MN, Colombo MI, Creutz C and Stahl PD (1994) Calcium-dependent fusion among endosomes. *J Biol Chem* 269, 30927–30934.

McCauley TC, Buhi WC, Wu GM, Mao J, Caamano JN, Didion BA and Day BN (2003) Oviduct-specific glycoprotein modulates sperm-zona binding and improves efficiency of porcine fertilization *in vitro*. *Biol Reprod* 69, 828–834.

Mehats C, Andersen CB, Filopanti M, Jin SL and Conti M (2002) Cyclic nucleotide phosphodiesterases and their role in endocrine cell signaling. *Trend Endocrinol Metab* 13, 29–35.

Michaut M, Tomes CN, De Blass G, Yunes R and Mayorga LS (2000) Calcium-triggered acrosomal exocytosis in human spermatozoa requires the coordinated activation of rab3A and N-ethylmaleimide-sensitive factor. *Proc Nat Acad Sci USA* 97, 9996–10001.

Miki K, Qu W, Goulding EH, Willis WD *et al.* (2004) Glyceraldehyde 3-phosphate dehydrogenase-S, a sperm-specific glycolytic enzyme, is required for sperm motility and male fertility. *Proc Natl Acad Sci USA* 101, 16501–16506.

Mitra K and Shivaji S (2004) Novel tyrosine-phosphorylated post-pyruvate metabolic enzyme, dihydrolipoamide dehydrogenase, involved in capacitation of hamster spermatozoa. *Biol Reprod* 70, 887–899.

Morisawa M and Suzuki K (1980) Osmolality and potassium ion: their roles in initiation of sperm motility in teleosts. *Science* 210, 1145–1147.

Mukai C and Okuno M (2004) Glycolysis plays a major role for adenosine triphosphate supplementation in mouse sperm flagellar movement. *Biol Reprod* 71, 540–547.

Munoz-Garay C, De la Vega-Beltran JL, Delgado R, Labarca P, Felix R and Darszon A (2001) Inwardly rectifying K(+) channels in spermatogenic cells: functional expression and implication in sperm capacitation. *Dev Biol* 234, 261–274.

Neill JM and Olds-Clarke P (1987) A computer-assisted assay for mouse sperm hyperactivation demonstrates that bicarbonate but not bovine serum albumin is required. *Gamete Res* 18, 121–140.

Nolan JP, Magargee SF, Posner RG and Hammerstedt RH (1995) Flow cytometric analysis of transmembrane phospholipid movement in bull sperm. *Biochemistry* 34, 3907–3915.

Nolan MA, Babcock DF, Wennemuth G, Brown W, Burton KA and McKnight GS (2004) Sperm-specific protein kinase A catalytic subunit Calpha2 orchestrates cAMP signaling for male fertility. *Proc Natl Acad Sci USA* 101, 13483–13488.

O'Farrell PH (1975) High resolution two-dimensional electrophoresis of proteins. *J Biol Chem* 250, 4007–4021.

Okamura N and Sugita Y (1983) Activation of spermatozoan adenylate cyclase by a low molecular weight factor in porcine seminal plasma. *J Biol Chem* 258, 13056–13062.

Okamura N, Tajima Y, Soejima A, Masuda H and Sugita Y (1985) Sodium bicarbonate in seminal plasma stimulates the motility of mammalian spermatozoa through direct activation of adenylate cyclase. *J Biol Chem* 260, 9699–9705.

Osheroff JE, Visconti PE, Valenzuela JP, Travis AJ, Alvarez J and Kopf GS (1999) Regulation of human sperm capacitation by a cholesterol efflux-stimulated signal transduction pathway leading to protein kinase A-mediated up-regulation of protein tyrosine phosphorylation. *Mol Human Reprod* 5, 1017–1026.

Overstreet JW and Cooper GW (1978) Sperm transport in the reproductive tract of the female rabbit: I. The rapid transit phase of transport. *Biol Reprod* 19, 101–114.

Parrish JJ, Susko-Parrish JL and First NL (1989) Capacitation of bovine sperm by heparin: inhibitory effect of glucose and role of intracellular pH. *Biol Reprod* 41, 683–699.

Pommer AC, Rutllant J and Meyers SA (2003) Phosphorylation of protein tyrosine residues in fresh and cryopreserved stallion spermatozoa under capacitating conditions. *Biol Reprod* 68, 1208–1214.

Pomorski T, Herrmann A, Zimmermann B, Zachowski A and Muller P (1995) An improved assay for measuring the transverse redistribution of fluorescent phospholipids in plasma membranes. *Chem Phys Lipids* 77, 139–146.

Quill TA, Sugden SA, Rossi KL, Doolittle LK, Hammer RE and Garbers DL (2003) Hyperactivated sperm motility driven by CatSper2 is required for fertilization. *Proc Natl Acad Sci USA* 100, 14869–14874.

Rajendran L and Simons K (2005) Lipid rafts and membrane dynamics. *J Cell Sci* 118, 1099–1102.

Ramalho-Santos J, Moreno RD, Sutovsky P et al. (2000) SNARE's in mammalian sperm: possible implications for fertilization. *Dev Biol* 223, 54–69.

Rathi R, Colenbrander B, Bevers MM and Gadella BM (2001) Evaluation of *in vitro* capacitation of stallion spermatozoa. *Biol Reprod* 65, 462–470.

Rathi R, Colenbrander B, Stout TA, Bevers MM and Gadella BM (2003) Progesterone induces acrosome reaction in stallion spermatozoa via a protein tyrosine kinase dependent pathway. *Mol Reprod Dev* 64, 120–128.

Ren D, Navarro B, Perez G et al. (2001) A sperm ion channel required for sperm motility and male fertility. *Nature* 413, 603–609.

Rochwerger L and Cuasnicu PS (1992) Redistribution of a rat sperm epididymal glycoprotein after *in vitro* and *in vivo* capacitation. *Mol Reprod Dev* 31, 34–41.

Romero MF and Boron WF (1999) Electrogenic Na+/HCO3− cotransporters: cloning and physiology. *Annu Rev Physiol* 61, 699–723.

Rotem R, Paz GF, Homonnai ZT, Kalina M and Naor Z (1990) Protein kinase C is present in human sperm: possible role in flagellar motility. *Proc Natl Acad Sci USA* 87, 7305–7308.

Roy S, Luetterforst R, Harding A et al. (1999) Dominant-negative caveolin inhibits H-Ras function by disrupting cholesterol-rich plasma membrane domains. *Nat Cell Biol* 1, 98–105.

San Agustin JT, Leszyk JD, Nuwaysir LM and Witman GB (1998) The catalytic subunit of the cAMP-dependent protein kinase of ovine sperm flagella has a unique amino-terminal sequence. *J Biol Chem* 273, 24874–24883.

Sassone-Corsi P (1997) Transcriptional checkpoints determining the fate of male germ cells. *Cell* 88, 163–166.

Schulz JR, Wessel GM and Vacquier VD (1997) The exocytosis regulatory proteins syntaxin and VAMP are shed from sea urchin sperm during the acrosome reaction. *Dev Biol* 191, 80–87.

Schulz JR, Saski JD and Vacquier VD (1998) Increased association of synaptosome associated protein of 25 kDa with syntaxin and vessicle-associated membrane protein following acrosomal exocytosis of sea urchin sperm. *J Biol Chem* 273, 24355–24359.

Setchell BP, Maddocks S and Brooks DE (1994) Anatomy, vasculature, innervation, and fluids of the male reproductive tract. In: *The Physiology of Reproduction*, eds E Knobil and JD Neill, Vol. 1. New York: Raven Press, pp. 1063–1175.

Shadan S, James PS, Howes EA and Jones R (2004) Cholesterol efflux alters lipid raft stability and distribution during capacitation of boar spermatozoa. *Biol Reprod* 71, 253–265.

Shalgi R, Matityahu A, Gaunt SJ and Jones R (1990) Antigens on rat spermatozoa with a potential role in fertilization. *Mol Reprod Dev* 25, 286–296.

Shi QX and Roldan ER (1995) Bicarbonate/CO2 is not required for zona pellucida- or progesterone-induced acrosomal exocytosis of mouse spermatozoa but is essential for capacitation. *Biol Reprod* 52, 540–546.

Simons K and Ikonen E (1997) Functional rafts in cell membranes. *Nature* 387, 569–572.

Simons K and Ikonen E (2000) How cells handle cholesterol. *Science* 290, 1721–1726.

Simons K and Toomre D (2000) Lipid rafts and signal transduction. *Nat Rev Mol Cell Biol* 1, 31–39.

Simons K and Vaz WL (2004) Model systems, lipid rafts, and cell membranes. *Annu Rev Biophys Biomol Struct* 33, 269–295.

Soskic V, Gorlach M, Poznanovic S, Boehmer FD and Godovac-Zimmermann J (1999) Functional proteomics analysis of signal transduction pathways of the platelet-derived growth factor beta receptor. *Biochemistry* 38, 1757–1764.

Suzuki F and Yanagimachi R (1989) Changes in the distribution of intramembranous particles and filipin-reactive membrane sterols during *in vitro* capacitation of golden hamster spermatozoa. *Gamete Res* 23, 335–347.

Tesarik J and Flechon JE (1986) Distribution of sterols and anionic lipids in human sperm plasma membrane: effects of *in vitro* capacitation. *J Ultrastruct Mol Struct Res* 97, 227–237.

Therien I, Soubeyrand S and Manjunath P (1997) Major proteins of bovine seminal plasma modulate sperm capacitation by high-density lipoprotein. *Biol Reprod* 57, 1080–1088.

Tombes RM and Shapiro BM (1985) Metabolite channeling: a phosphorylcreatine shuttle to mediate high energy phosphate transport between sperm mitochondrion and tail. *Cell* 41, 325–334.

Travis AJ, Vargas LA, Merdiushev T, Moss SB, Hunnicutt GR and Kopf GS (2000) Expression and localization of caveolin-1 in mouse and guinea pig spermatozoa. *Mol Biol Cell* 11, 121a.

Trevino CL, Serrano CJ, Beltran C, Felix R and Darszon A (2001) Identification of mouse trp homologs and lipid rafts from spermatogenic cells and sperm. *FEBS Lett* 509, 119–125.

Uma Devi K, Jha K, Patil SB, Padma P and Shivaji S (2000) Inhibition of motility of hamster spermatozoa by protein tyrosine kinase inhibitors. *Andrologia* 32, 95–106.

Verkleij AJ, Zwaal RF, Roelofsen B, Comfurius P, Kastelijn D and van Deenen LL (1973) The asymmetric distribution of phospholipids in the human red cell membrane. A combined study using phospholipases and freeze-etch electron microscopy. *Biochim Biophys Acta* 323, 178–193.

Vijayaraghavan S, Olson GE, NagDas S, Winfrey VP and Carr DW (1997) Subcellular localization of the regulatory subunits of cyclic adenosine 3′,5′-monophosphate-dependent protein kinase in bovine spermatozoa. *Biol Reprod* 57, 1517–1523.

Vijayaraghavan S, Mohan J, Gray H, Khatra B and Carr DW (2000) A role for phosphorylation of glycogen synthase kinase-3alpha in bovine sperm motility regulation. *Biol Reprod* 62, 1647–1654.

Visconti PE and Kopf GS (1998) Regulation of protein phosphorylation during sperm capacitation. *Biol Reprod* 59, 1–6.

Visconti PE, Muschietti JP, Flawia MM and Tezon JG (1990) Bicarbonate dependence of cAMP accumulation induced by phorbol esters in hamster spermatozoa. *Biochim Biophys Acta* 1054, 231–236.

Visconti PE, Bailey JL, Moore GD, Pan D, Olds-Clarke P and Kopf GS (1995a) Capacitation of mouse spermatozoa. I. Correlation between the capacitation state and protein tyrosine phosphorylation. *Development* 121, 1129–1137.

Visconti PE, Moore GD, Bailey JL *et al.* (1995b) Capacitation of mouse spermatozoa. II. Protein tyrosine phosphorylation and capacitation are regulated by a cAMP-dependent pathway. *Development* 121, 1139–1150.

Visconti PE, Olds-Clarke P, Moss SB, Kalab P, Travis AJ, de las Heras M and Kopf GS (1996) Properties and localization of a tyrosine phosphorylated form of hexokinase in mouse sperm. *Mol Reprod Dev* 43, 82–93.

Visconti PE, Johnson LR, Oyaski M, Fornes M, Moss SB, Gerton GL and Kopf GS (1997) Regulation, localization, and anchoring of protein kinase A subunits during mouse sperm capacitation. *Dev Biol* 192, 351–363.

Visconti PE, Galantino-Homer H, Moore GD, Bailey JL, Ning X, Fornes M and Kopf GS (1998) The molecular basis of sperm capacitation. *J Androl* 19, 242–248.

Visconti PE, Galantino-Homer H, Ning X *et al.* (1999a) Cholesterol efflux-mediated signal transduction in mammalian sperm. Beta-cyclodextrins initiate transmembrane signaling leading to an increase in protein tyrosine phosphorylation and capacitation. *J Biol Chem* 274, 3235–3242.

Visconti PE, Ning X, Fornes MW, Alvarez JG, Stein P, Connors SA and Kopf GS (1999b) Cholesterol efflux-mediated signal transduction in mammalian sperm: cholesterol release signals an increase in protein tyrosine phosphorylation during mouse sperm capacitation. *Dev Biol* 214, 429–443.

Visconti PE, Stewart-Savage J, Blasco A, Battaglia L, Miranda P, Kopf GS and Tezon JG (1999c) Roles of bicarbonate, cAMP, and protein tyrosine phosphorylation on capacitation and the spontaneous acrosome reaction of hamster sperm. *Biol Reprod* 61, 76–84.

Visconti PE, Westbrook VA, Chertihin O, Demarco I, Sleight S and Diekman AB (2002) Novel signaling pathways involved in sperm acquisition of fertilizing capacity. *J Reprod Immunol* 53, 133–150.

Wang D, King SM, Quill TA, Doolittle LK and Garbers DL (2003) A new sperm-specific Na+/H+ exchanger required for sperm motility and fertility. *Nat Cell Biol* 5, 1117–1122.

Ward CR and Kopf GS (1993) Molecular events mediating sperm activation. *Dev Biol* 158, 9–34.

Ward CR, Storey BT and Kopf GS (1992) Activation of a Gi protein in mouse sperm membranes by solubilized proteins of the zona pellucida, the egg's extracellular matrix. *J Biol Chem* 267, 14061–14067.

Wasco WM and Orr GA (1984) Function of calmodulin in mammalian sperm: presence of a calmodulin-dependent cyclic nuclearide phosphodiesterase associated with demembranated rat caudal epididymal sperm. *Biochem Biophys Res Comm* 118, 636–642.

Wiesner B, Weiner J, Middendorff R, Hagen V, Kaupp UB and Weyand I (1998) Cyclic nucleotide-gated channels on the flagellum control Ca2+ entry into sperm. *J Cell Biol* 142, 473–484.

Wolf DE and Cardullo RA (1991) Physiological properties of the mammalian sperm plasma membrane. In: *Comparative Spermatology 20 Years After*, ed. B Baccetti. New York: Raven Press, pp. 599–604.

Wolf DE, Hagopian SS and Ishijima S (1986) Changes in sperm plasma membrane lipid diffusibility after hyperactivation during *in vitro* capacitation in the mouse. *J Cell Biol* 102, 1372–1377.

Wu C, Stojanov T, Chami O, Ishii S, Shimuzu T, Li A and O'Neill C (2001) Evidence for the autocrine induction of capacitation of mammalian spermatozoa. *J Biol Chem* 276, 26962–26968.

Yanagimachi R (1970) The movement of golden hamster spermatozoa before and after capacitation. *J Reprod Fertil* 23, 193–196.

Yanagimachi R (1972) Penetration of guinea-pig spermatozoa into hamster eggs *in vitro*. *J Reprod Fertil* 28, 477–480.

Yanagimachi R (1994) Mammalian fertilization. In: *The Physiology of Reproduction*, eds. E Knobil and JD Neill, Vol. 1. New York: Raven Press, Ltd, pp. 189–317.

Yunes R, Michaut M, Tomes C and Mayorga LS (2000) Rab3A triggers the acrosome reaction in permeabilized human spermatozoa. *Biol Reprod* 62, 1084–1089.

Zachowski A (1993) Phospholipids in animal eukaryotic membranes: transverse asymmetry and movement. *Biochem J* 294(Pt 1), 1–14.

Zajchowski LD and Robbins SM (2002) Lipid rafts and little caves. Compartmentalized signalling in membrane microdomains. *Eur J Biochem* 269, 737–752.

Zeng Y, Clark EN and Florman HM (1995) Sperm membrane potential: hyperpolarization during capacitation regulates zona pellucida-dependent acrosomal secretion. *Dev Biol* 171, 554–563.

Zeng Y, Oberdorf JA and Florman HM (1996) pH regulation in mouse sperm: identification of Na(+)-, Cl(−)-, and HCO3(−)-dependent and arylaminobenzoate-dependent regulatory mechanisms and characterization of their roles in sperm capacitation. *Dev Biol* 173, 510–520.

7

Reactive oxygen species: friend or foe

R. John Aitken[1,2] and Liga Bennetts[2]

[1]ARC Centre of Excellence in Biotechnology and Development
[2]Discipline of Biological Sciences, The University of Newcastle, Callaghan, NSW, Australia

7.1 Introduction

Reactive oxygen species (ROS) not only play a key role in mediating the pathological consequences of oxidative stress but also drive the biochemical pathways that are central to the regulation of normal cell function. Thus, ROS are a two-edged sword: a friend when produced in the small quantities needed to promote cellular processes such as apoptosis and signal transduction and, because of their promiscuous reactivity, a foe when generated in excess. In this review we shall examine both sides of these biologically important molecules in the context of sperm cell biology. However, in order to set the scene, we shall first overview the fundamental chemistry of ROS and consider the difficulties encountered in detecting these short-lived but highly reactive molecules.

7.2 What are ROS?

The term ROS covers a range of metabolites that are derived from the reduction of oxygen, including free radicals, such as the superoxide anion ($O_2^{-\bullet}$) or the hydroxyl radical ($OH^{\bullet}$), as well as powerful oxidants such as hydrogen peroxide (H_2O_2). The term also covers molecular species derived from the reaction of carbon centred radicals with molecular oxygen including peroxyl radicals ($ROO^{\bullet}$), alkoxyl radicals ($RO^{\bullet}$) and organic hydroperoxides ($ROOH$). ROS may also include other powerful oxidants such as peroxynitrite ($ONOO^-$) or hypochlorous acid ($HOCl$) as well as the highly biologically active free radical, nitric oxide ($^{\bullet}NO$). Although NO has been implicated in the regulation of sperm function (Herrero and Gagnon, 2001), this chapter will confine itself to the major ROS, $O_2^{-\bullet}$ and H_2O_2.

The specific term 'free radicals' refers to any atom or molecule containing one or more unpaired electrons. As unpaired electrons are highly energetic, and seek out other electrons with which to pair, they confer upon free radicals considerable reactivity. Thus, free radicals and related 'reactive species' have the ability to react with and modify the structure of many different kinds of biomolecules including proteins, lipids and nucleic acids. The wide range of targets that can be attacked by ROS is a critical facet of their chemistry that contributes significantly to the pathological importance of these molecules.

As most chemical species in biological systems have only paired electrons, free radicals are also likely to be involved in chain reactions, whereby new free radical products are formed. A classical example of such a chain reaction is the peroxidation of lipids in biological membranes. In this process, a ROS-mediated attack on unsaturated fatty acids in the plasma membrane generates peroxyl (ROO$^{\bullet}$) and alkoxyl (RO$^{\bullet}$) radicals that, in order to stabilize, abstract a hydrogen atom from an adjacent carbon, generating the corresponding acid (ROOH) or alcohol (ROH). The abstraction of a hydrogen atom from an adjacent lipid creates a carbon centred radical that combines with molecular oxygen to create another lipid peroxide. In order to stabilize, the latter must abstract a hydrogen atom from a nearby lipid, creating yet another carbon radical that on reaction with molecular oxygen will generate more lipid peroxides. In this manner, a chain reaction is created that propagates the peroxidative damage throughout the plasma membrane (Halliwell and Gutteridge, 1999).

Since the hydrogen abstraction process is facilitated by the double bonds present in unsaturated fatty acids, membranes that are rich in the latter will be particularly vulnerable to oxidative stress. In this context, spermatozoa are especially susceptible because their plasma membranes are extremely rich in unsaturated fatty acids, notably 22:6 (Jones *et al.*, 1979). Such an abundance of unsaturated lipids is necessary to create the membrane fluidity required by the membrane fusion events associated with fertilization (acrosomal exocytosis and sperm–oocyte fusion); however their presence leaves these cells open to peroxidative attack. Termination of such lipid peroxidation chain reactions can be achieved with chain-breaking antioxidants such as vitamin E (α-tocopherol). The latter is extremely effective in terminating lipid peroxidation cascades in human spermatozoa (Aitken *et al.*, 1989a) and has been shown to improve the fertility of males selected on the basis of high levels of lipid peroxidation in their spermatozoa (Suleiman *et al.*, 1996).

Some of the major ROS considered important in biological systems are listed in Table 7.1. The most commonly encountered species are $O_2^{-\bullet}$ and H_2O_2. These molecules are capable of a range of rapid chemical reactions yielding a correspondingly broad range of reaction products. When in aqueous solution, $O_2^{-\bullet}$ has a short half-life (1 ms) and is relatively inert. The radical is more stable and reactive in the hydrophobic environment provided by cellular membranes. The charge associated with $O_2^{-\bullet}$ means that this molecule is generally incapable of passing across biological membranes, although there *are* reports of this molecule using voltage-dependent anion channels for this purpose (Han *et al.*, 2003). As a result of its lack of membrane permeability, $O_2^{-\bullet}$ may be more damaging if produced inside biological membranes than

Table 7.1. Nomenclature of ROS

Free radicals	Non-radicals
Reactive oxygen species	
Superoxide, $O_2^{\cdot-}$	Hydrogen peroxide, H_2O_2
Hydroxyl, $OH^{\cdot}$	Hypochlorous acid, $HOCl$
Hydroperoxyl $HO_2^{\cdot}$	Ozone, O_3
Peroxyl, $RO_2^{\cdot}$	Singlet oxygen, $^1O_2$
Alkoxyl, $RO^{\cdot}$	Organic peroxides, $ROOH$
Carbonate, $CO_3^{\cdot-}$	Peroxynitrite, $ONOO^-$
Carbon dioxide, $CO_2^{\cdot-}$	Peroxynitrous acid, $ONOOH$
Reactive nitrogen species	
Nitric oxide, $NO^{\cdot}$	Nitrous acid, HNO_2
Nitrogen dioxide, $NO_2^{\cdot}$	Nitrosyl cation, NO^+
	Nitroxyl anion, NO^-
	Dinitrogen tetroxide, N_2O_4
	Dinitrogen trioxide, N_2O_3
	Peroxynitrite, $ONOO^-$
	Peroxynitrous acid, $OHOOH$
	Nitronium (nitryl) cation, NO_2^+
	Alkyl peroxynitrites, $ROONO$
	Nitryl (nitronium) chloride, NO_2Cl

at other sites. It is also important to note that while $O_2^{-\cdot}$ can act as either a reducing agent or a weak oxidizing agent in aqueous solution, under the reducing conditions that characterize the intracellular environment, $O_2^{-\cdot}$ acts primarily as an oxidant. Many of the effects of $O_2^{-\cdot}$ are believed to arise from its conversion to more reactive oxidizing species (Fridovich, 1999; Halliwell and Gutteridge, 1999). For example, protonation of $O_2^{-\cdot}$ forms the hydroperoxyl radical ($HO_2^{\cdot}$), a much stronger oxidant (Equation (7.1)). It is therefore possible that many oxidations attributed to $O_2^{-\cdot}$ are in fact caused by $HO_2^{\cdot}$.

$$HO_2^{\cdot} \rightleftharpoons H^+ + O_2^{-\cdot} \tag{7.1}$$

The pH at which this reaction reaches equilibrium (pKa) is 4.8, with the result that at physiological pH, $HO_2^{\cdot}$ represents less than 1% of the $O_2^{-\cdot}$ present in a cell. However, given the considerable reactivity and membrane permeability of $HO_2^{\cdot}$ this radical is still believed to be a significant contributor to oxidative damage in biological systems (Fridovich, 1999) with the potential to initiate lipid peroxidation cascades (Bielski *et al.*, 1983; Storey, 1997).

Conversion of $O_2^{-\cdot}$ to other ROS also occurs. An important means by which this takes place is the dismutation reaction (Equation (7.2)), wherein $O_2^{-\cdot}$ reacts with itself, that is, superoxide is both oxidised and reduced. In this situation, one molecule of $O_2^{-\bullet}$ is oxidized to molecular oxygen, while the other is reduced to H_2O_2:

$$O_2^{-\bullet} + O_2^{-\bullet} + 2H^+ \rightarrow H_2O_2 + O_2 \tag{7.2}$$

Superoxide dismutase (SOD) catalyzes this conversion. SODs are metalloenzymes thought to be present in all oxygen-metabolizing cells (Gregory et al., 1974). The reaction can occur spontaneously without SOD, however, in its absence dismutation will proceed much more slowly due to the electrostatic repulsion of the anions (rate constant of about $5 \times 10^5 M^{-1}s^{-1}$ at physiological pH) (Fridovich, 1979; Halliwell and Gutteridge, 1999). SOD is an efficient catalyst that will drive the above reaction at a rate constant of about $1.6 \times 10^9 M^{-1}s^{-1}$ over a large pH range (5.3–9.5) (Halliwell and Gutteridge, 1999). In the human spermatozoon, there is sufficient SOD activity to account for all of the H_2O_2 produced by these cells (Alvarez et al., 1987).

Superoxide formation can also lead to the generation of other types of highly reactive species apart from H_2O_2. Many transition metal ions are able to participate in these processes, as they possess variable oxidation numbers, permitting them to change their redox status by either gaining or losing an electron. Consequently, transition metals act as very effective promoters of free radical reactions. For example, in the Fenton reaction (Equation (7.3)), H_2O_2 undergoes decomposition in the presence of ferrous ions to produce the pernicious hydroxyl radical ($OH^\bullet$):

$$H_2O_2 + Fe^{2+} \rightarrow Fe^{3+} + OH^- + OH^\bullet$$

$$Fe^{3+} + O_2^{-\bullet} \rightarrow Fe^{2+} + O_2 \tag{7.3}$$

The sum of these two reactions represents the iron-catalyzed Haber–Weiss reaction (Equation (7.4)):

$$H_2O_2 + O_2^{-\bullet} \xrightarrow{Fe^{2+}} O_2 + OH^- + OH^\bullet \tag{7.4}$$

Thus, $O_2^{-\bullet}$ also has a key role to play in the above reaction by serving as a reductant and facilitating the regeneration of reduced metal ions in the extracellular space. It is also well recognized that other transition metals may participate in these reactions. Thus, while iron is the major player (Toyokuni, 2002), copper is the other major candidate and cobalt, aluminium, chromium, nickel and titanium may also participate in such reactions (Halliwell and Gutteridge, 1999). Moreover in seminal plasma, both iron and copper are available in a free state and hence able to take part in $OH^\bullet$ production and the consequent promotion of oxidative stress in the ejaculate (Kwenang et al., 1987).

7.3 Detection of ROS in the male germ line

Given the importance of ROS and the apparent vulnerability of spermatozoa to oxidative stress, it might be anticipated that sophisticated methods have been developed to detect these intermediate oxygen metabolites for diagnostic purposes. In fact, this area has been severely compromised by the absence of sensitive, accurate analytical methods capable of confirming the presence of specific ROS in biological systems.

The most commonly used method for detecting ROS in an andrological context is chemiluminescence, using the probes lucigenin or luminol (Aitken *et al.*, 1992a, 2004a). Lucigenin (N,N'-dimethyl-9,9'-biacridinium dinitrate) carries a positive ionic charge; it is generally thought to be relatively membrane impermeant and to respond to O_2^-·, in the extracellular space. However, the positive charge associated with this molecule may also favour its partition into mitochondria, as a consequence of the electronegative mitochondrial membrane potential (Li *et al.*, 1999). Indeed, studies using rat spermatozoa as a model indicate that the lucigenin signal generated by these cells can reflect O_2^-· produced by the sperm mitochondria (Vernet *et al.*, 2001). However there are no data to suggest that the lucigenin signals generated by human spermatozoa are of mitochondrial origin, even though such signals are inversely correlated with sperm quality (Aitken *et al.*, 2003) and significantly elevated in cases of male infertility (McKinney *et al.*, 1996; Said *et al.*, 2004).

One of the key features of lucigenin is that this probe must undergo a one-electron reduction to the radical species (LH+·) before it becomes sensitized to the presence of O_2^-· (Fig. 7.1). In the case of mitochondrial O_2^-· production, this reductive process is accomplished by the organelle's electron transport chain. However, outside of the mitochondria, lucigenin reduction can be induced by reductases such cytochrome P_{450} reductase or cytochrome b_5 reductase (Baker *et al.*, 2004). This is particularly the case when exogenous nicotinamide adenine dinucleotide phosphate (NAD(P)H) is used to drive redox activity in populations of human spermatozoa (Aitken *et al.*, 1997). The LH+· generated on reduction then combines with O_2^-· to produce the dioxetane that, in turn, decomposes with the generation of light (chemiluminescence) (Fig. 7.1). Although this chemistry seems straightforward, complications may arise due to redox cycling reactions whereby LH+· combines with ground state oxygen (O_2) to create O_2^-· and regenerate the parent lucigenin molecule (Fig. 7.1). The O_2^-· artificially created in this manner will then combine LH+· to generate additional dioxetane and further the chemiluminescence response (Fig. 7.1). If such redox cycling does occur, the particularly intense NADPH-dependent lucigenin signals seen in defective human spermatozoa (Aitken *et al.*, 2003; Said *et al.*, 2005) may be as much an indication of excessive reductase activity as evidence for the overabundance of O_2^-·. This explanation would provide a link between the high levels of redox activity detected in defective spermatozoa by lucigenin chemiluminescence

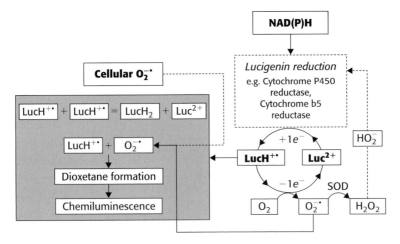

Figure 7.1   Schematic representation of the chemistry for lucigenin chemiluminescence; Luc^{2+}: lucigenin; $LH^{+\bullet}$: a lucigenin radical created by the one electron reduction of Luc^{2+}. The reaction of $LH^{+\bullet}$ with oxygen generates $O_2^{-\bullet}$. The latter then participates in an oxygenation reaction with $LH^{+\bullet}$ generating a dioxetane that decomposes with the generation of chemiluminescence. Any entity that can effect the one electron reduction of lucigenin can potentially create a redox cycle in the presence of oxygen that produces high levels of $O_2^{-\bullet}$ and chemiluminescence. It is impossible to distinguish the relative contribution of such probe-dependent and cell-dependent chemiluminescence. Hence data obtained with this probe should be interpreted with caution

and enhanced reductase activity due to the presence of excess residual cytoplasm. There is certainly a great deal of data to link cytoplasmic retention with defective sperm function (Gil-Guzman *et al.*, 2001; Gomez *et al.*, 1996; Ollero *et al.*, 2001; Zini *et al.*, 1998) so such an explanation would be fully compatible with our understanding of the aetiology of male infertility.

However it has also been argued that the reaction $LH+^{\bullet}$ with O_2 is thermodynamically unlikely (Afanas'ev *et al.*, 1999) and that redox cycling of this probe does not occur in biological systems. Given the high dose of lucigenin typically used to detect redox activity in human sperm samples ($\sim$250 μM) the possibility of redox cycling cannot be excluded. As a consequence, we currently do not know the extent to which the elevated lucigenin signals detected in defective human spermatozoa reflect primary $O_2^{-\bullet}$ production or the super-abundance of reductases due to the presence of excess cytoplasm. What we do know is that the activity of this probe correlates well with defective sperm function whether the activity is promoted by treatment with NAD(P)H or phorbol ester (Aitken *et al.*, 2003, 2004a; Said *et al.*, 2004, 2005).

A similar argument may apply to luminol. This probe has to undergo a one electron oxidation before it becomes sensitised to the presence of ROS. In a common

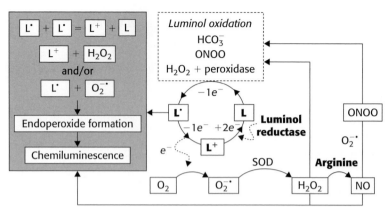

Figure 7.2   Schematic representation of the underlying chemistry for luminol-dependent chemiluminescence; L: luminol; L·: a luminol radical created by the one-electron oxidation of L. L^+: azaquinone formed by the further one electron oxidation of L· by oxygen, generating $O_2^{-\cdot}$ as a by-product. The reaction of L· with $O_2^{-\cdot}$ or L^+ with H_2O_2 generates an unstable endoperoxide whose decomposition leads to production of the chemiluminescence species, an electronically excited aminophthallate. Redox cycling of the probe could result if human spermatozoa possessed an appropriate reductase to convert L^+ back to the parent L. Any reactant that can achieve the univalent oxidation of luminol will generate chemiluminescence in this assay including H_2O_2 and $ONOO^-$

form of this assay, horseradish peroxidase is used to promote luminol oxidation in the extracellular space. In this form, the luminol assay largely reflects the presence of H_2O_2 released to the outside of the cell. In the absence of exogenous horseradish peroxidase the assay is dependent on the presence of intracellular peroxidases in order to activate the probe (Aitken et al., 1992a; Faulkner and Fridovich, 1993). The one electron oxidation of luminol leads to the creation of a radical species (L·). The latter then interacts with ground state oxygen to produce $O_2^{-\cdot}$ that induces the oxygenation of L· to create an unstable endoperoxide, which ultimately breaks down with the release of light (Fig. 7.2). According to this scheme, $O_2^{-\cdot}$ is an essential intermediate in the creation of luminol-dependent chemiluminescence and it is for this reason that SOD is such an effective inhibitor of this reaction cascade. However, the activity of this scavenger should never be taken to indicate the primary production of $O_2^{-\cdot}$ by human spermatozoa; $O_2^{-\cdot}$ is simply an artificially created intermediate that is essential for luminol-dependent chemiluminescence (Aitken et al., 1992a). Indeed, any univalent oxidant has the potential to generate $O_2^{-\cdot}$, and hence chemiluminescence, in the presence of luminol, including ferricyanide, persulphate, hypochlorite, $ONOO^-$ and xanthine oxidase (Fig. 7.2).

Hydrogen peroxide lies upstream of $O_2^{-\bullet}$ in the reaction scheme depicted in Figure 7.2 and its involvement in the initial oxidation of luminol, accounts for the inhibitory effects of catalase on this form of chemiluminescence. In addition, H_2O_2 will also react directly with the azaquinone (L+) and thereby contribute to the formation of excited aminophthalic acid, the chemiluminescent species (Nakamura and Nakamura, 1998). In species such as the rat and mouse, secondary radical species are created by the spermatozoa (NO, ONOO), possibly as a consequence of H_2O_2-mediated attacks on arginine, and this greatly increases the intensity of the spontaneous luminol–peroxidase signals detected during capacitation (Aitken *et al.*, 2004c). Such signals are not detected in suspensions of human spermatozoa for reasons that are, as yet, unclear (Aitken *et al.*, 2004c).

Fundamentally, luminol-based assays are measuring redox activity characterized by the cellular generation of oxidizing species capable of creating L'. Notwithstanding the reservations that might be expressed concerning the specificity of this probe, the luminol assay is robust and generates results that are highly correlated with sperm function. Thus Aitken and Clarkson (1987), using A23187-stimulated luminol-dependent chemiluminescence for assessment purposes, demonstrated a significant increase in the redox activities associated with defective human spermatozoa. This negative association between A23187-induced, luminol-dependent chemiluminescence and sperm quality has been found in patients with overt disruptions to their semen profile such as oligozoospermia (Aitken *et al.*, 1989b, 1992b), and in the low density, defective sperm populations recovered from Percoll gradients (Aitken and Clarkson, 1988; Aitken *et al.*, 1989a). The clinical significance of this assay has also been emphasized in a long-term prospective study of 139 couples characterized by a lack of detectable pathology in the female partners. In this cohort of patients, a negative association was observed between luminol-dependent chemiluminescence and the incidence of spontaneous pregnancy (Aitken *et al.*, 1991).

The addition of A23187 is probably not necessary for such luminol-based assays to yield diagnostic information because the basal and A23187-induced signals are highly correlated ($r = 0.805$; Aitken *et al.*, 1991). Indeed, recent studies have demonstrated that spontaneous, unstimulated luminol-dependent signals are, just like the A23187-stimulated version of the assay, perfectly capable of identifying the high levels of redox activity associated with defective sperm populations (Gil-Guzman *et al.*, 2001; Ollero *et al.*, 2001). In any case, a much more powerful stimulus for ROS generation by human spermatozoa in the presence of luminol/peroxidase is 12-myristate, 13-acetate phorbol ester (PMA), an activator of protein kinase C.

When sperm populations are isolated from the high density (80–90%) region of Percoll gradients and freed of detectable leucocyte contamination, the chemiluminescence elicited by PMA in the presence of luminol/peroxidase shows a very tight correlation with sperm quality as reflected by sperm morphology, movement

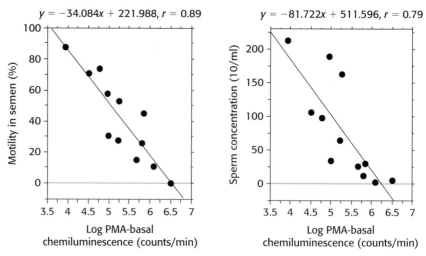

Figure 7.3   Relationship between the intensity of the PMA-induced chemiluminescence signals generated in leucocyte free sperm suspensions recovered from Percoll gradients and the quality of the original semen profile as reflected in both the percentage of motile cells and sperm concentration in the original semen sample (Gomez *et al.*, 1998)

characteristics and the capacity for sperm–oocyte fusion (Gomez *et al.*, 1998). Significantly, these PMA-induced signals are also negatively correlated with key attributes of the *original* semen profile, including sperm morphology, motility and total count (Gomez *et al.*, 1998; Fig. 7.3). In other words, the presence of defective spermatozoa exhibiting high levels of redox activity is not just telling us about the capacity of these cells to generate H_2O_2, they are also yielding important information about the underlying quality of the spermatogenic process. This conclusion is supported by Gil-Guzman *et al.* (2001) who also recorded a correlation between the luminol signals generated by defective spermatozoa recovered from Percoll gradients and the quality of sperm morphology in the original ejaculate. This association between ROS generation and overall semen quality may reflect the importance of cytoplasmic retention as both an indicator of spermatogenic quality and as a key factor in the origins of ROS production.

Apart from luminol and lucigenin there are currently no alternative techniques available for monitoring the production of ROS by human spermatozoa. These probes have an adequate level of sensitivity and generate data that is reflective of semen quality. However, as indicated above, the chemistry of probe activation and chemiluminescence generation is complex and requires careful interpretation (Aitken *et al.*, 2004a). Apart from the chemical complexities associated with luminol and lucigenin chemiluminescence, the very sensitivity of these probes means that they are susceptible to interference by a number of factors that have recently been reviewed (Aitken *et al.*, 2004a). These factors include:

(1) *Time to analysis*: The capacity of spermatozoa to generate chemiluminescence declines with time.

(2) *Semen liquefaction*: Chemiluminescence signals cannot be reliably obtained from samples that have not liquefied normally.

(3) *Bovine serum albumin*: Supplementation of media with this protein source is not recommended because such preparations are heavily contaminated with polyamine oxidase activity and can generate spurious signals on contact with the polyamines present in human seminal plasma.

(4) *Repeated centrifugation*: The mechanical shearing forces associated with centrifugation promote ROS generation.

(5) *Medium pH*: Chemiluminescence intensity is profoundly influenced by the pH of the medium, which must be standardized and tightly regulated.

(6) *Chemical interference*: Many chemicals will artificially promote or suppress chemiluminescence signals generated by luminol–peroxidase or lucigenin (e.g., phenol red, uric acid).

(7) *Leucocytes*: Probably the most common source of interference with these assays is leucocyte contamination. Leucocytes are professional generators of ROS and on a cell-for-cell basis are much more active than spermatozoa in stimulating chemiluminescence activity. It is therefore essential that every attempt is made to remove contaminating leucocytes before any attempt is made to measure redox activity in human sperm suspensions. Techniques for achieving this end have been described involving the use of CD45-coated magnetic beads (Aitken *et al.*, 1996b, 2004a). The effectiveness of this treatment can then been verified using leucocyte-specific agonists such FMLP (formyl methionyl leucyl phenylalanine) or opsonized zymosan in luminol–peroxidase detection systems (Krausz *et al.*, 1992).

Chemiluminescence aside, the field is in urgent need of more definitive techniques to specify and quantify the ROS generated by populations of human spermatozoa. Techniques such as electron spin resonance simply do not have the sensitivity necessary to detect the low level of ROS associated with normal human spermatozoa, although this technique has been used successfully with rabbit sperm (Chapman *et al.*, 1984). At the time of writing, chemiluminescence assays based on the use of luminol/ peroxidase or lucigenin, represent the state-of-the-art, inadequate as it may be.

7.4 Impact of oxidative stress on spermatozoa

The clinical significance of oxidative stress in the aetiology of defective sperm function was first indicated by Thaddeus Mann and colleagues at the University of Cambridge,

25 years ago (Jones *et al.*, 1979). These authors observed a correlation between the lipid peroxide content of human spermatozoa and severe motility loss. This relationship between motility loss and oxidative stress is striking and has been repeatedly demonstrated in independent studies (Aitken and Clarkson, 1988; Aitken and Fisher, 1994; Alvarez *et al.*, 1987; Sharma and Agarwal, 1996). Thus exposure of human spermatozoa to extracellularly generated ROS induces a loss of motility that is directly correlated with the level of lipid peroxidation experienced by the spermatozoa (Gomez *et al.*, 1998). Similarly, the loss of motility observed when spermatozoa are subjected to an overnight incubation is highly correlated with the lipid peroxidation status of the spermatozoa at the end of the incubation period (Gomez *et al.*, 1998). The prognostic value of stress tests based on the loss of motility observed when spermatozoa are incubated for defined periods of time in the presence of transition metals (Calamera *et al.*, 1998) is probably another reflection of the importance of lipid peroxidation in the modulation of sperm function. The ability of antioxidants such as α-tocopherol to rescue sperm motility *in vivo* and *in vitro* is yet more evidence that lipid peroxidation is a major cause of motility loss in populations of human spermatozoa (Aitken *et al.*, 1989a; Suleiman *et al.*, 1996). Indeed, measurements of lipid peroxidation have been used to select patients for antioxidant treatments incorporating α-tocopherol (Suleiman *et al.*, 1996).

The mechanisms by which lipid peroxidation leads to motility loss probably involves changes in the fluidity and integrity of the plasma membrane and a subsequent failure to maintain membrane functions critical to flagellar movement. In addition, lipid peroxidation will disrupt other sperm functions dependent on membrane activity including sperm–oocyte fusion and the ability to undergo a physiological acrosome reaction (Aitken *et al.*, 1993a, b; Jones *et al.*, 1978).

Oxidative stress is also a major cause of DNA damage in human spermatozoa. Using quantitative polymerase chain reaction (PCR) to calculate lesion frequency, the mitochondrial genome has been shown to be much more susceptible to DNA damage than the nuclear genome (Sawyer *et al.*, 2003). As a consequence, the integrity of the sperm mitochondrial genome is an excellent marker of oxidative stress, even though this genome is of no biological significance in its own right because sperm mitochondria do not generally replicate after fertilization. When quantitative PCR was used to compare the lesion frequencies induced in spermatozoa and a variety of other cell types following exposure to H_2O_2, the nuclear genome of the male gamete was shown to be particularly resistant to oxidative damage. This resistance is thought to mirror the unique manner in which nuclear chromatin is packaged in spermatozoa, as reflected in the high levels of irradiation required to damage sperm DNA compared with somatic cells (McKelvey-Martin *et al.*, 1997).

During the differentiation of spermatozoa, nuclear histones are progressively replaced with small positively charged molecules known as protamines. As a consequence of their small size and charge, protamines permit the packaging of sperm chromatin into an extremely small space. In Eutherian mammals, the protamines possess numerous cysteine residues that become oxidized during epididymal transit, establishing a series of inter- and intra-molecular disulphide bonds that serve to stabilize the nuclear chromatin structure. Such stabilization renders the DNA more resistant to oxidative damage. Marsupial spermatozoa cannot stabilize in this way because their protamines do not contain cysteine and, as a consequence, their nuclear DNA is significantly more susceptible to oxidative damage than Eutherian spermatozoa (Bennetts and Aitken, 2005).

Adequate compaction and stabilization of sperm nuclear DNA is therefore critical for protecting this material from oxidative stress. Amongst Eutherian mammals, human spermatozoa appear to be more susceptible to DNA damage than most other species. This is largely because the P2 protamine, characteristic of human spermatozoa, has a limited number of thiol groups for disulphide bonding (Jager, 1990). Furthermore the protamination of human spermatozoa is notably inefficient, with around 15% of the genome remaining histone rich, even in normal fertile men (Aoki and Carrell, 2003; Balhorn *et al.*, 1988; Belokopytova *et al.*, 1993). Failures in either the ability of the testes to adequately protaminate human sperm chromatin or the ability of the epididymis to support subsequent protamine cross-linkage, lead to imperfections in the state of chromatin stabilization. Such deficiencies in chromatin packaging have, in turn, been associated with an increased risk of DNA damage (Sakkas *et al.*, 1998).

In summary, while spermatozoa are vulnerable to oxidative stress and lipid peroxidation, the unique packaging of these cells normally renders the DNA resistant to such damage, particularly in Eutherian mammals. However in cases of male infertility, poor packaging of the sperm chromatin increases the vulnerability of these cells to oxidative DNA damage. This conclusion is in keeping with several studies showing that spermatozoa from infertile men not only exhibit more basal DNA damage but are also more susceptible to damage from both H_2O_2 and X-irradiation (Hughes *et al.*, 1998; McKelvey-Martin *et al.*, 1997).

Thus, even though the nuclear DNA of human spermatozoa is theoretically protected from oxidative damage by virtue of its compact assembly, the reality is that spontaneous DNA damage is observed more frequently in spermatozoa than somatic cells and, moreover, is observed in spermatozoa that have retained their capacity for fertilization (Aitken *et al.*, 1998a). This situation is clinically critical since it explains how male-mediated toxicology can occur, that is, how DNA damage originating in the paternal germ line, through such factors as age (Singh *et al.*, 2003), occupation (Knight and Marrett, 1997; Olshan and Mattison, 1994) and smoking (Ji *et al.*, 1997), can have impacts on the health and well-being of children, as a result of its transmission to the zygote at fertilization.

There is now abundant evidence indicating an increased incidence of conditions such as cancer, schizophrenia or dominant genetic mutation in the children of men with DNA damage in their spermatozoa because of their age, lifestyle or occupation (Lewis and Aitken, 2005). Since spontaneous mutation rates in the male germ line are extremely low (Hill *et al.*, 2004), it has been hypothesized that male-mediated pathology arises because of the aberrant repair of DNA damage in the early embryo, rather than the direct transfer of mutations from the male germ line to the offspring (Aitken, 1999; Aitken and Krausz, 1991; Aitken and Marshall Graves, 2002; Aitken *et al.*, 2004b) (Fig. 7.4). Clearly, such fundamental issues merit further attention.

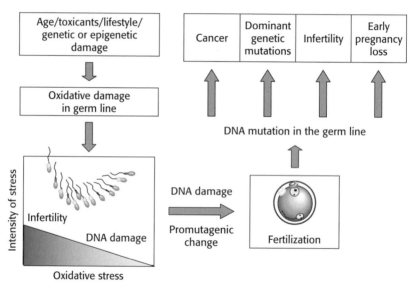

Figure 7.4   Proposed mechanisms by which oxidative stress in the male germ line can lead to genetic disease in the offspring. According to this model, a variety of intrinsic and extrinsic factors conspire to generate oxidative stress in the male germ line. Oxidative stress is not held to induce mutagenic change in male germ cells but creates non-specific DNA damage (strand breaks, oxidative DNA base change, abasic sites) as well as peroxidative damage to the sperm plasma membrane. At high levels of oxidative stress, the latter predominates and the spermatozoa lose their capacity for fertilization. At lower levels of oxidative stress, the DNA-damaged spermatozoa are still able to fertilize the oocyte and the latter must then repair the damaged DNA brought in by the fertilizing spermatozoon before the initiation of the first cleavage division. Aberrant DNA repair by the oocyte is then hypothesized to create mutations in the newly formed zygote, with the potential to impair the progress of pregnancy and induce genetic disease in the offspring

7.5 Origins of oxidative stress associated with defective sperm function

The oxidative damage detected in human spermatozoa may originate from several potential sources. Firstly, the leucocytes that contaminate every human semen sample are largely comprised of neutrophils that are commonly in an activated state. Thus the levels of spontaneous luminol-dependent chemiluminescence recorded in (unfractionated) human semen samples are highly correlated with the levels of leucocyte contamination (Aitken *et al.*, 1995a; Fig. 7.5). The presence of free-radical generating leucocytes in human ejaculates might therefore create a degree of oxidative stress. Much depends on the types of leucocytes that are present, their state of activation and their origin (Aitken and Baker, 1995). If the leucocytes originate in secondary sexual organs, such as the prostate and seminal vesicles, then their ability to cause oxidative damage to the spermatozoa will be counteracted by the powerful antioxidant properties of human seminal plasma. These antioxidants include small molecular mass free radical scavengers, such as ascorbic or uric acid, as well as antioxidant enzymes including SOD and glutathione peroxidase (Aitken and Baker, 1995; Aitken *et al.*, 1996a). As a consequence of the protective action of seminal plasma, neutrophil concentrations in the range normally encountered in human semen samples (~40,000/ml) do not adversely affect sperm function (Aitken *et al.*, 1994, 1995a). If however the seminal plasma is removed, and spermatozoa are compacted with leucocytes by centrifugation in the absence of antioxidant protection, then oxidative damage to the spermatozoa can result, impairing both the functional and genomic integrity of these cells (Aitken

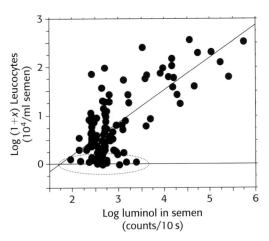

Figure 7.5   Positive correlation between the luminol signals generated in unfractionated human semen and leucocyte (CD45 positive) contamination (Aitken *et al.*, 1995a). Encircled area indicates that luminol-dependent chemiluminescence can vary by a log order of magnitude in the absence of detectable leucocyte contamination, emphasizing the underlying contribution of spermatozoa to the luminol signals obtained

and Clarkson, 1988; Aitken *et al.*, 1995a; Twigg *et al.*, 1998b). This situation can arise, for example, if spermatozoa are swum-up from a washed pellet in the course of assisted conception therapy. Such a sperm-preparation strategy will not invariably impair sperm function but, if infiltrating leucocytes are present, there is every chance that it will do so (Aitken and Clarkson, 1988). Of course, if the leucocytes infiltrate the male reproductive system proximal to the origin of the vas deferens, in the testes or epididymis, then there is ample opportunity for the ROS generated by activated white cells to damage the spermatozoa. Under these circumstances relatively small numbers of activated leucocytes could be harmful to the spermatozoa. Unfortunately, because it is impossible to determine the origin of seminal leucocytes, their pathological significance is frequently difficult to determine.

Another potential source of ROS is the spermatozoa themselves (Aitken and West, 1990; Aitken *et al.*, 1992b). Thus when all of the leucocytes have been carefully removed from human sperm suspensions using magnetic beads coated with anti-CD45 antibodies, the remaining spermatozoa are frequently capable of generating chemiluminescent signals with probes such as luminol or lucigenin. Moreover the intensity of these signals is inversely related to sperm function (Gomez *et al.*, 1998). Indeed, these signals are the most effective biochemical markers of defective sperm function that have been identified to date. Because of the complex chemistry that underpins these chemiluminescence responses there is uncertainty about whether they actually represent the excessive generation of ROS or the excessive presence of enzymes (reductases and peroxidases) capable of activating these probes. (Aitken *et al.*, 2004a). However the existence of correlations between the chemiluminescence signals generated by human spermatozoa, lipid peroxidation and DNA damage (Aitken *et al.*, 1993b; Gomez *et al.*, 1998; Said *et al.*, 2005) is strongly suggestive that these signals are reflecting ROS generation and oxidative stress.

Oxidative stress may also arise in the male germ line as a consequence of deficiencies in the antioxidant protection proffered by the male reproductive tract (Sharma and Agarwal, 1996). Measurements of total antioxidant activity in seminal plasma can be readily made and are relevant to sperm function, particularly in the protection of these cells during sperm preparation for assisted conception (Twigg *et al.*, 1998a, b; Sikka, 2004). However such measurements are not reflective of the protection provided to the spermatozoa prior to ejaculation, during their prolonged sojourn in the male reproductive tract. And it is at this phase of their life cycle that these cells are at their most vulnerable (Aitken *et al.*, 2004b).

7.6 The physiological role of ROS

If ROS are so dangerous to spermatozoa, then why have these cells evolved a capacity to generate these highly reactive molecules? The answer appears to lie in a poorly understood physiological process that is characteristic of mammalian spermatozoa–capacitation. Capacitation is a maturational process that spermatozoa must undergo if they are to interact successfully with the oocyte and commence the cascade of intercellular interactions leading to fertilization. As a biological phenomenon, capacitation has been acknowledged for more than 50 years since the pioneering work of Austin (1951) and Chang (1951). However, as a biochemical entity, the nature of capacitation has only become apparent in the past decade. The most significant finding over that period has been the discovery that sperm capacitation involves a dramatic increase in the overall level of tyrosine phosphorylation (Visconti *et al.*, 1995). This signal transduction pathway is driven by cAMP and modulated by the redox status of the cells (Aitken *et al.*, 1995b, 1998b; de Lamirande and Gagnon, 1993, 1995; Leclerc *et al.*, 1998). ROS generation is thought to exert a positive influence on tyrosine phosphorylation in spermatozoa through its ability to influence the intracellular levels of cAMP. The case for ROS involvement in cAMP generation and tyrosine phosphorylation has now been made for human (Aitken *et al.*, 1995b, 1998b), rat (Lewis and Aitken, 2001), mouse (Ecroyd *et al.*, 2003), bovine (Rivlin *et al.*, 2004) and equine (Baumber *et al.*, 2003) spermatozoa, via mechanisms that involve the stimulation of adenylyl cyclase activity (Aitken *et al.*, 1998b; Lewis and Aitken, 2001; Rivlin *et al.*, 2004; Zhang and Zheng, 1996). It is also possible that ROS, particularly H_2O_2, may enhance tyrosine phosphorylation through the selective suppression of tyrosine phosphatase activity. The latter enzyme contains a key cysteine residue in the catalytic domain that must be in a reduced state for phosphatase activity to be expressed. Direct exposure of tyrosine phosphatase enzymes to H_2O_2 leads to oxidation of this cysteine and a dramatic decline in enzyme activity. (Hecht and Zick, 1992).

The precise nature of the ROS triggering this cascade is still uncertain. A pivotal role for H_2O_2 generation has been suggested by experiments demonstrating that direct addition of this oxidant to suspensions of human, hamster or bovine spermatozoa, leads to the stimulation of tyrosine phosphorylation and capacitation (Aitken *et al.*, 1998b; Bize *et al.*, 1991; Rivlin *et al.*, 2004). Similarly, the artificial creation of oxidizing conditions by exposing spermatozoa to extracellularly generated ROS using the glucose oxidase or xanthine oxidase systems, has been shown to stimulate capacitation and tyrosine phosphorylation in several species (man, hamster, bull and horse) via mechanisms that can be reversed by the addition of catalase (Aitken *et al.*, 1995b; Baumber *et al.*, 2003; Bize *et al.*, 1991; Rivlin *et al.*, 2004). Even the incubation of spermatozoa in the presence of phorbol ester-activated leucocytes has been shown to stimulate human sperm capacitation via mechanisms that can be reversed by the antioxidants present in seminal plasma (Villegas *et al.*, 2003). The biological importance of H_2O_2 has been further emphasized by the ability of catalase to inhibit the spontaneous induction of tyrosine phosphorylation in capacitating mammalian spermatozoa (Aitken *et al.*, 1995b). In addition, catalase has been shown to suppress sperm functions such as hyperactivation, the acrosome reaction and sperm–oocyte fusion that are all ultimately dependent on the attainment of a capacitated state (Aitken et al., 1995b; Bize et al., 1991; Griveau et al., 1994).

The stimulation of intense redox activity in spermatozoa by the addition of exogenous NADPH has also been shown to stimulate tyrosine phosphorylation and/or sperm capacitation in a variety of species including man (Aitken et al., 1998b), rat (Lewis and Aitken, 2001), bull (Rivlin et al., 2004) and horse (Baumber et al., 2003). Measurements of $O_2^{-\bullet}$ production using a sensitive chemiluminescent probe failed to reveal any evidence for the production of this free radical when mammalian spermatozoa were exposed to NADPH (de Lamirande et al., 1998). However the fact that catalase can inhibit the ability of NADPH to stimulate capacitation and tyrosine phosphorylation suggests that the active oxygen metabolite generated under these circumstances is H_2O_2 rather than $O_2^{-\bullet}$ (Aitken et al., 1998b; Rivlin et al., 2004).

The physiological importance of NADPH-induced free radical generation has been emphasized in studies of hexose monophosphate shunt activity during capacitation. The hexose monophosphate shunt is required to generate the NADPH needed by a putative, ROS-generating sperm NADPH oxidase. Involvement of hexose monophosphate shunt activity in ROS generation and sperm capacitation has been emphasized by a number of different studies. Firstly, both the tyrosine phosphorylation cascade associated with sperm capacitation and ROS generation are dependent on the presence of glucose (Aitken et al., 1998b). Secondly tyrosine phosphorylation, capacitation and ROS generation can all be blocked by the presence of a non-metabolizable glucose analogue, 2-deoxyglucose via mechanisms that can be reversed with NADPH (Aitken et al., 1998b; Urner and Sakkas, 2005). Thirdly, inhibition of shunt activity with 6 amino nicotinamide also suppresses sperm capacitation via mechanisms that can be reversed by NADPH (Urner and Sakkas, 2005). Fourthly, ROS generation by spermatozoa is highly correlated with the presence of G6PDH (glucose-6-phosphate-dehydrogenase), a key enzyme in the control of hexose monophosphate shunt activity (Gomez et al., 1996). Finally, in permeabilized spermatozoa, ROS generation can be triggered by the concomitant presence of glucose-6 phosphate and NADP+, the substrates required for activation of the hexose monophosphate shunt (unpublished observations).

The minimal cytoplasmic volume associated with mature spermatozoa ensures limited production of ROS via this hexose monophosphate shunt-driven mechanism. Under these circumstances the shunt is generating just enough NADPH to fuel the glutathione reductase system, one of the major protective mechanisms present in mammalian spermatozoa. However, if cytosolic volume is increased because of the incomplete extrusion of residual cytoplasm during the terminal stages of spermiation, then excess NADPH will be generated and ROS production will be increased. In keeping with this suggestion, clear correlations have been observed between cytoplasmic volume, G6PDH content and redox activity in populations of human spermatozoa (Aitken *et al.*, 2004a; Gomez *et al.*, 1996). Moreover, as discussed above, the presence of excess residual cytoplasm, as indicated by high levels of cytoplasmic enzymes such as LDH, SOD and creatine kinase, has frequently been correlated with functional deficiencies in human spermatozoa (Aitken *et al.*, 1996a; Casano *et al.*, 1991; Huszar *et al.*, 1988; Ollero *et al.*, 2001). Similarly, subpopulations of defective immature spermatozoa associated with the retention of excess residual cytoplasm (Said *et al.*, 2005) exhibit significantly elevated levels of DNA damage following exposure to exogenous NADPH (Aitken *et al.*, 1998a; Said *et al.*, 2005; Twigg *et al.*, 1998a).

7.7 Conclusions

In conclusion, ROS represent a two edged sword as far as spermatozoa are concerned. On the one hand they are critical for the physiological programming of spermatozoa for fertilization through the facilitation of sperm capacitation. This effect involves stimulation of tyrosine phosphorylation through the ability of ROS to enhance the availability of intracellular cAMP and, possibly, suppress tyrosine phosphatase activity. In order to achieve this beneficial effect it is imperative that only limited amounts of ROS are generated. This is ensured by the limited availability of cytoplasm in mature functional cells, as a consequence of which spermatozoa produce just enough NADPH to fuel their glutathione reductase–peroxidase cycle. If, however, excess cytoplasm is present then there is the potential for excessive ROS to be produced because of the enhanced availability of both substrate and putative oxidase. Excessive ROS generation, and/or defects in the antioxidant systems designed to protect spermatozoa from oxidative damage, leads to a pathological loss of sperm function. Lipid peroxidation of unsaturated fatty acids in the sperm plasm membrane disrupts all membrane-dependent functions in these cells including motility and sperm–oocyte fusion. In addition, oxidative stress can damage the integrity of DNA in the sperm nucleus and mitochondria. Such damage has been associated with failures of fertilization as well as abnormal embryonic development and premature pregnancy loss (Lewis and Aitken, 2005). Given the important clinical consequences of oxidative stress in the male germ line, it is imperative that further research is undertaken to determine the source(s) of ROS and the development of safe, effective procedures to ameliorate pathologies based on the aberrant regulation of redox activity in these highly specialized cells.

REFERENCES

Afanas'ev IB, Ostrachovich EA and Korkina LG (1999) Lucigenin is a mediator of cytochrome C reduction but not of superoxide anion production. *Arch Biochem Biophys* 366, 267–274.

Aitken RJ (1999) The human spermatozoon – a cell in crisis? The Amoroso Lecture. *J Reprod Fertil* 115, 1–7.

Aitken RJ and Baker HW (1995) Seminal leukocytes: passengers, terrorists or good samaritans? *Human Reprod* 10, 1736–1739.

Aitken RJ and Clarkson JS (1987) Cellular basis of defective sperm function and its association with the genesis of reactive oxygen species by human spermatozoa. The Walpole Lecture. *J Reprod Fertil* 83, 459–469.

Aitken RJ and Clarkson (1988) Significance of reactive oxygen species and antioxidants in defining the efficacy of sperm preparation techniques. *J Androl* 9, 367–376.

Aitken RJ and Fisher H (1994) Reactive oxygen species generation and human spermatozoa, the balance of benefit and risk. *Bioessays* 16, 259–268.

Aitken RJ and Krausz CG (2001) Oxidative stress, DNA damage and the Y chromosome. *Reproduction* 122, 497–506.

Aitken RJ and Marshall Graves JA (2002) The Y chromosome, oxidative stress and the future of sex. *Nature* 415, 963.

Aitken RJ and West K (1990) Relationship between reactive oxygen species generation and leucocyte infiltration in fractions isolated from the human ejaculate on Percoll gradients. *Int J Androl* 13, 433–451.

Aitken RJ, Clarkson JS and Fishel S (1989a) Generation of reactive oxygen species, lipid peroxidation and human sperm function. *Biol Reprod* 40, 183–197.

Aitken RJ, Clarkson JS, Hargreave TB, Irvine DS and Wu FCW (1989b) Analysis of the relationship between defective sperm function and the generation of reactive oxygen species in cases of oligozoospermia. *J Androl* 10, 214–220.

Aitken RJ, Irvine DS and Wu FC (1991) Prospective analysis of sperm–oocyte fusion and reactive oxygen species generation as criteria for the diagnosis of infertility. *Am J Obstet Gynec* 164, 542–551.

Aitken RJ, Buckingham DW and West KM (1992a) Reactive oxygen species and human spermatozoa: analysis of the cellular mechanisms involved in luminol- and lucigenin-dependent chemiluminescence. *J Cell Physiol* 151, 466–477.

Aitken RJ, Buckingham D, West K, Wu FC, Zikopoulos K and Richardson DW (1992b) Differential contribution of leucocytes and spermatozoa to the high levels of reactive oxygen species recorded in the ejaculates of oligozoospermic patients. *J Reprod Fertil* 94, 451–462.

Aitken, RJ, Harkiss D and Buckingham DW (1993a) Analysis of lipid peroxidation mechanisms in human spermatozoa. *Mol Reprod Dev* 35, 302–315.

Aitken RJ, Harkiss D and Buckingham D (1993b) Relationship between iron-catalysed lipid peroxidation potential and human sperm function. *J Reprod Fertil* 98, 257–265.

Aitken RJ, West K and Buckingham D (1994) Leukocyte infiltration into the human ejaculate and its association with semen quality, oxidative stress and sperm function. *J Androl* 15, 343–352.

Aitken RJ, Buckingham DW, Brindle J, Gomez E, Baker HW and Irvine DS (1995a) Analysis of sperm movement in relation to the oxidative stress created by leukocytes in washed sperm preparations and seminal plasma. *Human Reprod* 10, 2061–2071.

Aitken RJ, Paterson M, Fisher H, Buckingham DW and van Duin M (1995b) Redox regulation of tyrosine phosphorylation in human spermatozoa and its role in the control of human sperm function. *J Cell Sci* 108, 2017–2025.

Aitken RJ, Buckingham DW, Carreras A and Irvine DS (1996a) Superoxide dismutase in human sperm suspensions: relationships with cellular composition, oxidative stress and sperm function. *Free Radic Biol Med* 21, 495–504.

Aitken RJ, Buckingham W, West K and Brindle J (1996b) On the use of paramagnetic beads and ferrofluids to assess and eliminate the leukocytic contribution to oxygen radical generation by human sperm suspensions. *Am J Reprod Immunol* 35, 541–551.

Aitken RJ, Fisher H, Fulton N, Knox W and Lewis B (1997) Reactive oxygen species generation by human spermatozoa is induced by exogenous NADPH and inhibited by the flavoprotein inhibitors diphenylene iodonium and quinacrine. *Mol Reprod Dev* 47, 468–482.

Aitken RJ, Gordon E, Harkiss D, Twigg JP, Milne P, Jennings Z and Irvine DS (1998a) Relative impact of oxidative stress on the functional competence and genomic integrity of human spermatozoa. *Biol Reprod* 59, 1037–1046.

Aitken RJ, Harkiss D, Knox W, Paterson M and Irvine DS (1998b) A novel signal transduction cascade in capacitating human spermatozoa characterised by a redox-regulated, cAMP-mediated induction of tyrosine phosphorylation. *J Cell Sci* 111, 645–656.

Aitken RJ, Ryan AL, Curry BJ and Baker MA (2003) Multiple forms of redox activity in populations of human spermatozoa. *Mol Human Reprod* 9, 645–661.

Aitken RJ, Baker MA and O'Bryan MK (2004a) Shedding light on chemiluminescence: the application of chemiluminescence in diagnostic andrology. *J Androl* 25, 455–465.

Aitken RJ, Koopman P and Lewis SE (2004b) Seeds of concern. *Nature* 432, 48–52.

Aitken RJ, Ryan AL, Baker MA and McLaughlin EA (2004c) Redox activity associated with the maturation and capacitation of mammalian spermatozoa. *Free Rad Biol Med* 36, 994–1010.

Alvarez JG, Touchstone JC, Blasco L and Storey BT (1987) Spontaneous lipid peroxidation and production of hydrogen peroxide and superoxide in human spermatozoa. *J Androl* 8, 338–348.

Aoki VW and Carrell DT (2003) Human protamines and the developing spermatid: their structure, function, expression and relationship with male infertility. *Asian J Androl* 5, 315–324.

Austin CR (1951) Observations on the penetration of the sperm into the mammalian egg. *Aust J Sci Res* B 4, 581–596.

Baker MA, Krutskikh A, Curry BJ, McLaughlin EA and Aitken RJ (2004) Identification of cytochrome P450-reductase as the enzyme responsible for NADPH-dependent lucigenin and tetrazolium salt reduction in rat epididymal sperm preparations. *Biol Reprod* 71, 307–318.

Balhorn R, Reed S and Tanphaichitr N (1988) Aberrant protamine 1/protamine 2 ratios in sperm of infertile human males. *Experientia* 44, 52–55.

Baumber J, Sabeur K, Vo A and Ball BA (2003) Reactive oxygen species promote tyrosine phosphorylation and capacitation in equine spermatozoa. *Theriogenology* 60, 1239–1247.

Belokopytova IA, Kostyleva EI, Tomilin AN and Vorob'ev VI (1993) Human male infertility may be due to a decrease of the protamine P2 content in sperm chromatin. *Mol Reprod Dev* 34, 53–57.

Bennetts LE and Aitken RJ (2005) A comparative study of oxidative DNA damage in mammalian spermatozoa. *Mol Reprod Dev* 71, 77–87.

Bielski BHJ, Arudi RL and Sutherland MW (1983) A study of the reactivity of $HO_2/O_2^{-\cdot}$ with unsaturated fatty acids. *J Biol Chem* 258, 4759–4761.

Bize I, Santander G, Cabello P, Driscoll D and Sharpe C (1991) Hydrogen peroxide is involved in hamster sperm capacitation *in vitro*. *Biol Reprod* 44, 398–403.

Calamera JC, Doncel GF, Brugo Olmedo S, Kolm P and Acosta AA (1998) Modified sperm stress test: a simple assay that predicts sperm-related abnormal *in vitro* fertilization (1998) *Human Reprod* 13, 2484–2488.

Casano R, Orlando C, Serio M and Forti G (1991) LDH and LDH-X activity in sperm from normospermic and oligozoospermic men. *Int J Androl* 14, 257–263.

Chang MC (1951) Fertilizing capacity of spermatozoa deposited into the Fallopian tubes. *Nature* 168, 697–698.

Chapman DA, Killian GJ, Gelerinter E and Jarrett MT (1984) Reduction of the spin label TEMPONE by ubiquinol in the electron transport chain of intact rabbit spermatozoa. *Biol Reprod* 32, 884–893.

de Lamirande E and Gagnon C (1993) Human sperm hyperactivation and capacitation as parts of an oxidative process. *Free Radic Biol Med* 14, 157–166.

de Lamirande E and Gagnon C (1995) Capacitation-associated production of superoxide anion by human spermatozoa. *Free Radic Biol Med* 18, 487–495.

de Lamirande E, Harakat A and Gagnon C (1998) Human sperm capacitation induced by biological fluids and progesterone, but not by NADH or NADPH, is associated with the production of superoxide anion. *J Androl* 19, 215–225.

Ecroyd H, Jones RC and Aitken RJ (2003) Endogenous redox activity in mouse spermatozoa and its role in regulating the tyrosine phosphorylation events associated with sperm capacitation. *Biol Reprod* 69, 347–354.

Faulkner K and Fridovich I (1993) Luminol and lucigenin as detectors for $O_2^{\cdot-}$. *Free Radic Biol Med* 15, 447–451.

Fridovich I (1999) Fundamental aspects of reactive oxygen species, or what's the matter with oxygen? *Ann NY Acad Sci* 893, 13–18.

Gil-Guzman E, Ollero M, Lopez MC, Sharma RK, Alvarez JG, Thomas Jr., AJ and Agarwal A (2001) Differential production of reactive oxygen species by subsets of human spermatozoa at different stages of maturation. *Human Reprod* 16, 1922–1930.

Gomez E, Buckingham DW, Brindle J, Lanzafame F, Irvine DS and Aitken RJ (1996) Development of an image analysis system to monitor the retention of residual cytoplasm by human spermatozoa: correlation with biochemical markers of the cytoplasmic space, oxidative stress and sperm function. *J Androl* 17, 276–287.

Gomez E, Irvine DS and Aitken RJ (1998) Evaluation of a spectrophotometric assay for the measurement of malondialdehyde and 4-hydroxyalkenals in human spermatozoa: relationships with semen quality and sperm function. *Int J Androl* 21, 81–94.

Gregory E, Goscin S and Fridovich I (1974) Superoxide dismutase and oxygen toxicity in a eukaryote. *J Appl Bacteriol* 117, 456.

Griveau JF, Renard P and Le Lannou D (1994) An *in vitro* promoting role for hydrogen peroxide in human sperm capacitation. *Int J Androl* 17, 300–307.

Halliwell B and Gutteridge JMC (1999) Free Radicals in Biology and Medicine. New York: Oxford University Press.

Han D, Antunes F, Canali R, Rettori D and Cadenas E (2003) Voltage-dependent anion channels control the release of the superoxide anion from mitochondria to cytosol. *J Biol Chem* 278, 5557–5563.

Hecht D and Zick Y (1992) Selective inhibition of protein tyrosine phosphatase activities by H_2O_2 and vanadate *in vitro*. *Biochem Biophys Res Commun* 188, 773–779.

Herrero MB and Gagnon C (2001) Nitric oxide: a novel mediator of sperm function. *J Androl* 22, 349–356.

Hill KA, Buettner VL, Halangoda A, Kunishige M, Moore SR, Longmate J, Scaringe WA and Sommer SS (2004) Spontaneous mutation in Big Blue® mice from fetus to old age: tissue-specific time courses of mutation frequency but similar mutation types. *Env Mol Mut* 43, 110–120.

Hughes CM, Lewis SE, McKelvey-Martin VJ and Thompson W (1998) The effects of antioxidant supplementation during Percoll preparation on human sperm DNA integrity. *Human Reprod* 13, 1240–1247.

Huszar G, Vigue L and Corrales M (1988) Sperm creatine phosphokinase quality in normospermic, variablespermic and oligospermic men. *Biol Reprod* 138, 1061–1066.

Jager S (1990) Sperm nuclear stability and male infertility. *Arch Androl* 25, 253–259.

Ji BT, Shu XO, Linet MS, Zheng W, Wacholder S, Gao YT, Ying DM and Jin F (1997) Paternal cigarette smoking and the risk of childhood cancer among offspring of non-smoking mothers. *J Natl Cancer Inst* 89, 238–244.

Jones R, Mann T and Sherins RJ (1978) Adverse effects of peroxidized lipid on human spermatozoa. *Proc R Soc Lond* B 201, 413–417.

Jones R, Mann T and Sherins RJ (1979) Peroxidative breakdown of phospholipids in human spermatozoa: spermicidal effects of fatty acid peroxides and protective action of seminal plasma. *Fertil Steril* 31, 531–537.

Knight JA and Marrett LD (1997) Parental occupational exposure and the risk of testicular cancer in Ontario. *J Occup Environ Med* 39, 333–338.

Krausz C, West K, Buckingham D and Aitken RJ (1992) Analysis of the interaction between N-formylmethionyl-leucyl phenylalanine and human sperm suspensions, development of a technique for monitoring the contamination of human semen samples with leucocytes. *Fertil Steril* 57, 1317–1325.

Kwenang A, Krous MJ, Koster JF and Van Eijk HG (1987) Iron, ferritin and copper in seminal plasma. *Human Reprod* 2, 387–388.

Leclerc P, de Lamirande E and Gagnon C (1998) Interaction between Ca^{2+}, cyclic $3',5'$ adenosine monophosphate, the superoxide anion, and tyrosine phosphorylation pathways in the regulation of human sperm capacitation. *J Androl* 19, 434–443.

Lewis B and Aitken RJ (2001) A redox-regulated tyrosine phosphorylation cascade in rat spermatozoa. *J Androl* 22, 611–622.

Lewis SEM and Aitken RJ (2005) Sperm DNA damage, fertilization and pregnancy. *Cell Tissue Res* (in press).

Li Y, Stansbury KH, Zhu H and Trush MA (1999) Biochemical characterization of lucigenin (bis-N-methylacridinium) as a chemiluminescent probe for detecting intramitochondrial superoxide anion radical production. *Biochem Biophys Res Commun* 262, 80–87.

McKelvey-Martin VJ, Melia N, Walsh IK, Johnson SR, Hughes CM, Lewis SEM and Thompson W (1997) Two potential clinical applications of the alkaline single cell gel electrophoresis assay: i. Human bladder washings and transitional cell carcinoma of the bladder, ii. Human sperm and male infertility. *Mut Res* 375, 93–104.

McKinney KA, Lewis SE and Thompson W (1996) Reactive oxygen species generation in human sperm: luminol and lucigenin chemiluminescence probes. *Arch Androl* 36, 119–125.

Nakamura M and Nakamura S (1998) One- and two-electron oxidations of luminol by peroxidase systems. *Free Radic Biol Med* 24, 537–544.

Ollero M, Gil-Guzman E, Lopez MC, Sharma RK, Agarwal A, Larson K, Evenson D, Thomas Jr., AJ and Alvarez JG (2001) Characterization of subsets of human spermatozoa at different stages of maturation: implications in the diagnosis and treatment of male infertility. *Human Reprod* 16, 1912–1921.

Olshan AF and Mattison DR (1994) Male Mediated Developmental Toxicity. New York: Plenum Press.

Rivlin J, Mendel J, Rubinstein S, Etkovitz N and Breitbart H (2004) Role of hydrogen peroxide in sperm capacitation and acrosome reaction. *Biol Reprod* 70, 518–522.

Said TM, Agarwal A, Sharma RK, Mascha E, Sikka SC and Thomas Jr., AJ (2004) Human sperm superoxide anion generation and correlation with semen quality in patients with male infertility. *Fertil Steril* 82, 871–877.

Said TM, Agarwal A, Sharma RK, Thomas AJ and Sikka S (2005) Impact of sperm morphology on DNA damage caused by oxidative stress induced by β-nicotinamide adenine dinucleotide phosphate. *Fertil Steril* 83, 95–103.

Sakkas D, Urner F, Bizzaro D, Manicardi G, Bianchi PG, Shoukir Y and Campana A (1998) Sperm nuclear DNA damage and altered chromatin structure: effect on fertilization and embryo development. *Human Reprod* 13, 11–19.

Sawyer DE, Mercer BG, Wiklendt AM and Aitken RJ (2003) Analysis of gene-specific DNA damage and single-strand DNA breaks induced by pro-oxidant treatment of human spermatozoa *in vitro*. *Mut Res* 529, 21–34.

Sharma RK and Agarwal A (1996) Role of reactive oxygen species in male infertility. *Urology* 48, 835–850.

Sikka SC (2004) Role of oxidative stress and antioxidants in andrology and assisted reproductive technology. *J Androl* 25, 5–18.

Singh NP, Muller CH and Berger RE (2003) Effects of age on DNA double-strand breaks and apoptosis in human sperm. *Fertil Steril* 80, 1420–1430.

Storey BT (1997) Biochemistry of the induction and prevention of lipoperoxidative damage in human spermatozoa. *Mol Human Reprod* 13, 203–214.

Suleiman SA, Elamin Ali M, Zaki ZMS, El-Malik EMA and Nasr MA (1996) Lipid peroxidation and human sperm motility: protective role of vitamin E. *J Androl* 17, 530–537.

Toyokuni S (2002) Iron and carcinogenesis: from Fenton reaction to target genes. *Redox Report* 7, 189–197.

Twigg J, Fulton N, Gomez E, Irvine DS and Aitken RJ (1998a) Analysis of the impact of intracellular reactive oxygen species generation on the structural and functional integrity of human spermatozoa, lipid peroxidation, DNA fragmentation and effectiveness of antioxidants. *Human Reprod* 13, 1429–1437.

Twigg JP, Irvine DS, Houston P, Fulton N, Michael L and Aitken RJ (1998b) Iatrogenic DNA damage induced in human spermatozoa during sperm preparation: protective significance of seminal plasma. *Mol Human Reprod* 4, 439–445.

Urner F and Sakkas D (2005) Involvement of the pentose phosphate pathway and redox regulation in fertilization in the mouse. *Mol Reprod Dev* 70, 494–503.

Vernet P, Fulton N, Wallace C and Aitken RJ (2001) Analysis of reactive oxygen species generating systems in rat epididymal spermatozoa. *Biol Reprod* 65, 1102–1111.

Villegas J, Kehr K, Soto L, Henkel R, Miska W and Sanchez R (2003) Reactive oxygen species induce reversible capacitation in human spermatozoa. *Andrologia* 35, 227–232.

Visconti PE, Moore GD, Bailey JL, Leclerc P, Connors SA, Pan D, Olds-Clarke P and Kopf GS (1995) Capacitation of mouse spermatozoa. II. Protein tyrosine phosphorylation and capacitation are regulated by a cAMP-dependent pathway. *Development* 121, 1139–1150.

Zhang H and Zheng R-L (1996) Promotion of human sperm capacitation by superoxide anion. *Free Rad Res* 24, 261–268.

Zini A, O'Bryan MK, Israel L and Schlegel PN (1998) Human sperm NADH and NADPH diaphorase cytochemistry: correlation with sperm motility. *Urology* 51, 464–468.

8

Testing sperm manufacturing quality: the sperm–zona binding assay

Sergio Oehninger[1] and Daniel Franken[2]

[1]Department of Obstetrics and Gynecology, The Jones Institute for Reproductive Medicine, Eastern Virginia Medical School, Norfolk, VA, USA

[2]Department of Obstetrics and Gynecology, Reproductive Biology Unit, Tygerberg Hospital, University of Stellenbosch, Capetown, Republic of South Africa

8.1 Introduction

Infertility in general and the proportion of cases where a male factor can be identified as the cause (alone or in combination with female factors) are prevalent conditions (Centers for Disease Control and Prevention, 1997; Hull *et al.*, 1985; Mosher and Pratt, 1990). Although diagnostic problems make it difficult to establish the extent of the male partner's contribution with certainty, a number of studies suggest that male problems represent the commonest single defined cause of infertility (Irvine, 1998).

Current treatment options for male infertility include a variety of urological procedures (surgical and non-surgical), medical–pharmacological interventions, low complexity assisted reproductive procedures (such as intrauterine insemination (IUI) therapy), and the more advanced and complex assisted reproductive technologies (ARTs). Among the latter, *in vitro* fertilization (IVF) and embryo transfer, augmented with intracytoplasmic sperm injection (ICSI) in the moderate and severe male factor cases, constitute validated and successful ways to assist fertilization. The national statistics from the USA (Centers for Disease Control and Prevention, 2004) reported a 44% incidence of ICSI in 115,392 ART cycles performed during 2002, a figure that highlights the impact that this assisted fertilization technique has recently had on infertility management.

Other lines of investigation have recently provided further reasons for concern in the area of human male reproduction. First, some researchers have reported an overall decline in the quantity and quality of spermatozoa present in semen, perhaps caused by reproductive bio-hazards, for example, environmental estrogens (Irvine, 1997). Second, it has been shown that spermatozoa from infertile men may carry chromosomal and/or genetic abnormalities. Such findings are in agreement with a slight but significant increase in the incidence of chromosomal anomalies in babies born after ICSI (Bonduelle *et al.*, 1999). Although ICSI represents a 'boom' in the treatment of men with various degrees of sperm anomalies, its use may increase the risk of chromosomal/genetic disease transmission. Third, we also have to keep in mind that in most situations ARTs are 'palliative' as opposed to 'curative' of the underlying pathology. The truth of the matter is that in a very large proportion of male infertility cases (probably over 50% of the cases) the reason of the underlying disease is unknown or idiopathic. Consequently, there is a fundamental need to carry out research directed towards increasing our understanding of the underlying pathophysiology as well as to be able to prevent those conditions resulting in infertility (i.e., sexually transmitted diseases, reproductive bio-hazards and others). These steps should lead to the development of simpler, safer, more cost-efficient and universally applicable therapies.

Recent work derived from the clinical arena has demonstrated that ejaculated spermatozoa from subfertile men carry other numerous structural and functional abnormalities. Principally, these include: an abnormal capacity to achieve capacitation, an inability to bind to the zona pellucida (ZP) and/or to undergo acrosomal exocytosis, as well as the presence of a variety of nuclear/chromatin defects such as DNA fragmentation and aberrations of nuclear proteins. These findings can be observed in the presence of normal, subnormal or overtly abnormal basic sperm parameters. The presence of these abnormal features is typically associated with an inability to conceive naturally as well as fertilization failure or low rates of fertilization during IVF therapy, thereby decreasing chances of pregnancy. The application of ICSI, on other hand, appears to circumvent most of these deficiencies. However, more research is needed to determine the true paternal effects and contributions of the normal and abnormal male gamete to early embryogenesis (Oehninger *et al.*, 1998).

As a consequence, it follows that there is a real need to assess sperm functional competence in an 'extended' evaluation of the infertility work-up. There is a fundamental gap in the knowledge of the pathogenic mechanisms that impair spermatogenesis, spermiogenesis, sperm storage and gamete interaction in the human. Although the cellular and molecular mechanisms involved in sperm–oocyte interaction are beginning to be unraveled in several animal species little is known in the human.

Within this defying clinical scenario, important practical questions that arise are: Which tests of sperm function are validated and predictive of *in vivo* and/or *in vitro* conception? Can sperm function tests be used to guide clinical management?

8.2 Assessment of the subfertile patient: the andrological examination and the basic semen analysis

The clinical andrological investigation of the male partner in an infertile couple relies on a thorough history and physical examination. Additionally, urological, endocrinological and genetic investigations should be implemented as needed. Nonetheless, the semen analysis still remains the cornerstone of the diagnostic management. We and others promoted a sequential, multi-step diagnostic approach for the evaluation of the various structural, dynamic and functional sperm characteristics when abnormalities are found in the initial evaluation (Amann and Hammerstedt, 1993; Oehninger *et al.*, 1991a, 1997a). This diagnostic scheme should include: (i) assessment of the 'basic' semen analysis and (ii) functional testing of spermatozoa. A comprehensive semen analysis following the World Health Organization (WHO) Guidelines (WHO, 1999) is fundamental at the primary care level to make a rational initial diagnosis and to select the appropriate clinical management. The collection and analysis of the semen must be undertaken by properly trained technologists using standardized procedures in accredited laboratories (De Jonge, 2000).

8.3 The extended semen evaluation

If abnormalities are found during the basic investigation, or if the couple is diagnosed with unexplained infertility, the work-up should progress to the examination of specific structural features, biochemical characteristics and sperm functions.

Sperm from subfertile men often contain multiple structural and biochemical alterations. Anatomically they can be divided into: membrane alterations, that can be assessed, for example, by tests of resistance to osmotic stress, translocation of phosphatidylserine; nuclear aberrations, such as abnormal chromatin condensation, retention of histones and presence of DNA fragmentation; cytoplasmic lesions as evidenced, for example, by excessive generation of reactive oxygen species, loss of mitochondrial membrane potential, cytoplasmic retention, or presence of caspases and flagellar disturbances, such as abnormalities in the microtubules and/or the fibrous sheath. Some of these alterations are indicative of immaturity, presence of an apoptosis phenotype, infection-necrosis, or other unknown causes (reviewed in Aitken and Baker, 2004; Baccetti *et al.*, 1996, 2002; Barroso *et al.*, 2000; Huszar *et al.*, 2004; Marchetti *et al.*, 2002; Oehninger *et al.*, 2003).

Notwithstanding their occurrence and correlation with clinical outcomes, it is not clear how these abnormalities directly impact sperm function, particularly motility, fertilization and contribution to embryogenesis. Furthermore, many assays are still experimental and more research is needed to validate their results in the clinical setting and to determine their true capacity to predict male fertility potential.

On the other hand, there are other specific and critical sperm functional capacities that can be more reliably examined *in vitro*. These functions include: motility, ability to capacitate, ZP binding, acrosome reaction, oolemma binding, nuclear decondensation and pronuclear formation. The assessment of some of these features is what is typically considered as sperm functional testing (Fig. 8.1).

Crucial sperm functions

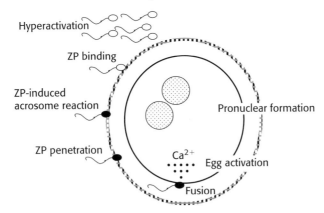

Figure 8.1   Sperm functions that are critical for fertilization to ensue. ZP binding: tight binding of
sperm to the ZP is tested with the HZA or a zona binding assay. ZP-induced acrosome
reaction: acrosomal exocytosis triggered by the ZP is tested with the ZIAR microassay

8.3.1 Sperm function tests

The categories of assays that are usually considered include: (i) bioassays of
gamete interaction, that is, the heterologous zona-free hamster oocyte test and the
homologous sperm–ZP binding assays, (ii) induced-acrosome reaction testing
and (iii) computer-aided sperm motion analysis (CASA) for evaluating sperm
motion characteristics (Burkman *et al.*, 1988; Cross *et al.*, 1986; Fraser *et al.*, 1997;
Liu *et al.*, 1988; Mortimer, 1990; Mortimer *et al.*, 1990; WHO, 1992; Yanagimachi
et al., 1976).

We reported a meta-analysis on 34 published and prospectively designed, controlled studies. The aim was carried out through the examination of the predictive
value of four categories of sperm functional assays (computer-aided sperm motion
analysis or CASA, induced-acrosome reaction testing, sperm penetration assay or
SPA, and sperm–ZP binding assays) for IVF outcome (Oehninger *et al.*, 2000).
Results demonstrated a high predictive power of the sperm–ZP binding and the
induced-acrosome reaction assays for IVF outcome. On the other hand, the findings indicated a poor clinical value of the SPA as predictor of fertilization and a real
need for standardization and further investigation of the potential clinical utility of
CASA systems. Although this study provided objective evidence in which clinical
management and future research may be directed, the analysis also pointed out
limitations of the current tests and the need for standardization of present methodologies and development of novel technologies. It is important to note that there
are no studies addressing the validity and predictive power of these assays for
natural conception.

8.3.2 Sperm–ZP binding assays

The two most common zona binding tests currently used are the hemizona assay (HZA) (Burkman *et al.*, 1988) and a ZP-binding test (Liu *et al.*, 1988, 1989). The HZA is a diagnostic bioassay testing the binding of human spermatozoa to human ZP to predict fertilization potential (Burkman *et al.*, 1988). In the HZA, two matched zona hemispheres are created by microbisection of the human oocyte providing three main advantages: (1) the two halves (hemizonae) are functionally equal surfaces allowing controlled comparison of binding and reproducible measurements of sperm binding from a single egg; (2) the test is internally controlled test by being performed on a single oocyte and (3) because the oocyte is split microsurgically, even fresh oocytes cannot lead to inadvertent fertilization and pre-embryo formation (Burkman *et al.*, 1988; Hodgen *et al.*, 1988).

Sperm–ZP binding tests evaluate the first crucial step of sperm–oocyte interaction that leads to fertilization, and that is tight binding of spermatozoa to the ZP (Yangimachi, 1994). Overstreet and Hembree (1976) were the first to develop an assay for evaluating penetration of ZP by human spermatozoa using human oocytes recovered from the ovaries of cadavers. Both the HZA and the zona binding test have the advantage of providing a functional homologous test for sperm binding to the zona comparing populations of fertile and infertile spermatozoa within the same assay. The internal control offered by the HZA represents an advantage by diminishing the intra-assay variation and decreasing the number of oocytes needed during the assay (Burkman *et al.*, 1988; Franken *et al.*, 1989a, 1991a, b; Hodgen *et al.*, 1988; Oehninger *et al.*, 1991a, b).

Before a spermatozoon can penetrate the ZP there is a specific need for firm attachment between the gametes. Tight gamete binding is attributed to the presence of complimentary binding sites or receptors on the surface of the gametes and typically these receptors manifest a high degree of species specificity (Ahuja, 1985; Oehninger, 2001a; Yanagimachi, 1994).

For the last two decades, investigators have sought to identify an individual protein or carbohydrate side chain as the 'sperm receptor'. Using 'knockout mice', in the absence of either ZP protein 2 (ZP2) or ZP protein 3 (ZP3) expression, a ZP fails to assemble around growing oocytes and females are infertile. In the absence of ZP protein 1 (ZP1) expression, a disorganized zona assembles around growing oocytes and females exhibit reduced fertility. These observations are consistent with the current model for ZP structure in which ZP2 and ZP3 form long zona filaments crosslinked by ZP1 (reviewed in Wassarman *et al.*, 2004).

However, recent genetic data in mice appear to be more consistent with the three-dimensional structure of the ZP, rather than a single protein (or carbohydrate), determining sperm binding. Collectively, the genetic data indicate that no single mouse ZP protein is obligatory for taxon-specific sperm binding and that two human proteins are not sufficient to support human sperm binding. An observed post-fertilization persistence of mouse sperm binding to 'humanized' ZP corre-lates with uncleaved ZP2. These observations are consistent with a model for sperm binding in which the supramolecular structure of the ZP necessary for sperm binding is modulated by the cleavage status of ZP2 (Castle and Dean, 1999; Hoodbhoy and Dean, 2004; Rankin et al., 1998, 2003).

Because binding of gametes is a critical step in fertilization and pre-embryo development; the HZA has many potential uses in reproductive medicine. Initially developed as a test to investigate male infertility and predict fertilization potential, this bioassay has been used to assess sperm function after contraceptive treatment (Burkman et al., 1988; Hodgen et al., 1988; Oehninger et al., 1991a, b). As is often the case, new findings in reproductive medicine can usually be equally applied to infer-tility or contraception technology depending on the focus of interest.

Human oocytes derived from different sources can be used for the HZA, such as surgically removed ovaries, post-mortem ovarian tissue and surplus oocytes from the IVF program. Since fresh oocytes are not always available for the test, different methods for storage have been developed. Overstreet and Hembree (1976) described the storage of human oocytes in dimethylsulfoxide (DMSO) at ultra low tempera-tures. Additionally, Yanagimachi and colleagues showed that highly concentrated salt solutions provided effective protection and storage of hamster and human oocytes, such that the integrity of sperm-binding characteristics of the ZP was pre-served (Yanagimachi et al., 1979; Yoshimatsu et al., 1988). In developing the HZA, the binding ability of fresh, DMSO and salt-stored (under controlled pH condi-tions) human oocytes was examined and sperm-binding characteristics of the ZP remained intact under all these conditions (Franken et al., 1989a; Kruger et al., 1991). Subsequently, the kinetics of sperm binding to the zona was assessed. Maximum binding occurred at 4–5 h of gamete coincubation with binding curves similar for fertile and infertile semen samples (Burkman et al., 1988; Franken et al., 1989a).

Detailed description of oocyte collection, handling and micromanipulation, as well as semen processing and sperm preparations for the HZA have been described (Burkman et al., 1988; Franken et al., 1989a). The assay has been standardized to a 4 h gamete coincubation, exposing each hemizona to a post swim-up sperm droplet of 500,000 motile sperm/ml. Human tubal fluid medium supplemented with synthetic serum substitute or human serum albumin is typically used for sperm preparation and gamete coincubation. After coincubation, the hemizona are subjected to pipetting through a glass pipet in order to dislodge loosely attached sperm. The number of tightly bound spermatozoa on the outer surface of the zona is counted using phase contrast microscopy ($\times$200). Results are expressed as the number of sperm tightly bound to the hemizona for control and patient, and also as hemizona index (HZI) the number of sperm tightly bound for the control sample ($\times$100) (Burkman et al., 1988).

The HZA has been validated by a clear-cut definition of the factors effecting data interpretation: that is, kinetics of binding, egg variability and maturation status, intra-assay variation and influence of sperm concentration, morphology, motility and acrosome reaction status (Coddington et al., 1990, 1991; Franken et al., 1989a; 1991a, b; Oehninger et al., 1991b). Definition of the assay's limitations and its small intra-assay variation (less than 10%) has maximized the power of discrimination of the HZA. Conversely, several oocytes have to be used for other sperm–zona binding tests because of the high inter-egg variation. In fact, a high intra-assay coefficient of variation (CV) has been reported (Liu et al., 1988, 1989).

Inter-egg variability is high for oocytes at different stages of maturation (immature versus mature eggs) and eggs at the same maturation stage. Egg variability is internally controlled in the HZA assay by using the bisected, matching hemizona. This allows for direct comparison of fertile versus infertile semen sample binding in the same assay and under the same oocyte quality conditions. We have been able to determine the intra-egg (intra-assay viability) of human oocytes by incubating matching hemizona from eggs at the same maturational stage with homologous spermatozoa from the same fertile ejaculate (Oehninger et al., 1989, 1991b, 1992). Overall, the mean intra-egg variation between the two matching halves for all categories of egg nuclear maturation is approximately 10%. Additionally, we have shown that full meiotic competence of human and monkey oocytes are associated with an increased binding potential of ZP. It would appear that zona maturation is associated with the nuclear development in parallel with cytoplasmic and membrane maturation leading to a fully fertilizable status.

The specificity of the interaction between human spermatozoa and the human ZP under HZA conditions is strengthened by the fact that sperm tightly bound to the zona are acrosome reacted (Coddington et al., 1990; Franken et al., 1991a). Results from interspecies experiments using human, cynomolgus monkey and hamster gametes have demonstrated high species specificity of human sperm/ZP functions under HZA conditions providing further support for the use of this bioassay in infertility and contraception testing (Oehninger et al., 1993).

In prospective blinded studies, we have investigated the relationship between sperm binding to the hemizona and IVF outcome (Franken et al., 1989b; Oehninger et al., 1989, 1991a, 1992, 1997a). Results show that the HZA successfully identifies male-factor patients at risk for failed or poor fertilization. Using either a cut-off value of fertilization rate of 65% (mean − 2SD of the overall fertilization rate in the Norfolk Program for non-male-factor patients), or distinguishing between failed versus successful fertilization (0% versus 1–100%), the HZA results expressed as HZI provide a valuable means to separate these categories of patients (Oehninger et al., 1992, 1997a).

Powerful statistical results confirm the utility of the HZA for the predicting IVF rates (Franken et al., 1993; Gamzu et al., 1994; Oehninger, 1997a, b). Therefore, the

HZA can distinguish a population of male-factor patients that will encounter low fertilization rates in IVF and, when combined with other sperm parameters (morphology and motion characteristics), gives reliable and useful clinical information. Of the classical sperm parameters, sperm morphology is the best predictor of the ability of spermatozoa to bind to the ZP. Patients with severe teratozoospermia ('poor prognosis' pattern or less than 4% normal sperm scores as judged by strict criteria) have an impaired capacity to bind the zona under HZA conditions perhaps indicating membrane/receptor defects. We agreed with Liu *et al.* that the ability of sperm to achieve tight binding to the ZP might reflect multiple functions of human spermatozoa (Liu *et al.*, 1988, 1989).

In our studies, when the HZA was removed from regression analysis in order to identify the predictive value of other sperm parameters (sperm concentration, morphology and motion characteristics), the percentage of progressive motility was the second best predictor of fertilization outcome (Oehninger *et al.*, 1992). We speculated that the relationship between sperm morphology and IVF results depends upon an effect on zona binding. On the other hand, motility seems to affect the prediction of fertilization rate outside the prediction of the HZA. It would appear that although important in achieving binding, motility may be more important for cumulus penetration and ZP penetration, factors not directly evaluated in the HZA. Logistic regression analysis provided a robust HZI range predictive of the oocytes potential to be fertilized. This HZI cut-off value is approximately 35%. Overall, for failed versus successful and poor versus good fertilization rate, the correct predictive ability (discriminative power) of the HZA was 80% and 85%, respectively. The information gained may be extremely valuable for counseling patients in the IVF setting (i.e., considering a HZI below 35% the chances of poor fertilization are 90–100%; whereas for the HZI over 35%, the chances of good fertilization are 80–85%) (Franken *et al.*, 1993; Oehninger *et al.*, 1992, 1997a, b).

Overall, the HZA has demonstrated an excellent sensitivity and specificity with a low incidence of false positive results. For an HZI of 35%, the positive predictive value of the HZA is 79% and its negative predictive value is 100% (considering good versus poor fertilization rates). In the HZA, false positive results can be expected, since other functional steps follow the tight binding of sperm to the ZP and are essential for fertilization and pre-embryo development (Table 8.1).

8.3.3 Acrosome reaction assays

The acrosome reaction is a pre-requisite for fertilization in mammalian spermatozoa (Yanagimachi, 1994). In the mouse, one of the species best characterized so far, acrosomal exocytosis is physiologically induced by components of the ZP, particularly the ZP3 (Bleil and Wassarman, 1980, 1983; Florman and Storey, 1982; Florman and Wassarman, 1985). Binding of ZP3 to putative complementary receptor(s) on

Table 8.1. Predictive value of the HZA for IVF outcome considering an HZI cut-off of 35% (data compiled from references of Franken *et al.*, 1993; Oehninger *et al.*, 1997a, 2000a). Predictive power was calculated for failed (0% of oocytes fertilized/inseminated) versus successful (>1%) fertilization and also for good (>65%) versus poor (⩽65%) fertilization rate

	Failed versus successful fertilization in IVF (%)	Poor versus good fertilization in IVF (%)
Hemizona index		
Positive predictive value	82	79
False positive rate	12	13
False negative rate	6	0
Negative predictive value	73	100

the sperm surface activates transmembrane signals that trigger cellular cascades resulting in the acrosome reaction (Wassarman, 1990a, b, 1999).

Several cellular pathways are involved in the stimulation of the acrosome reaction (Fig. 8.2). It has been demonstrated that activation of pertussis toxin-sensitive heterotrimeric G proteins (G_i-class) is necessary for the ZP-induced acrosome reaction in the murine model (Kopf *et al.*, 1986; Kopf, 1990). G_i-protein acts as a signal transducing element downstream of ZP3-receptor interactions and couples receptor occupancy to changes in ionic conductance and/or a variety of intracellular second messenger cascade systems whose activation in turn results in release of acrosomal contents (Kopf, 1990). One of such elements is likely to be a pH regulator, resulting in a transient alkanization of intracellular pH (Florman *et al.*, 1989, 1998; Kopf, 1990). Second messengers include the adenylate cyclase-cAMP system resulting in activation of protein kinase A (PKA) leading to phosphorylation of specific, putative proteins resulting in exocytosis. Also, the activation of phospholipase C (PLC) may lead to 1,2-diacylglycerol (DAG) and inositol 1,4,5-trisphosphate (IP3) formation. Diacylglycerol may stimulate protein phosphorylation through protein kinase C (PKC) whereas IP3 may activate intracellular calcium release through modulation of IP3-sensitive intracellular calcium stores (Florman *et al.*, 1998; Kopf, 1990; Wassarman, 1999).

It has also been proposed that the ZP may alternatively activate a low voltage-activated T type calcium channel that is pertussis toxin-insensitive (Florman *et al.*, 1992, 1998; O'Toole *et al.*, 2000). Activation of pertussis toxin-sensitive and -insensitive mechanisms leads to significant and sustained changes in intracellular calcium levels, a prerequisite for the acrosome reaction (Florman *et al.*, 1998; Kopf, 1990).

Progesterone, present in high concentrations in the follicular fluid, is also a known stimulator of the acrosome reaction. It has been shown that progesterone exerts a priming effect on the ZP-stimulated acrosome reaction in the mouse (Roldan *et al.*,

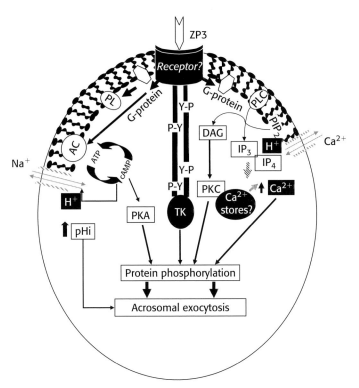

Figure 8.2 Diagram of putative intracellular cascades leading to the acrosome reaction. The scheme is based on data compiled from the references (Baldi *et al.*, 2000; Burks *et al.*, 1995; Doherty *et al.*, 1995; Florman *et al.*, 1998; Kopf, 1990). Upon binding of ZP3 with its putative receptor, one (or all) of three main phosphorylation systems may be activated resulting in acrosomal exocytosis. These second messenger systems are: activation of a tyrosine kinase, G-protein–cAMP–protein kinase A, and phospholipase C-diacylglycerol-protein kinase C. In addition, increased intracellular calcium levels may result after mobilization from internal stores and following influx from activated membrane channels. An efflux of H^+, which in turn determines a rise of intracellular pH, may also accompany this event

1994) and in the human (Schuffner *et al.*, 2002). In the former studies, treatment with progesterone followed by ZP led to maximal generation of DAG and maximal breakdown of phosphatidylinositol-4,5-bisphosphate (PIP$_2$) signaling a priming role for progesterone in the initiation of exocytosis.

Relatively few studies have addressed the role of the physiologic, homologous inducer of the acrosome reaction, the ZP, in human spermatozoa. This is probably due to the difficulty in obtaining human material (oocytes) to perform such experiments. ZP can be obtained from oocytes recovered from ovarian tissue (post-surgical or post-mortem) or from IVF treatment following appropriate patients' consent for donation.

Cross *et al.* (1988) were the first to report that treatment of human spermatozoa in suspension with acid-disaggregated human ZP (2–4 ZP/μl) increased the incidence of acrosome reacted spermatozoa. Lee *et al.* (1992) demonstrated that pertussis toxin treatment of human spermatozoa inhibited the (solubilized) ZP-induced acrosome reaction. In contrast, acrosomal exocytosis induced by the calcium ionophore A-23187 was not inhibited by pertussis toxin pre-treatment. Studies by Franken *et al.* (1996) showed a dose-dependent effect of solubilized human ZP on the acrosome reaction in the range of 0.25–1 ZP/μl and also confirmed the involvement of G_i-protein during ZP-induced acrosome reaction of human spermatozoa.

Capacitated human spermatozoa also respond to a progesterone stimulus *in vitro* by a rapid increase in intracellular free calcium due to promotion of calcium influx (Blackmore *et al.*, 1990, 1991; Thomas and Meizel, 1989). Progesterone activates a calcium channel that has yet to be defined at the molecular level in the human (Blackmore and Eisoldt, 1999). Recent findings have revealed the molecular structure of such ion channel in the murine species (Ren *et al.*, 2001). The entire increase in intracellular calcium levels induced by progesterone is abolished when the extracellular calcium is removed by the addition of the calcium chelator glycol bis(2-aminoethyl ether)-N,N,N′N′-tetraacetic acid (EGTA) to the extracellular medium (Blackmore *et al.*, 1990). There is evidence for both L- and T-type calcium channels in mouse and human spermatozoa (Arnoult *et al.*, 1996; Benoff *et al.*, 1994; Blackmore *et al.*, 1990, 1991; Blackmore and Eisoldt, 1999; Florman *et al.*, 1998). It has been proposed that progesterone reacts with a multi-receptor system on the sperm surface and that this system cooperates with that used by the ZP to control the physiological acrosome reaction (Fraser *et al.*, 1997; Mendoza *et al.*, 1995). In human spermatozoa, progesterone effects are not associated with G_i-protein activation (Tesarik *et al.*, 1993).

The first signal transduction-second messenger pathway demonstrated to have a role in human sperm acrosome reaction involved the cAMP/PKA system (De Jonge *et al.*, 1991a). Also, the PLC–PKC system was demonstrated to play a role in human sperm exocytosis (De Jonge *et al.*, 1991b; Doherty *et al.*, 1995). However, it is unclear which of such mechanisms is the most significant under physiologic conditions and how the various systems cross talk.

Although transmission electron microscopy still represents the gold standard for the evaluation of acrosomal status, this method is expensive and laborious and cannot be therefore used routinely (Kohn *et al.*, 1997; Zaneveld *et al.*, 1991). Other well-established methods are currently being used to assess the acrosome reaction in the human. The most widely used method involves lectins (e.g., *Pisum sativum* agglutinin or PSA, and others) labeled with fluorescence (e.g., fluorescein isothiocynate or FITC). The inducibility of the acrosome reaction following calcium ionophore challenge (ARIC) using PSA-FITC has been recommended as the presently available optimal way to assess this physiologic event under *in vitro* conditions to test human spermatozoa (Cummins *et al.*, 1991; Fraser *et al.*, 1997; Tesarik, 1985, 1989; Kohn *et al.*, 1997; Oehninger, 2000; Oehninger *et al.*, 2000).

Recently, Franken *et al.* (2000) reported on the validation of a new 'micro assay' using minimal volumes of solubilized, human ZP to test the physiological induction of the acrosome reaction in human spermatozoa (ZIAR or zona-induced acrosome reaction). In such studies, a dose-dependent effect of solubilized ZP on acrosomal exocytosis was observed reaching maximal induction using 0.25–2.5 ZP/µl for both the micro assay and the standard (macro) assay. Furthermore, the inducibility of the acrosome reaction by a calcium ionophore was similar in both assays.

It is imperative to evaluate technician proficiency and variability of results according to sperm samples in order to establish intra- and inter-assay/technician CVs for PSA-FITC staining during ZIAR testing. Intra-assay and technician variation should be determined by evaluating at least 100 cells on 5 different microscopic fields (total 500 cells) from the same semen specimen by each technician responsible for acrosome reaction testing. CVs for both intra-and inter-assay and intra-and inter-technician values must be calculated by dividing the mean with standard deviation × 100% for each observation. The inter-and intra-assay as well as inter-and intra-technician CV should be <15% among the different slides and technicians.

Typically, we mix 20 µl of the zonae solution and 20 µl prepared sperm (5×10^6 motile sperm/ml) in a microplate (Greiner, Lab and Scientific Equipment, North Riding, Republic of South Africa). The mixture is then aspirated into a Hamilton Pipette Tip (R84254, Hamilton) using a 1.0 ml sterile, non-pyrogenic latex free syringe (Becton Dickinson). The tip containing the sperm–zonae solution is incubated in a Falcon dish (Falcon 3003, Becton Dickinson) for 60 minutes at 37°C and 5% CO_2. After the incubation period the spermatozoa are expelled onto the glass slide and coded 'test' sperm, while 'control' sperm are aspirated from the Dulbeccos phosphate-buffered saline (DPBS) resuspended sample described above. Pilot studies indicated that NaOH neutralized acid Tyrode's solution had a similar effect on the percentage of acrosome reaction compared to that recorded with DPBS, namely $13.7 \pm 2\%$ for neutralized acid Tyrode's compared to $14.6 \pm 3\%$, for DPBS ($P > 0.5$). We therefore used DPBS to resuspend the control sperm in all ZIAR experiments.

Slides are air dried and fixed in 100% ethanol for 24 h. Previous experiments in our laboratory also indicated that prolonged exposure of sperm to ethanol during the fixation period increased the sensitivity of the PSA-FITC staining. This allowed us to record acrosome reactions mediated by lower ZP concentrations (0.3 ZP/µl) generally reported in the literature, that is, 2 ZP/µl (Liu and Baker, 1996). Thereafter the spermatozoa are stained for 2 hours at room temperature with 30 µg/ml PSA labeled with fluorescein-isothiocyanate (FITC) (L-0770, Sigma Aldrich). Finally, slides are washed in DPBS and mounted. A minimum of 100 spermatozoa are counted under a Nikon fluorescent microscope (Nikon Labophot 2), Filter Ex 465-495 0 with 400× magnification. In general, the following staining patterns are diagnosed as acrosome reacted spermatozoa: (i) patchy staining on acrosomal region, (ii) distinct staining in the equatorial region occurring as an equatorial bar and (iii) no staining observed over entire sperm surface. Motile sperm fractions after swim-up separation are used and consequently, the progressive motility in all cases is typically >80%. Acrosome reaction data are presented as recorded for live sperm. Spermatozoa with patchy FITC-PSA staining are classified as a population of sperm showing initiation of the acrosome reaction and are classified as acrosome reacted. The zona-induced acrosome reaction is calculated as the difference between the zona-induced acrosomal exocytosis minus the spontaneous (unstimulated) acrosome reaction results.

8.4 Clinical use of sperm function tests: directing treatment to a defined therapy and predictive value for IVF and pregnancy outcome

Our results indicated that the interaction between spermatozoa and the ZP is a critical event leading to fertilization and reflects multiple sperm functions (i.e., completion of capacitation as manifested by the ability to bind to the ZP and to undergo ligand-induced acrosome reaction) (Oehninger et al., 1992, 1997a, 2000; Oehninger, 2000). As mentioned above, the two most common sperm–ZP binding tests currently utilized are the HZA (Burkman et al., 1988) and a competitive intact-zona binding assay (Liu et al., 1988). The high positive and negative predictive values, but more importantly, the low false negative rate (i.e., robust power to identify patients at high risk for fertilization failure) underscore the predictive ability of these tests.

The induced-acrosome reaction assays appear to be equally predictive of fertilization outcome and are simpler in their methodologies (Oehninger et al., 2000). Although the use of a calcium ionophore to induce acrosome reaction is at the present time the most widely used methodology (Cummins et al., 1991; Tesarik, 1989), the assay uses non-physiological conditions that may not accurately represent fertilization potential. The recent implementation of assays using small volumes of human solubilized zonae pellucidae (ZIAR) (Franken et al., 1996, 2000), biologically active recombinant human ZP3 (Chapman and Barratt, 1996; Dong et al., 2001; van Duin et al., 1994) or active, synthetic ZP3 peptides (Hinsch et al., 1998) will probably allow for the design of improved, physiologically oriented acrosome reaction assays.

Franken et al. (2000) devised a new micro assay that is easy and rapid to perform, and facilitates the use of minimal volumes of solubilized ZP (even a single zona)

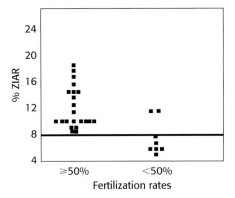

Figure 8.3   Interactive dot diagram of randomly selected IVF patients (*n* = 30) showing results of ZIAR and IVF rate. This prospective study was performed using a cut-off threshold of 50% of oocytes fertilized/inseminated. When ZIAR results were >8% (percentage of acrosome reacted sperm), the sensitivity and specificity of the test to predict fertilization success (>50% of oocytes) were 100% and 75%, respectively. For the group of patients with fertilization rate ⩾50%, the ZIAR range was 9–23% acrosome reacted sperm (mean: 13.5%, *n* = 22), whereas for the group of patients with fertilization rate <50% the ZIAR range was 4–13% (mean: 7.1, *n* = 8)

for assessment of human acrosome reaction. The micro assay has been validated as compared to standard macro assays and consequently offers a unique arena to test for the physiological induction of acrosomal exocytosis by the homologous ZP. Moreover, initial clinical studies using the micro assay have demonstrated that the ZIAR can predict fertilization failure in the IVF setting (Fig. 8.3). The micro assay ZIAR can therefore refine the therapeutic approach for male infertility prior to the onset of therapy (Esterhuizen *et al.*, 2001a, b). Bastiaan *et al.* (2002) prospectively evaluated the relationship between sperm morphology, acrosome responsiveness to solubilized ZP using the micro assay, sperm–zona binding potential (HZA) and IVF outcome. Receiver operator characteristics (ROC) curve analyses indicated ZIAR to be a robust indicator for fertilization failure during IVF therapy with a sensitivity of 81% and specificity of 75%.

Liu *et al.* (2004) reported that sperm defects associated with low sperm–ZP binding or impaired ZP-induced acrosome reaction and sperm–ZP penetration, are the major causes of failure of fertilization when all or most oocytes from a couple do not fertilize in standard IVF. These authors further demonstrated that there is a high frequency of defective sperm–ZP interaction in men with oligozoospermia (<20 × 10^6/ml) and severe teratozoospermia (strict normal sperm morphology ⩽5%). According to these authors, sperm morphology correlates with sperm–ZP binding, and sperm concentration correlates with ZP-induced acrosome reaction in infertile men with sperm concentrations >20 × 10^6/ml. A defective ZP-induced acrosome reaction may be the cause of infertility in up to 25% men with idiopathic infertility. These patients would therefore require ICSI despite the presence of an otherwise normal standard semen analyses (Liu and Baker, 1994, 2000, 2003, 2004; Liu et al., 2004).

Before offering treatment to the infertile man, it is mandatory to examine the female counterpart. The simultaneous presence of female factors is frequently observed and such abnormalities may have an impact on the decision-making process. Pregnancy success varies among different therapies, but the presence of multi-factorial (male and female) infertility and/or a female age >35 years may direct the couple earlier to the more advanced and successful techniques (such as ICSI) rather than recommending less efficient (albeit less expensive) approaches.

It is at this time that sperm function/biochemical tests may be of highest value in order to direct the couple to ART. Assisted reproduction can be indicated as a result of (a) failure of urological/medical treatments; (b) the diagnosis of 'unexplained' infertility in the couple; (c) the presence of 'basic' sperm abnormalities of moderate-high degree or (d) abnormalities of sperm function as diagnosed by predictive bio-assays (such as the HZA or ZIAR).

Currently recommended ART options include: 'low complexity' IUI therapy, 'standard' IVF and embryo transfer, and IVF augmented with ICSI. If the female partner is <35 years, typically 4–6 cycles of IUIs using husband's sperm are recommended as a simple (low complexity) ART approach.

Although there are no established sperm cut-off levels, it is preferable to perform IUI if >5 million total motile spermatozoa can be used per insemination (particularly if sperm morphology is normal or only slightly abnormal). Pregnancy results for IUI in male infertility are higher with concomitant ovarian stimulation. Such regimens include use of clomiphene citrate, a combination of clomiphene and gonadotropins, or gonadotropins alone. Sperm preparation techniques involve a simple washing step (in a capacitating medium) or washing/separation of the motile fraction (typically using a gradient centrifugation method). The latter will result in a better selection of functional cells at the price of a decreased total number of spermatozoa (reviewed in Duran et al., 2002).

Patients with oligo-astheno-teratozoospermia but with >1.5 million motile spermatozoa following swim-up or gradient centrifugation should be offered 'standard' IVF therapy versus ICSI. Although in many of these cases, good fertilization and pregnancy rates are achieved with increased sperm insemination concentration, ICSI may frankly decrease the likelihood of fertilization failure. An abnormal sperm function test should direct therapy to ICSI.

Typically patients are selected for ICSI under the following scenarios: (1) poor sperm parameters (i.e., $<1.5 \times 10^6$ total spermatozoa with adequate progressive motility after separation, and/or severe teratozoospermia with <4% normal forms in the presence of a borderline to low total motile fraction); (2) a poor sperm–ZP binding capacity with a HZA index <30%, and/or low ZIAR (Bastiaan *et al.*, 2002; Oehninger *et al.*, 1997a, b); (3) failure of IUI therapy in cases presenting with abnormal sperm parameters including presence of anti-sperm antibodies; (4) previous failed fertilization in IVF; and (5) presence of obstructive or non-obstructive azoospermia, where ICSI is combined with sperm extraction from the testes or the epididymis (Oehninger, 2000, 2001b; Oehninger *et al.*, 2000; Oehninger and Gosden, 2002). In the presence of severe oligo-astheno-teratozoospermia or if the outcome of sperm function testing indicates a significant impairment of fertilizing capacity, couples should be immediately directed to ICSI. This approach is probably more cost-effective and will avoid loss of valuable time, particularly in women >35 years (Monzó *et al.*, 2001; Oehninger, 2001b).

8.5 Conclusions

The examination of the semen should be performed following a sequential multi-step diagnostic scheme including the analysis of the seminal plasma and basic sperm parameters followed by sperm function testing. There are a variety of fundamental sperm functions acquired after completion of capacitation that are essential for a successful sperm–oocyte interaction. The HZA and the ZIAR are validated and useful functional tests to predict the outcome of fertilization under *in vitro* conditions. CASA allows for the identification of sperm populations showing hyperactivation but the clinical value in the prediction of fertilization or pregnancy outcomes remains to be validated.

Consequently, the HZA, ARIC and ZIAR tests should be added to the diagnostic armamentarium in the clinical arena to assess male fertility potential. Used as part of the sequential diagnostic scheme presented herein, these bioassays offer the clinician useful means to direct therapy in clinical assisted reproduction.

Notwithstanding their confirmed value to predict fertilization potential *in vitro*, it is important to emphasize that more prospectively designed studies are needed to establish the value of these tests to predict pregnancy outcome in the IUI and natural reproduction settings. Moreover, all these assays demand skilful technicians and can be time-consuming. Owing to this, and due to the difficulties generally encountered to obtain donated oocytes or ovarian specimens to perform the assays, only a few centers throughout the world have incorporated them in the extended semen evaluation.

It is therefore estimated that new assays based on biotechnological advances, such as (i) the use of cloned and *in vitro* expressed ZP proteins used as recombinant vectors in solid or liquid phase assays, or (ii) the production of agonistic molecules and identification of complementary gamete receptors involved in the crucial sperm functions, may soon be developed to provide simpler and more universally applicable diagnostic tools.

REFERENCES

Aitken RJ and Baker MA (2004) Oxidative stress and male reproductive biology. *Reprod Fertil Dev* 16, 581–588.

Ahuja KK (1985) Carbohydrate determinants involved in mammalian fertilization. *Am J Anat* 174, 207–223.

Amann RP and Hammerstedt RH (1993) *In vitro* evaluation of sperm quality: an opinion. *J Androl* 14, 397–406.

Arnoult C, Cardullo RA, Lemos JR and Florman HM (1996) Activation of mouse sperm T-type Ca^{2+} channels by adhesion to the egg zona pellucida. *Proc Natl Acad Sci USA* 93, 13004–13009.

Baccetti B, Collodel G and Piomboni P (1996) Apoptosis in human ejaculated sperm cells (notulae seminologicae 9). *J Submicrosc Cytol Pathol* 28, 587–596.

Baccetti B, Capitani S, Collodel G, Strehler E and Piomboni P (2002) Recent advances in human sperm pathology. *Contraception* 65, 283–287.

Baldi E, Luconi M, Bonaccorsi L, Muratori M and Forti G (2000) Intracellular events and signaling pathways involved in sperm acquisition of fertilizing capacity and acrosome reaction. *Front Biosci* 5, E110–E123.

Barroso G, Morshedi M and Oehninger S (2000) Analysis of DNA fragmentation, plasma membrane translocation of phosphatidylserine and oxidative stress in human spermatozoa. *Human Reprod* 15, 1338–1345.

Bastiaan HS, Menkveld R, Oehninger S and Franken DR (2002) Zona pellucida induced acrosome reaction, sperm morphology, and sperm–zona pellucida binding assessments among subfertile men. *J Assist Reprod Genet* 19, 329–334.

Benoff S, Cooper GW, Hurley I *et al.* (1994) The effect of calcium ion channel blockers on sperm fertilization potential. *Fertil Steril* 62, 606–617.

Blackmore PF and Eisoldt S (1999) The neoglycoprotein mannose-bovine serum albumin, but not progesterone, activates T-type calcium channels in human spermatozoa. *Mol Human Reprod* 5, 498–506.

Blackmore PF, Beebe SJ, Danforth DR and Alexander N (1990) Progesterone and 17α-hydroxyprogesterone. *J Biol Chem* 265, 1376–1380.

Blackmore PF, Neulen J, Lattanzio FA and Beebe SJ (1991) Cell surface receptors for progesterone mediated calcium uptake in human sperm. *J Biol Chem* 266, 18655–18659.

Bleil JD and Wassarman PM (1980) Mammalian sperm-egg interaction: identification of a glycoprotein in mouse egg zonae pellucidae possessing receptor activity for sperm. *Cell* 20, 873–882.

Bleil JD and Wassarman PM (1983) Sperm-egg interactions in the mouse: sequence of events and induction of the acrosome reaction by a zona pellucida glycoprotein. *Dev Biol* 95, 317–324.

Bonduelle M, Camus M, De Vos A *et al.* (1999) Seven years of intracytoplasmic sperm injection and follow-up of 1987 subsequent children. *Human Reprod* 14, 243–264.

Burkman LJ, Coddington CC, Franken DR *et al.* (1988) The hemizona assay (HZA): development of a diagnostic test for the binding of human spermatozoa to the human hemizona pellucida to predict fertilization potential. *Fertil Steril* 49, 688–697.

Burks DJ, Carballada R, Moore HD and Saling PM (1995) Interaction of a tyrosine kinase from human sperm with the zona pellucida at fertilization. *Science* 269, 83–86.

Castle PE and Dean J (1999) Manipulating the genome to study reproduction. Mice with 'humanized' zonae pellucidae. *Human Reprod* 14, 1927–1939.

Centers for Disease Control and Prevention (1997) *Fertility, Family Planning and Women's Health: New Data from the 1995 National Survey of Family Growth*, U.S. Department of Health and Human Services, pp. 1–11.

Centers for Disease Control and Prevention (2004) *2002 Assisted Reproductive Technology Success Rates*. U.S. Department of Health and Human Services.

Chapman NR and Barratt CLR (1996) The role of carbohydrate in sperm-ZP3 adhesion. *Mol Human Reprod* 2, 767–774.

Coddington CC, Fulgham DL, Alexander NJ, Johnson D, Herr JC and Hodgen GD (1990) Sperm bound to zona pellucida in hemizona assay demonstrate acrosome reaction when stained with T-6 antibody. *Fertil Steril* 54, 504–508.

Coddington CC, Franken DR, Burkman LJ, Oosthuizen WT, Kruger T and Hodgen GD (1991) Functional aspects of human sperm binding to the zona pellucida using the hemizona assay. *J Androl* 12, 1–8.

Cross NL, Morales P, Overstreet JW *et al.* (1986) Two simple methods for detecting acrosome-reacted human sperm. *Gamete Res* 15, 213–226.

Cross NL, Morales P, Overstreet J and Hanson FW (1988) Induction of acrosome reaction by the human zona pellucida. *Biol Reprod* 38, 235–244.

Cummins J, Pember S, Jequier A, Yovich JL and Hartmann PE (1991) A test of the human sperm acrosome reaction following ionophore challenge. *J Androl* 12, 98–103.

De Jonge C (2000) Commentary: forging a partnership between total quality management and the andrology laboratory. *J Androl* 21, 203–205.

De Jonge CJ, Han H, Lawrie H, Mack SR and Zaneveld LJ (1991a) Modulation of the human sperm acrosome reaction by effectors of the adenylate cyclase/cyclic AMP second messenger pathway. *J Exp Zool* 258, 113–125.

De Jonge CJ, Han H, Mack SR and Zaneveld LJ (1991b) Effect of phorbol diesters, synthetic diacylglycerols, and a protein kinase inhibitor on the human sperm acrosome reaction. *J Androl* 12, 62–70.

Doherty C, Tarchala S, Radwanska E and De Jonge CJ (1995) Characterization of two second messenger pathways and their interactions in eliciting the human sperm acrosome reaction. *J Androl* 16, 36–46.

Dong KW, Chi TF, Juan YW *et al.* (2001) Characterization of the biological activities of a recombinant human zona pellucida protein 3 (ZP3) expressed in human ovarian (PA-1) cells. *Am J Obstet Gynecol* 184, 835–844.

Duran HE, Morshedi M, Kruger T and Oehninger S (2002) Intrauterine insemination: a systematic review on determinants of success. *Human Reprod Update* 8, 373–384.

Esterhuizen AD, Franken DR, Lourens JGH and Van Rooyen LH (2001a) Clinical importance of a micro-assay for the evaluation of sperm acrosome reaction using homologus zona pellucida. *Andrologia* 33, 87–93.

Esterhuizen AD, Franken DR, Lourens JGH *et al.* (2001b) Clinical importance of zona pellucida induced acrosome reaction (ZIAR test) in cases of failed human fertilization. *Human Reprod* 16, 136–144.

Florman HM and Storey BT (1982) Mouse gamete interactions: the zona pellucida is the site of the acrosome reaction leading to fertilization *in vitro*. *Dev Biol* 91, 121–130.

Florman HM and Wassarman PM (1985) O-linked oligosaccharides of mouse eggs ZP3 account for its sperm receptor activity. *Cell* 41, 313–324.

Florman HM, Tombes RM, First NL and Babcock DF (1989) An adhesion-associated agonist from the zona pellucida activates G protein-promoted elevations of internal Ca and pH that mediate mammalian sperm acrosomal exocytosis. *Dev Biol* 135, 133–146.

Florman HM, Corron ME, Kim TD and Babcock DF (1992) Activation of voltage-dependent calcium channels of mammalian sperm is required for zona pellucida-induced acrosomal exocytosis. *Dev Biol* 152, 304–314.

Florman HM, Arnoult C, Kazam IG, Li C and O'Toole CM (1998) A perspective on the control of mammalian fertilization by egg-activated ion channels in sperm: a tale of two channels. *Biol Reprod* 59, 12–16.

Franken D, Kruger T, Oehninger S, Coddington CC, Lombard C, Smith K and Hodgen GD (1993) The ability of the hemizona assay to predict human fertilization *in vitro* in different and consecutive IVF/GIFT cycles. *Human Reprod* 8, 1240–1244.

Franken DR, Burkman LJ, Oehninger SC, Coddington CC, Veeck LL, Kruger TF, Rosenwaks Z and Hodgen GD (1989a) Hemizona assay using salt-stored human oocytes: evaluation of zona pellucida capacity for binding human spermatozoa. *Gamete Res* 22, 15–26.

Franken DR, Oehninger S, Burkman LJ, Coddington CC, Kruger TF, Rosenwaks Z, Acosta AA and Hodgen GD (1989b) The hemizona assay (HZA): a predictor of human sperm fertilizing potential in *in vitro* fertilization (IVF) treatment. *J In Vitro Fert Embryo Transf* 6, 44–50.

Franken DR, Coddington CC, Burkman LJ, Oosthuizen WT, Oehninger SC, Kruger TF and Hodgen GD (1991a) Defining the valid hemizona assay: accounting for binding variability within zonae pellucidae and within semen samples from fertile males. *Fertil Steril* 56, 1156–1161.

Franken DR, Windt ML, Kruger TF, Oehninger S, and Hodgen GD (1991b) Comparison of sperm binding potential of uninseminated, inseminated- unfertilized, and fertilized-noncleaved human oocytes under hemizona assay conditions. *Mol Reprod Dev* 30, 56–61.

Franken DR, Morales PJ and Habenicht UF (1996) Inhibition of G protein in human sperm and its influence on acrosome reaction and zona pellucida binding. *Fertil Steril* 66, 1009–1011.

Franken DR, Bastiaan HS and Oehninger S (2000) Physiological induction of the acrosome reaction in human sperm: validation of a microassay using minimal volumes of solubilized, homologous zona pellucida. *J Assist Reprod Genet* 17, 374–378.

Fraser L, Barratt CL, Canale D, Cooper T, De Jonge C, Irvine S, Mortimer D, Oehninger S and Tesarik J (1997) Consensus workshop on advanced diagnostic andrology techniques. ESHRE Andrology Special Interest Group. *Human Reprod* 12, 873.

Gamzu R, Yogev L, Amit A, Lessing J, Homonnai ZT and Yavetz H (1994) The hemizona assay is of good prognostic value for the ability of sperm to fertilize oocytes *in vitro*. *Fertil Steril* 62, 1056–1059.

Hinsch E, Oehninger S and Hinsch K (1998) ZP3-6 peptide and acrosome reaction. Semen evaluation, testing and selection: a new look in the 2000s. In: *Andrology in the Nineties Precongress Training Course*. Belgium: Genk, pp. 25–30.

Hodgen GD, Burkman LJ, Coddington CC, Franken DR, Oehninger SC, Kruger TF and Rosenwaks Z (1988) The hemizona assay (HZA): finding sperm that have the 'right stuff'. *J In Vitro Fert Embryo Transf* 5, 311–313.

Hull MGR, Glazener CMA and Kelly NJ (1985) Population study of causes, treatment, and outcome of infertility. *J Br Med* 291, 1693–1697.

Hoodbhoy T and Dean J (2004) Insights into the molecular basis of sperm-egg recognition in mammals. *Reproduction* 127, 417–422.

Huszar G, Celik-Ozenci C, Cayli S, Kovacs T, Vigue L and Kovanci E (2004) Semen characteristics after overnight shipping: preservation of sperm concentrations, HspA2 ratios, CK activity, cytoplasmic retention, chromatin maturity, DNA integrity, and sperm shape. *J Androl* 25, 593–604.

Irvine DS (1997) Declining sperm quality: a review of facts and hypotheses. *Bailliere Clin Obstet Gynaecol* 11, 655–671.

Irvine DS (1998) Epidemiology and etiology of male infertility. *Human Reprod* 13 (Suppl. 1), 33–44.

Kohn FM, Mack SR, Schill WB and Zaneveld LJ (1997) Detection of human sperm acrosome reaction: comparison between methods using double staining, Pisum sativum agglutinin, concanavalin A and transmission electron microscopy. *Human Reprod* 12, 714–721.

Kopf GS (1990) Zona pellucida-mediated signal transduction in mammalian spermatozoa. *J Reprod Fertil* 42, 33–49.

Kopf GS, Woolkalis MJ and Gerton GL (1986) Evidence for a guanine nucleotide-binding regulatory protein in invertebrate and mammalian sperm: identification by islet-activating protein-catalyzed ADP-ribosylation and immunochemical methods. *J Biol Chem* 261, 7327–7331.

Kruger TF, Oehninger S, Franken DR and Hodgen GD (1991) Hemizona assay: use of fresh versus salt-stored human oocytes to evaluate sperm binding potential to the zona pellucida. *J In Vitro Fert Embryo Transf* 8, 154–156.

Lee MA, Check LH and Kopf GA (1992) Guanine nucleotide-binding regulatory protein in human sperm mediates acrosomal exocytosis induced by the human zona pellucida. *Mol Reprod* 31, 78–86.

Liu DY and Baker HWG (1994) Disordered acrosome reaction of spermatozoa bound to the zona pellucida: a newly discovered sperm defect causing infertility with reduced sperm–zona penetration and reduced fertilization *in vitro*. *Human Reprod* 9, 1694–1700.

Liu DY and Baker HW (1996) A simple method for assessment of the human acrosome reaction of spermatozoa bound to the zona pellucida: lack of relationship with ionophore A23187-induced acrosome reaction. *Human Reprod* 11, 551–557.

Liu DY and Baker HW (2000) Defective sperm–zona pellucida interaction: a major cause of failure of fertilization in clinical *in-vitro* fertilization. *Human Reprod* 15, 702–708.

Liu DY, Lopata A, Johnston WIH *et al.* (1988) A human sperm–zona pellucida binding test using oocytes that failed to fertilize *in vitro*. *Fertil Steril* 50, 782–788.

Liu DY, Clarke GN, Lopata A, Johnston WI and Baker HW (1989) A sperm–zona pellucida binding test and *in vitro* fertilization. *Fertil Steril* 52, 281–287.

Liu de Y and Baker HW (2003) Frequency of defective sperm–zona pellucida interaction in severely teratozoospermic infertile men. *Human Reprod* 18, 802–807.

Liu de Y and Baker HW (2004) High frequency of defective sperm–zona pellucida interaction in oligozoospermic infertile men. *Human Reprod* 19, 228–233.

Liu de Y, Garrett C and Baker HW (2004) Clinical application of sperm–oocyte interaction tests in *in vitro* fertilization – embryo transfer and intracytoplasmic sperm injection programs. *Fertil Steril* 82, 1251–1263.

Marchetti C, Obert G, Deffosez A, Formstecher P and Marchetti P (2002) Study of mitochondrial membrane potential, reactive oxygen species, DNA fragmentation and cell viability by flow cytometry in human sperm. *Human Reprod* 17, 1257–1265.

Mendoza C, Soler A and Tesarik J (1995) Nongenomic steroid action: independent targeting of plasma membrane calcium channel and a tyrosine kinase. *Biochem Biophys Res Commun* 210, 518–523.

Monzó A, Kondylis F, Lynch D *et al.* (2001) Outcome of ICSI in azoospermic patients: stressing the liason between the urologist and reproductive medicine. *Urology* 58, 69–75.

Mortimer D (1990) Objective analysis of sperm motility and kinematics. In: *Handbook of the Laboratory Diagnosis and Treatment of Infertility*, eds BA Keel and BW Webster. Boca Raton: CRC Press, pp. 97–133.

Mortimer D, Curtis EF and Camenzind AR (1990) Combined use of fluorescent peanut agglutinin lectin and Hoechst 33258 to monitor the acrosomal status and vitality of human spermatozoa. *Human Reprod* 5, 99–103.

Mosher WD and Pratt WF (1990) Fecundity and infertility in the United States, 1965–1988. *Advance Data from Vital and Health Statistics*. Public Health Service, Hyattsville, MD, (DHHA publication no. (PHS) 91-1250).

Oehninger S (2000) Clinical and laboratory management of male infertility: an opinion on its current status. *J Androl* 21, 814–821.

Oehninger S (2001a) Molecular basis of human sperm–zona pellucida interaction. *Cells Tissues Organs* 168, 58–64.

Oehninger S (2001b) Place of intracytoplasmic sperm injection in clinical management of male infertility. *Lancet* 357, 2068–2069.

Oehninger S and Gosden RG (2002) Should ICSI be the treatment of choice for all cases of *in-vitro* conception? No, not in light of the scientific data. *Human Reprod* 17, 2237–2242.

Oehninger S, Coddington CC, Scott R, Franken DA, Burkman LJ, Acosta AA and Hodgen GD (1989). Hemizona assay: assessment of sperm dysfunction and prediction of *in vitro* fertilization outcome. *Fertil Steril* 51, 665–670.

Oehninger S, Acosta AA and Veeck L (1991a) Recurrent failure of *in vitro* fertilization: role of the hemizona assay (HZA) in the sequential diagnosis of specific sperm/oocyte defects. *Am J Obstet Gynecol* 164, 1210–1215.

Oehninger S, Veeck L, Franken D, Kruger TF, Acosta AA and Hodgen GD (1991b) Human preovulatory oocytes have a higher sperm-binding ability than immature oocytes under hemizona assay conditions: evidence supporting the concept of 'zona maturation'. *Fertil Steril* 55, 1165–1170.

Oehninger S, Toner JP, Muasher SJ, Coddington C, Acosta AA and Hodgen GD (1992) Prediction of fertilization *in vitro* with human gametes: Is there a litmus test? *Am J Obstet Gynecol* 167, 1760–1767.

Oehninger S, Mahony MC, Swanson JR and Hodgen GD (1993) The specificity of human spermatozoa/zona pellucida interaction under hemizona assay conditions. *Mol Reprod Dev* 35, 57–61.

Oehninger S, Mahony M, Ozgur K, Kolm P, Kruger T and Franken D (1997a) Clinical significance of human sperm–zona pellucida binding. *Fertil Steril* 67, 1121–1127.

Oehninger S, Franken D and Kruger T (1997b) Approaching the next millennium: how should we manage andrology diagnosis in the intracytoplasmic sperm injection era? *Fertil Steril* 67, 434–436.

Oehninger S, Chaturvedi S, Toner J, Morshedi M, Mayer J, Lanzendorf S and Muasher S (1998) Semen quality: is there a paternal effect on pregnancy outcome in *in-vitro* fertilization/intracytoplasmic sperm injection? *Human Reprod* 13, 2161–2164.

Oehninger S, Franken DR, Sayed E, Barroso G and Kolm P (2000) Sperm function assays and their predictive value for fertilization outcome in IVF therapy: a meta-analysis. *Human Reprod Update* 6, 160–168.

Oehninger S, Morshedi M, Weng SL, Taylor S, Duran H and Beebe S (2003) Presence and significance of somatic cell apoptosis markers in human ejaculated spermatozoa. *Reprod Biomed Online* 7, 469–476.

Oehninger SC (1995) An update on the laboratory assessment of male fertility. *Human Reprod* 10(Suppl. 1), 38–45.

O'Toole C, Arnoult C, Darszon A, Steinhardt RA and Florman HM (2000) Ca^{2+} entry through store-operated channels in mouse sperm is initiated by egg ZP3 and drive the acrosome reaction. *Mol Biol Cell* 11, 1571–1584.

Overstreet JW and Hembree WC (1976) Penetration of the zona pellucida of nonliving human oocytes by human spermatozoa *in vitro*. *Fertil Steril* 27, 815–831.

Rankin TL, Tong ZB, Castle PE, Lee E, Gore-Langton R, Nelson LM and Dean J (1998) Human ZP3 restores fertility in Zp3 null mice without affecting order-specific sperm binding. *Development* 125, 2415–2424.

Rankin TL, Coleman JS, Epifano O *et al.* (2003) Fertility and taxon-specific sperm binding persist after replacement of mouse sperm receptors with human homologs. *Dev Cell* 5, 33–43.

Ren D, Navarro B, Perez G, Jackson AC, Hsu S, Shi Q, Tilly JL and Clapham DE (2001) A sperm ion channel required for sperm motility and male fertility. *Nature* 413, 603–609.

Roldan ERS, Murase T and Shi Qi-Xian (1994) Exocytosis in spermatozoa in response to progesterone and zona pellucida. *Science* 266, 1578–1581.

Schuffner AA, Bastiaan HS, Duran HE, Lin LY, Morshedi M, Franken DR and Oehninger S (2002) Zona pellucida-induced acrosome reaction in human sperm: dependency on activation of pertussis toxin-sensitive G(i) protein and extracellular calcium, and priming effect of progesterone and follicular fluid. *Mol Human Reprod* 8, 722–727.

Tesarik J (1985) Comparison of acrosome reaction-inducing activities of human cumulus oophorus, follicular fluid and ionophore A23187 in human sperm populations of proven fertilizing ability *in vitro*. *J Reprod Fertil* 74, 383–388.

Tesarik J (1989) Appropriate timing of the acrosome reaction is a major requirement for the fertilizing spermatozoon. *Human Reprod* 4, 957–961.

Tesarik J, Carrera A and Mendoza C (1993) Differential sensitivity of progesterone and zona pellucida-induced acrosome reactions to pertussis toxin. *Mol Reprod Dev* 34, 183–189.

Thomas P and Meizel S (1989) Phosphatidylinositol 4,5-bisphosphate hydrolysis in human sperm stimulated with follicular fluid or progesterone is dependent upon Ca^{2+} influx. *Biochem J* 264, 539–546.

van Duin M, Polman J and De Breet IT (1994) Recombinant human zona pellucida protein ZP3 produced by Chinese Hamster Ovary cells induces the human sperm acrosome reaction and promotes sperm-egg fusion. *Biol Reprod* 51, 607–617.

Wassarman PM (1990a) Profile of a mammalian sperm receptor. *Development* 108, 1–17.

Wassarman PM (1990b) Regulation of mammalian fertilization by zona pellucida glycoproteins. *J Reprod Fertil* 42, 79–87.

Wassarman PM (1999) Mammalian fertilization: molecular aspects of gamete adhesion, exocytosis and fusion. *Cell* 96, 175–183.

Wassarman PM, Jovine L and Litscher ES (2004) Mouse zona pellucida genes and glycoproteins. *Cytogenet Genome Res* 105(2–4), 228–234.

World Health Organization (1992) *WHO Laboratory Manual for the Examination of Human Semen and Sperm–Cervical Mucus Interaction*, 3rd edn. Cambridge: Cambridge University Press, pp. 23–26.

World Health Organization (1999) *WHO Laboratory Manual for Examination of Human Semen and Semen–Cervical Mucus Interaction*, 2nd edn. Cambridge: Cambridge University Press, pp. 14–17.

Yanagimachi R, Yanagimachi H and Rogers BJ (1976) The use of zona-free animal ova as a test-system for the assessment of the fertilizing capacity of human spermatozoa. *Biol Reprod* 15, 471–476.

Yanagimachi R, Lopata A, Odom CB, Bronson RA, Mahi CA and Nicolson GL (1979) Retention of biologic characteristics of zona pellucida in highly concentrated salt solution: the use of salt-stored eggs for assessing the fertilizing capacity of spermatozoa. *Fertil Steril* 31, 562–574.

Yanagimachi R (1994) Mammalian fertilization. In: *The Physiology of Reproduction*, eds N Knobil N and JD Neill. New York: Raven Press, pp. 189–317.

Yoshimatsu N, Yanagimachi R and Lopata A (1988) Zonae pellucidae of salt-stored hamster and human eggs: their penetrability by homologous and heterologous spermatozoa. *Gamete Res* 21, 115–126.

Zaneveld L, De Jonge C, Anderson R and Mack SR (1991) Human sperm capacitation and the acrosome reaction. *Human Reprod* 6, 1265–1274.

Genetics: a basic science perspective

Peter H. Vogt

Section Molecular Genetics and Infertility, Department of Gynecology Endocrinology and Reproductive Medicine, University of Heidelberg, Heidelberg, Germany

9.1 Introduction

From mouse and Drosophila knock out experiments it has been deduced that the products of more than 3000 genes are involved in the genetic control regulating the expression of male (and female) fertility (Cooke and Saunders, 2002, Hackstein *et al.*, 2000; Matzuk and Lamb, 2002). In human, the molecular identification of male fertility genes is hampered by the fact that human is not an experimental species. An infertile man is only recognised after the couple desiring for a child has asked for some therapeutic treatments in an infertility clinic.

Genetic lesions causing male infertility can be roughly grouped in three classes: (I) Chromosomal aneuploidies and rearrangements where batteries of genes on specific chromosomes have increased or decreased their expression dosage or have changed their normal nuclear territorium; (II) submicroscopic deletions (i.e. the genomic AZF deletions) where deletions or rearrangements of multiple genes – mapped in a molecular neighbourhood – have lost or altered their normal expression pattern and (III) single gene defects where the expression of a single gene is changed or lost causing then male infertility (e.g. the *CFTR* gene). This chapter offers a basic science perspective to the molecular genetic principles causing male infertility in the three different genetic-abnormality groups. Thereby one aim is to point to the practical prerequisites which will be needed for their proper analysis in the infertility clinic reducing time and costs and increasing the patient's success rate for conceiving a child without an inherited genetic abnormality.

9.1.1 Chromosome abnormalities in infertile men

Aneuploidies or structural aberrations are found in about 14% of azoospermic men (i.e. infertile patients with no spermatozoa in their semen fluid) and 5% of oligozoospermic men (i.e. infertile patients with a severe reduction in the number of spermatozoa in their semen fluid) (Van Assche *et al.*, 1996). Most chromosome abnormalities causing male infertility include one of the sex chromosomes, X and Y.

The karyotype 47XXY, associated with the Klinefelter syndrome, is the largest homogenous group. Since Klinefelter patients with the same karyotpye are not always azoospermic (Tournaye *et al.*, 1996), and there are also reports of Klinefelters' men who naturally fathered a child (Foss and Lewis, 1971), it can be concluded that the extra X-chromosome in the cell nuclei of these men has individually a variable genetic expression profile and that a variable number of X genes exist that are imprinted, that is, inactivated. It is not yet known why Klinefelter patients are infertile, and why in about 20% of cases a mosaic karyotype 46XY/47XXY is observed.

It has also been speculated that the reduction of postmeiotic germ cells, generally observed in this patient group, is probably due to an interference of the premeiotic sex chromosomes' pairing process where the second X chromosome would compete with the Y chromosome in the same nuclear territorium also known as 'sex vesicle'. Mouse animal models, however, suggest interference beginning in the male germ line already during foetal life (Mroz *et al.*, 1999). This indicates that indeed the expression of homologous genes on the sex chromosomes (X and Y) with a putative function in male gonadogenesis and germ cell formation (Fig. 9.1) can contribute to the individual Klinefelter phenotypes, if they are overexpressed in men with the 47,XXY karyotype (triple dose of gene product).

A second Klinefelter syndrome candidate group of X-genes are the seven X-chromosomal spermatogonia genes (*FTHL17, USP26, TKTL1, TEX11, TAF2Q/TAF7L, NXF2, TEX13A/B*) isolated by Wang *et al.* (2001) and the male gonad genes encoding the androgen receptor (*AR*), the *Double-dose Associated sex-reversal* (*DAX*) gene, the *Fragile X-Mental Retardation 1* (*FMR-1*) gene and the X-linked *Helicase 2* (*XH2*) located only on the X chromosome (Fig. 9.1). Indeed Klinefelter patients with increasing numbers of X chromosomes in their karyotype (48,XXXY; 49,XXXXY) shift their sexual phenotype to the female side. Penis development is reduced and cryptorchidism is found in most cases.

In 143 patients analysed for mutations in the X-chromosome *USP26* gene, the same variant sequence (370–371insACA; 494 T>C and 1423 C>T) causing three amino acid changes in the *USP26* coding sequence was found in eight individuals (Stouffs *et al.*, 2005). These were not found in the 152 control samples. Interestingly this triple *USP26* sequence variant seemed to be associated with the occurrence of the Sertoli-cell-only (SCO) syndrome (8/111; 7.2%) and was not found in 32 patients with maturation arrest (Stouffs *et al.*, 2005). Since the homologous mouse gene *Usp26* was shown to be expressed predominantly in spermatogonia (Wang *et al.*, 2001), it can be speculated about an overexpression of this human X gene in the germ cells of men with Klinefelter karyotype which contribute to the testicular pathology of this patient group. The USP26 protein contains a conserved ubiquitin C-terminal hydrolase domain like the *USP9Y* gene in AZFa and its X homologue, *USP9X* (see below). These proteins are probably involved in the control of the stability of other germ cell proteins.

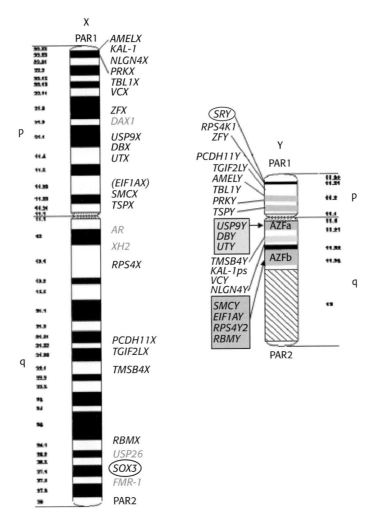

Figure 9.1   Schematic view on current map of functional X-Y homologous genes (black colour) and X-linked genes (grey colour) mapped to distinct chromosome G-bands which are known to be involved in male germ cell and gonad development (the X-chromosomal germ line genes: *FTHL17, TKTL1, TEX11, TAF2Q/TAF7L, NXF2, TEX13A/B* isolated by Wang *et al.* (2001) are not yet mapped to distinct G-bands). The putative X-chromosomal homologue of the male sex determining *SRY* gene, *SOX3* (Foster and Graves, 1994) is circled like *SRY*. Boxes stained with different grey-tones in Yq11 mark the X-homologous Y genes mapped to the two AZF regions, AZFa and AZFb (see also Fig. 9.2). The map site of the *EIF1AX* gene is put in brackets because not yet confirmed. PAR1 and PAR2 at both tips of the X and Y chromosome mark the pseudoautosomal regions paired during male meiosis

Other chromosomal abnormalities associated with male infertility are deletions and rearrangements of the euchromatic part of the long arm of the human Y-chromosome (Yq11) therefore also considered as AZF (AZoospermia Factor) deletions. This is based on the belief that the complete genomic Yq11 sequence is functionally involved in the process of human spermatogenesis. Another hypothesis is that the Y chromosome is a genetic desert, escaping step by step from the male chromosome constitution. The Y gene for male sex determination *SRY* is considered to be an exception on a generally desolate human Y-chromosome (Marshall Graves, 2000, 2002).

Both assumptions were established with the identification of the first cytogenetically visible deletions of the long Y arm (Yq-) in men with oligozoospermia and azoospermia (Kjessler, 1965; Neu *et al.*, 1973) and with the detection of an extremely variable length of the human Y-chromosome also in fertile men (Unnerus *et al.*, 1967). By fluorescent chromosome staining experiments with quinacrine it was recognised that most of the Y variability was caused by a polymorphic length of the distal heterochromatic part of its long arm (Yq12) although length variations of the non-fluorescent euchromatic Yq11 region were reported as well (Soudek *et al.*, 1973). Surprisingly, these chromosome variabilities are stable in family pedigrees and used to assign individuals to specific populations (for review see Vogt, 2005b).

The mosaic karyotype 45X/46XY leads to mixed gonad dysgenesis and male infertility. Men with this karyotype are recognised in the clinic by a streak gonad on one side and a dysgenic gonad on the other side. Outer genitalia might be normal or presented with micropenis, hypospadia and small testis volumes. The occurrence of female phenotypes with the same karyotype points again to the delicate balance of developmental decision(s) towards the male or female sexual pathway in early embryogenesis. Although the karyotype usually displays a normal sized Y chromosome in this patient group, it often lacks the fluorescent staining block after banding with quinacrine, which marks the Yq12 heterochromatin in the distal part of the Y long arm. The 'non-fluorescent' Y chromosome (Ynf) has been created after breakage in Yq11 with subsequent fusion of a second Y-chromosome also broken in Yq11, both forming the dicentric iso-Yp-chromosome (Daniel, 1985). Meiotic pairing of the Y to the X chromosome is inhibited because of self-pairing of the iso-Yp between its doubled short arms (Chandley *et al.*, 1989). Men with azoospermia and the karyotype 45,X have an unbalanced karyotype because the distal part of the euchromatic long Y arm (Yq11) is lost. The other part of the Y chromosome including the *SRY* gene locus is translocated to an autosome (most frequently to the short arm of one of the acrocentric chromosomes 13, 14, 15, 21 or 22).

The impact of balanced Y-A translocations on male fertility is variable because the same karyotypes were observed in fertile and sterile men sometimes even in the same pedigree (Fryns *et al.*, 1985). In most familial cases, the distal heterochromatic part of the Y long arm (Yq12) is translocated to the short arm of an acrocentic chromosome and the Y chromosome is broken in Yq11. Since these Y-chromosomal abnormalities were all associated with male infertility a chromosomally based Y fertility factor was proposed (Vogt *et al.*, 1995) which might be functionally linked to the AZF mapped in distal Yq11 (Tiepolo and Zuffardi, 1976). That means an "AZF chromatin code" functional involved in the X-Y pairing process during male meiosis and located in Yq11 should be part of the Y chromosomal spermatogenesis function. Indeed a functionally active chromatin domain in Yq11 was indicated in nuclei spreading experiments where the Y chromosome was shown to decondense in the nuclei of spermatogonia before pairing with the X chromosome to form the condensed X-Y chromatin structure ('sex vesicle') in the spermatocyte nuclei (Speed *et al.*, 1993).

Chromosomal aneuploidies and translocations between autosomes (Robertsonian and reciprocal) were found less frequently than sex chromosomal abnormalities in infertile men. In particular pericentric inversions in chromosome 1, 3, 5, 6, 10 seem to interfere with meiosis leading to a reduced rate of postmeiotic sperm numbers or even azoospermia. In 60% of cases with Robertsonian translocations the two acro-centric chromosomes, 13 and 14, were involved (Vogt, 1997). Autosome aneuploidies like trisomies of chromosome 21 (Downs syndrome), have individual effects on male fertility. For more details of structural chromosome abnormalities associated with male infertility see also the following chapter of P. Turek.

9.1.2 Genomic AZF gene deletions in infertile men

Sequence analysis of the male specific region of the human Y chromosome (MSY) has subdivided this Y sequence in three different classes: Y-specific, X-degenerate, X-homologous (Skaletsky *et al.*, 2003). The Y-specific repetitive block structures (also called 'amplicon structures') in Yq11 can now easily explain the high frequency of the intrachromosomal AZFa, AZFb and AZFc deletions mapped in this Y region by molecular deletion mapping (Fig. 9.2A, Color plate 8). Most interesting, the amplicons were structurally assembled in eight different long structures with oppo-site polarities called 'palindrome arms' (P1–P8), with the largest palindrome (P1: 2.9 Mb) in distal AZFc (Fig. 9.2B, Color plate 8). The other palindromes, P2–P8, were mapped, from distal to proximal (towards the Y centromere) in distal AZFb (P2: 246 kb; P3: 736 kb), in proximal AZFb (P4: 419 kb; P5: 996 kb) and between the AZFa and AZFb deletion intervals (P6: 266 kb; P7: 30 kb; P8: 75 kb) respectively. These eight palindromes are highly symmetrical and comprise ~25% of the complete Y-specific sequence class, that is 5.7 Mb of the genomic Yq11 sequence. Sequence analyses of the homologous amplicons mapped in the different palindrome arms revealed extensive homologies between 99.94 and 99.997% along the complete amplicon sequence (Kuroda-Kawaguchi *et al.*, 2001; Skaletsky *et al.*, 2003). They contain nine families of Y-specific protein coding genes all found to be expressed specifically in testis (Table 9.1A). Their functional integrity is probably maintained by frequent gene conversion events between the homologous palindrome arms (Rozen *et al.*, 2003). Y-sequence analysis has now also confirmed that the distal part of the AZFb deletion interval and

AZF locus in Yq11 sequence of Y haplogroup R*

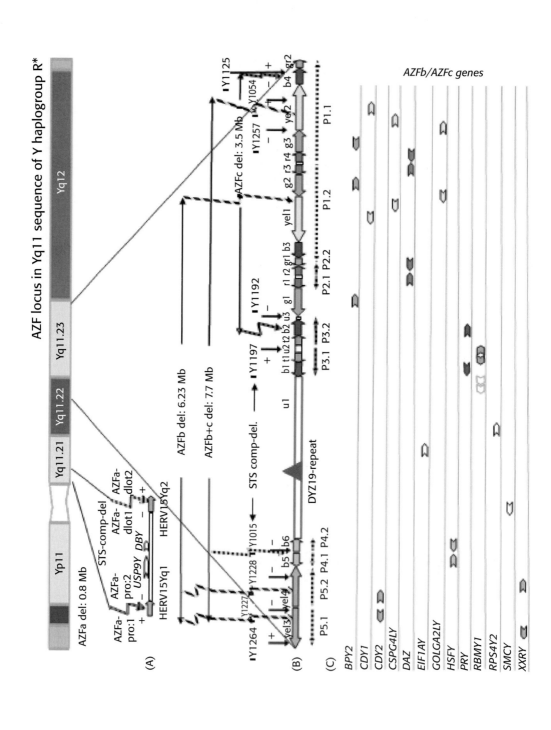

Figure 9.2   Schematic view on the AZF locus structure in Yq11 from men with haplogroup R*. (A) The AZF locus first marked by three distinct molecular deletion intervals (AZFa, AZFb, AZFc; Vogt et al., 1996) has now been sequenced. The AZFa deletion caused by recombination of two homologous HERV15 sequence blocks (HERV15Yq1/q2) is marked by a 0.8 Mb genomic DNA fragment in proximal Yq11. It contains the two AZFa genes, USP9Y and DBY. The AZFb deletion (extension 6.23 Mb) is largely overlapping with the AZFc deletion interval (extension 3.5 Mb) as indicated. Additionally a still larger AZFb deletion exists (coined AZFb+c del: 7.7 Mb; Repping et al., 2002), which however is not the sum of a complete AZFb + AZFc deletion interval. The indicated STS comp-del. markers can be used to diagnose complete AZFa, AZFb, AZFb+c, and AZFc deletions by a distinct deletion pattern. For example the sY1054 marker in distal AZFc is present in men with an AZFb+c deletion but absent in men with a complete AZFc deletion. (B) The approximate extension of the different palindromes formed by the AZFb/c amplicon structure is drawn below the amplicon blocks. Only the large P1 palindrome and the P3 palindrome include more than one amplicon type. (C) A schematic map of the location of all protein coding genes with a recognizable function (listed in Table 9.1A) are given for the AZFb and AZFc sequence interval. Their 5′–3′ polarity is indicated by the direction of the arrows marking the location of the different gene copies. Further pseudogene copies and the Testis-specific Transcript Y (TTY) genes (see Table 9.1B) mapping in the same sequence region (Skaletsky et al., 2003) are excluded to reduce the complexity of this map The colour code of the genes and associated arrows indicates in which amplicon block the gene copies are located. Only the EIF1AY, RPS4Y2, and SMCY gene and two copies of the RBMY1 gene family are located outside the amplicon blocks. One copy of the duplicated CDY2 and XKRY gene is located proximal to the AZFb deletion interval (Repping et al., 2002). Please note that the ampliconic structure of the AZFb and AZFc sequence with its gene content as shown here is based on the GenBank Y chromosome sequence (http://www.ensembl.org/Homo_sapiens/mapview?chr=Y) and that this sequence belong to a Y chromosome of the R* lineage. Thus it can be different in men with another Y chromosomal haplogroup (for more details see Vogt, 2005b) (see Color plate 8)

Table 9.1A. Human Y genes with putative spermatogenesis function mapped to the AZFa, AZFb, AZFc deletion intervals[1]

Gene symbol	Gene name	Number of copies and code	Protein homologue to	Tissue RNA expression	Copies in Yp interval?	Location in Yq11	X chromosome homologue	Autosome homologue
BPY2	Basic Protein Y 2	BPY2.1–3	Novel	Only testis	No	AZFc	No	No
CDY1	Chromo Domain Y1/2	CDY1.1–2	Chromatin-Protein and histone-acetyltransferases	Only testis	No	AZFb +	No	6p24; CDYL1
CDY2		CDY2.1–2		Only testis	No	Yq11-D11 (CDY2) AZFc (CDY1)		16q23; CDYL2
CSPG4LY	Chondroitin sulphate proteoglycan 4 Like Y	CSPG4LY.1 CSPG4LY.2	Cadherins	Only testis	No	AZFc	No	15q24; CSPG4
DAZ	Deleted in Azoospermia	DAZ1, DAZ2, DAZ3, DAZ4	RNA binding RRM proteins	Only testis	No	AZFc	No	3p24; DAZL 2q33; BOULE
DBY aka DDX3Y	DEAD box Y	1	DEAD box RNA helicases	Multiple[2]	No	AZFa	DBX aka DDX3X	No
EIF1AY	Essential Initiation Translation. Factor 1A Y	1	Translation Initiation Factor	Multiple	No	AZFb	EIF1AX	No
GOLGA2LY	Golgi autoantigen, golgin subfamily a2 Like Y	GOLGA2LY.1 GOLGA2LY.2	CIS GOLGI Matrix Protein GM130	Only testis	No	AZFc	No	9q34; GOLGA2

						AZF		
HSFY	Heat-Shock transcription Factor Y-linked	HSFY.1–2	HSP- 2 like	Testis, brain kidney, pancreas	No	AZFb	LW-1[4]	22p11–q11; HSYFL[3]
PRY	PTP–BL Related Y	PRY.1–2	Protein tyrosine Phosphatase	Only testis	Proximal Yp11 pseudogenes	AZFb AZFc: pseudogenes	No	No
RBMY	RNA binding motif Y-linked	RBMY1.1–6	RNA binding RRM–Proteins	Only testis	Proximal Yp11 pseudogenes	AZFb AZFc: pseudogenes	RBMX	HNRNP G-T retrogene
RPS4Y2	Ribosomal Protein S4 Y-linked 2	1	S4 ribosomal protein	Multiple	Distal Yp11 RPS4Y1	AZFb	RPS4X	No
SMCY	Selected mouse C DNA Y	1	H–Y antigen HLA B7	Multiple	No	AZFb	SMCX	No
USP9Y	Ubiquitin specific protease 9 Y	1	Ubiquitin-specific protease	Multiple	No	AZFa	USP9X aka DFFRX	No
XKRY	X–Kell blood group precursor related Y	XKRY.1–2	Putative membrane transport protein	Only testis	No	AZFb + Yq11–D11	No	No

[1] According to Vogt (2005a) with permission from Reproductive Healthcare Ltd. Data primarily extracted from Vogt et al. (1997); Kuroda-Kawaguchi et al. (2001); Repping et al. (2002); Skaletzky et al. (2003).

[2] Additional RNA populations with smaller lengths were found only in testis tissue (Lahn and Page, 1997; Ditton et al., 2004).

[3] According to Tessari et al. (2004).

[4] According to Shinka et al. (2004).

Table 9.1B. Human Y-genes in AZFb and AZFc with and without putative protein coding potential[1]

Gene symbol	Gene name	Protein homologue to	Tissue RNA expression	Copies in Yp interval	Yq11 interval	X chromosome homologue
CYorf15A	Chromosome Y open reading frame 15A	Unknown	Multiple	No	AZFb	Yes; cXorf 15
CYorf15B	Chromosome Y open reading frame 15B	Unknown	Multiple	No	AZFb	Yes; cXorf 15
TTY1	Testis Transcript Y1	No-protein encode RNA	Only testis	Proximal Yp11	No	No
TTY2	Testis Transcript Y2	No-protein encode RNA	Only testis	Proximal Yp11	AZFb	No
TTY3	Testis Transcript Y3	No-protein encode RNA	Only testis	No	AZFc	No
TTY4	Testis Transcript Y4	No-protein encode RNA	Only testis	No	AZFc	No
TTY5	Testis Transcipt Y5	No-protein encode RNA	Only testis	No	AZFb	No
TTY6	Testis Transcript Y6	No-protein encode RNA	Only testis	No	AZFb	No
TTY9	Testis Transcript Y9	No-protein encode RNA	Only testis	No	AZFb	No
TTY10	Testis Transcript Y10	No-protein encode RNA	Only testis	No	AZFb	No
TTY12	Testis Transcript Y12	No-protein encode RNA	Only testis	No	AZFb	No
TTY13	Testis Transcript Y13	No-protein encode RNA	Only testis	No	AZFb	No
TTY14	Testis Transcript Y14	No-protein encode RNA	Only testis	No	AZFb	No
TTY15 AZFaT1[2] Phex152[3]	Testis Transcript Y15	No-protein encode RNA	Testis, brain	No	AZFa	No
TTY17	Testis Transcript Y17	No-protein encode RNA	Only testis	No	AZFc	No
TTY16	Testis Transcript Y16	No-protein encode RNA	Only testis	No	AZFb	No

[1]According to Vogt (2005a) with permission from Reproductive Healthcare Ltd. Although Skaletzky *et al.* (2003) described 23 TTY genes (TTY1–TTY23) only the 14 listed here are mapped on the Y sequence.

[2] Sargent *et al.* (1999) in: *J Med Genet* 36: 670–677.

[3] Ditton, Hirschmann, Vogt (1999) unpublished results.

the proximal part of the AZFc deletion interval are largely overlapping. This was first deduced from an extensive YAC (Yeast Artificial Chromosomes) analysis in distal Yq11 also indicating the duplication of the gene content of the proximal AZFc region (Kirsch *et al.*, 1996).

The genomic DNA of each AZF deletion interval contains multiple genetic elements which are probably part of the AZF locus, that is, are functioning for spermatogenesis or male fertility. Extensive testes cDNA screening programs (Lahn and Page 1997; Vogt *et al.*, 1997), and the structural analysis of the GenBank AZF sequences (AZFa and AZFb in contig: NT_011875; AZFc in contig: NT_011903) by predictive gene analyses programs have now identified the putative complete gene content of each AZF microdeletion. 31 Y genes expressed in human testis and located in one of the AZF deletion intervals are registered. They are subdivided in Table 9.1 in a list of genes with a recognizable function because of one or more conserved functional peptide domains (Table 9.1A) and in a list of genes with non-identified function because similar sequences have not yet been found in the data base (Table 9.1B).

The functional AZFa locus contains the X-Y homologous genes: *USP9Y* and *DBY*, and might include the *UTY* gene mapped closely to the distal AZFa deletion HERV border line because the same gene triplet has been found structurally conserved on the mouse and cat Y chromosomes (Murphy *et al.*, 1999). AZFb which overlaps with the proximal part of AZFc contains 23 putative functional Y genes (Repping *et al.*, 2002): 16 Y genes were mapped in the unique AZFb interval: *CDY2, CYorf14, CYorf15A/B, EIF1AY, HSFY, PRY, RBMY1, RPS4Y2, SMCY, TTY5, TTY6, TTY9, TTY10, TTY13, TTY14, XKRY* (Table 9.1A, B). Three *AZFb* genes (*CDY2, RPS4Y2, XKRY*) have more copies also proximal to AZFb and the seven *AZFb* genes that are located in the AZFb-AZFc overlapping interval (*BPY2.1, CDY1.1, DAZ1, DAZ2, TTY3.1, TTY4.1, TTY17.1*) have more copies distal to AZFb in the unique part of the AZFc deletion interval (Fig. 9.2C). Thus most AZFc gene families have a copy in the AZFb deletion interval (*BPY2, CDY1, DAZ, TTY3, TTY4, TTY17*) and only the *CSPG4LY* and *GOLGA2LY* gene families are located in the unique part of AZFc. This might explain the more severe testicular pathology associated with complete AZFb deletions when compared with the testicular pathology of men with only a pure AZFc deletion. AZFb deletions include deletion of 13 Y genes completely and of 10 Y genes partially because more copies are located proximal and distal to the AZFb deletion interval (Fig. 9.2C), whereas complete AZFc deletions include only the deletion of 8 Y gene families.

Interestingly, all AZFa genes and many AZFb genes have an X-chromosomal counterpart (Fig. 9.1), and some of them are conserved on the mouse Y chromosome (*Dby, Smcy, Rbm, Uty, Usp9y*). However, to date their function in mouse spermatogenesis looks different from that in human spermatogenesis. Deletion of most mouse *Rbm* genes does not cause male infertility but only some sperm dysmorphology (Mahadevaiah *et al.*, 1998). In human, *RBM* genes are expressed during meiosis and their deletion causes meiotic arrest (Elliot *et al.*, 1997). In mouse, *Usp9y* is expressed in brain and testis tissue (Xu *et al.*, 2002), whereas the human homologue *USP9Y* is expressed in all tissues analysed (Lahn and Page, 1997). In mouse, the *Dby* gene seems not to be required for the premeiotic spermatogenesis phase whereas in human, DBY proteins were found predominantly in spermatogonia (Ditton *et al.*, 2004). In mice, expression of the *Eif2y* gene restores the proliferation phase of spermatogonia suggesting that this gene is the functional gene of the genetically AZFa-related mouse Spy locus (Mazeyrat *et al.*, 2001). In human, there is no homologous *EIF2Y* gene on the Y chromosome.

The distinct spermatogenesis functions of the *DBY* gene and its mouse homologues can be probably explained by the presence of a functional autosomal retrogene (*PL10*, *D1Pas1*) which maps on mouse chromosome 1 and which displays a testis-specific transcription profile (Leroy *et al.*, 1989; Session *et al.*, 2001). The creation of intron-less retrogenes originating from their progenitor genes by retroposition of their transcripts in the genome seem to be a common mechanism for male germ line genes when they are located on the sex chromosomes and have a function at meiosis (Wang, 2004). Accordingly, D1Pas1 protein is expressed predominantly in the nuclei of germ cells undergoing meiosis (Session *et al.*, 2001) whereas transcription of the mouse *Dby* and its X homologue (*Dbx*) is repressed because of the *Meiotic Sex Chromosomes' Inactivation* (MSCI) and formation of the sex vesicle (Fernandez-Capetillo *et al.*, 2003). In mouse, *D1Pas1* might therefore have complemented or even taken over the spermatogenic *Dby* gene function. A similar functional *DBY* retrogene has not been found in the human genome (Kim *et al.*, 2001) and may be not necessary, since the *DBY* function seems to be restricted to the premeiotic germ cell phase and its X homologue (*DBX*), is expressed predominantly in spermatids (Ditton *et al.*, 2004).

In the AZFb interval a testis-specific function before after or at meiosis has been described for the *HSFY*, *PRY*, and *RBMY* genes. The *HSFY* (H*eat-Shock* F*actor* Y) gene contains seven exons spanning 42 kb of the genomic DNA in proximal AZFb (Tessari *et al.*, 2004). This gene structure is duplicated in the P4 palindrome (Fig. 9.2) and three transcripts are generated by alternative splicing processes of which two (*HSFYT-2*; *HSFYT-3*) were testis-specific (Tessari *et al.*, 2004). Besides testis, only *HSFYT-1* transcripts are expressed in brain, kidney and pancreas tissue, contain the DNA-binding domain typical for other heat-shock proteins, and are related to the same domain of the autosomal *HSF2* gene (Repping *et al.*, 2002). The *HSF2* gene was however found to be not functional in the male germ line (McMillan *et al.*, 2002). Interestingly, another group claimed that the functional *HSFY* DNA-binding peptide sequence is most conserved to that of the *LW-1* heat-shock gene and that *HSFY* has not its evolutionary origin from chromosome 22 but from *LW-1* located in Xq28 of the X chromosome (Shinka *et al.*, 2004). A polyclonal antiserum raised against an HSFY-peptide from the conserved DNA-binding sequence was shown to mark a number of different germ cells and the Sertoli cells, suggesting the presence of the *HSFY* protein at multiple phases of human spermatogenesis. *HSFY* gene deletions, as found in all patients with a complete AZFb deletion, should therefore cause disruption of spermatogenesis at different phases depending on the patients' individual genotypes. This, however, has not been found, complete AZFb deletions usually display a meiotic arrest (Krausz *et al.*, 2003; Vogt, 2005a). However, partial AZFb deletions, that is not including the *PRY* and *RBMY* genes showed variable testicular pathologies, including hypospermatogenesis in four infertile men from Italy (Ferlin *et al.*, 2003). This would suggest that the *HSFY* gene is indeed functionally expressed in the male germ line but that the *PRY* and/or *RBMY* genes, if disrupted, are the major *AZFb* genes causing meiotic arrest.

The *PRY* gene family in AZFb consists of two full-length copies (*PRY1* and *PRY2*) with five exons. Additional pseudogene copies with deletion of the first two exons were mapped in AZFc and between AZFa and AZFb, a repeat structure of only exons 1 and 2 were found on the short and long Y arm (Stouffs *et al.*, 2001). That means functional *PRY* gene copies are only located in the AZFb region (Fig. 9.2C). *PRY* encodes a protein phosphatase probably involved in the apoptotic degradation of non-functional spermatozoa (Stouffs *et al.*, 2004). In men with normal spermatogenesis the PRY protein was found in some spermatids and spermatozoa but the fraction of PRY positively-staining spermatozoa increased from 1.5% to 51.2% in sperm samples with increased apoptotic DNA degradation as visualised using the TUNEL assay. PRY protein was not detected in premeiotic germ cells. Its contribution to the testicular pathology of men with AZFb deletion (meiotic arrest) is therefore questionable.

The *RBMY* gene is homologous to *RBMX* on the X chromosome (Fig. 9.1) and to a functional retrogene *HNRNP G-T* on chromosome 11 (11p15) that is predominantly expressed in pachytene spermatocytes (Elliott *et al.*, 2000). A spermatogenic function of HNRNP G-T proteins has been recently illustrated by the identification of two '*de novo*' exon mutations causing loss of a conserved arginine (R100H) and deletion of a C-terminal glycine (G388del), respectively, in some men with severe impairment of spermatogenesis (Westerveld *et al.*, 2004). Expression of the RBMY protein has been shown in the nuclei of both type A and B spermatogonia, spermatocytes and round spermatids. This suggests a role of this *AZFb* gene in the nuclear metabolism of newly synthesised RNAs in the germ cell at different phases (Elliot *et al.*, 1997).

The structural and functional organisation of the *RBMY/RBMX/HNRNP-G-T* genes in human is reminiscent of that of the *Dby/Dbx/D1Pas1* genes in the mouse genome (see above); different members of the *RBMY* gene family have obviously subdivided their germ line function to different spermatogenic phases, as was also found for the *DBY* and *DBX* genes (Ditton *et al.*, 2004) and the *DAZ* gene family (Xu *et al.*, 2002). This would then also explain why the lack of RBMY proteins of men with AZFb deletions cannot become compensated in spermatogenesis by the presence of RBMX and/or HNRNP G-T proteins.

In summary, it can be assumed that the spermatogenic functions of the human *AZFa* and *AZFb* genes and their homologous counterparts on the mouse Y chromosomes are probably divergent because of a species-specific adaptation of their different germ line expression profiles, similarly, as found earlier for a number of autosomal genes functioning in the genetic network controlling male fertility (Wyckoff *et al.*, 2000).

Recently, some peptides encoded from *AZFa* and *AZFb* genes (*USP9Y*, *DBY*, *UTY*, and *SMCY*) were identified as putative male specific minor histocompatibility antigens (H-Y antigens) recognised from gene products encoded in different classes of the large Major Histocompatibility Locus (MHC) on the short arm of chromosome 6 (3.6 Mb in 6p21.3) (MHC sequencing consortium, 1999): the HLA-A1 class (USP9Y) (Vogt *et al.*, 2000a), the HLA-DQ5 class (DBY) (Vogt *et al.*, 2002), the HLA-B8 and -B60 class (UTY; Vogt *et al.*, 2000b; Warren *et al.*, 2000) and the HLA-B7 and -A2 class (SMCY) (Meadows *et al.*, 1997; Wang *et al.*, 1995). Indeed, the influence of some H-Y antigens on human (and mouse) testicular organisation and spermatogenesis has long been predicted (Ohno *et al.*, 1979) and molecular deletion mapping has localised an H-Y antigen locus on the human Y-chromosome in the proximal part of the long Y arm (O'Reilly *et al.*, 1992) overlapping with the AZFa and AZFb intervals. The only receptor for H-Y antigens was identified in the membranes of Sertoli cells (Ohno *et al.*, 1979) and their expression occurred in early embryogenesis (Goldberg, 1988). Y-chromosomal H-Y antigens might therefore be considered as early male-specific cell markers probably contributing as positive signals for the first steps of male sexual and germ line development during early embryogenesis.

The *AZFc* locus can be considered as an evolutionarily very young spermatogenesis locus because no *AZFc* gene family has been found on the mouse Y-chromosome. The *BPY2* gene family might have evolved only recently during primate evolution. It contains three gene copies (*BPY2.1–3*), which were mapped with an identical exon structure (nine exons spanning ~25 kb) to the green amplicons (Fig. 9.2C). *BPY2* encodes a basic protein of 13.9 kDa, is transcriptional active in spermatids and spermatozoa, and the protein probably involved in the cytoskeletal network of microtubules formed during the postmeiotic elongation phase of the male germ cell (Wong *et al.*, 2003). The *DAZ* gene family has been transposed from chromosome 3 (3p25; *DAZL1* locus) on to the Y chromosome after divergence of the Old world monkey line of primates, that is not before ~35 million years ago (Seboun *et al.*, 1997; Shan *et al.*, 1996). The two gene copies in proximal AZFc (*DAZ1/DAZ2*) form the P2 palindrome, whereas the two other gene copies (*DAZ3/DAZ4*) are located 1.47 Mb more distal in the center of the large P1 palindrome in distal AZFc (Fig. 9.2B, C). In contrast to *BPY2*, and also *CDY* gene family (see below), the exon structures of the *DAZ* gene copies are rather variable especially in the number of the exon 7 variants also called '*DAZ-repeat*' (Fernandes *et al.*, 2002; Saxena *et al.*, 2000).

Most likely, the *DAZ* gene family evolved and became established on the Y chromosome following a duplication–diversification process similar to that proposed by Hughes (1994). It would suggest that the *DAZ* genes are extending or improving the functional profile of their autosomal homologues, *DAZL1* on chromosome 3 and *BOULE* on chromosome 2 (Xu *et al.*, 2001).

Classical theories predict that the evolutionary route towards functional divergence of two given gene copies starts first with a functional redundancy of the duplicated genes that still serve identical functions. However, this state is transient because it is usually not selected for over long evolutionary times. Functional divergence will occur by further exon mutations leading to the novel function of one or both duplicates (neo-functionalisation) or to a division of the ancestral function among the duplicated paralogs (sub-functionalisation). The last is also known as the 'Duplication–Degeneration–Complementation' (DDC) hypothesis (Force *et al.*, 1999).

Unfortunately, it is not yet possible to distinguish the spermatogenic function of the *DAZ* genes on the Y chromosomes from that of the autosomal *DAZL1* gene. While some authors assert an essential function of the *DAZ* genes in multiple cellular compartments at multiple phases of male germ cell development (Reijo *et al.*, 2000) others have found a restriction of *DAZ* gene products to the postmeiotic germ cell phase with transcripts only in early spermatids and protein in late spermatids and spermatozoa (Habermann *et al.*, 1998). Some of these discordant findings can probably be explained by the use of different polyclonal DAZ-antisera and others by the use of gene probes not able to distinguish between transcripts or proteins of the *DAZ* or its autosomal ancestors, *BOULE* and *DAZL1*. In any case, one can assume that the complete *DAZ* gene family, that is including *BOULE* and *DAZL1*, is functionally essential for human spermatogenesis, encoding different testis specific RNA-binding proteins probably involved in the translational control of transcripts of other germ line genes (Yen, 2004). These downstream-genes might be expressed as early as during foetal germ cell development like Pumilio-2 (PUM2) which proteins are functionally interacting with DAZ-like proteins (Moore *et al.*, 2003), or at meiosis where the translation of CDC25 transcripts is probably controlled by BOULE protein (Luetjens *et al.*, 2004), or in late spermatids where DAZL1 and DAZ proteins, both immunohistochemically identified, although with different antisera (Habermann *et al.*, 1998; Reijo *et al.*, 2000), are functionally interacting with the DAZAP1 protein (Vera *et al.*, 2002).

The *CDY* gene family in AZFb and AZFc originates from a polyadenylated mRNA of the *CDYL* locus on chromosome 6 that has been then retrotransposed to the Y chromosome (Lahn and Page, 1999). In contrast to its autosomal homologue expressed in all tissues analysed, the *CDY* gene is expressed only in testis tissue.

Interestingly, the *CDY1* gene copies in AZFc have evolved into a two exon gene structure forming four alternatively spliced transcripts encoding three different protein isoforms (Fig. 9.3). Since only the major *CDY1* transcript is identical in sequence to the *CDY2* transcript, the *CDY1* gene is considered to be a different paralog of the autosomal *CDYL* gene. All CDY isoforms are nuclear proteins with an N-terminal Chromo-domain probably involved in chromatin binding and a C-terminal domain that catalyses histone-acetylation reactions. Accordingly, CDY proteins were recently identified as histone acetyltransferases with a strong preference for histone H4 and localised in the nuclei of maturing spermatids (Lahn *et al.*, 2002). Histone hyperacetylation in late spermatids results in a more open chromatin structure that facilitates not only the spermatogenic histone replacement but also provides easier access of transcriptional regulatory proteins to the postmeiotic sperm DNA. Interestingly, the *CDY* autosomal homologue, *CDYL*, does not encode a testis-specific RNA population, as found with the mouse homologue (*Cdyl*), but expresses its housekeeping transcripts retained during primate evolution. This suggests selection for functional diversification of the autosomal and Y gene copies during primate evolution, similarly as discussed for the *DAZ* gene family above. Interestingly, although the *CDYL* gene encodes a histone acetyltransferases its protein sequence is only 63% homologous to

(A) *CDY1* gene has evolved novel two-exon structure

(B) Alternative spliced *CDY1* transcripts with different poly A sites

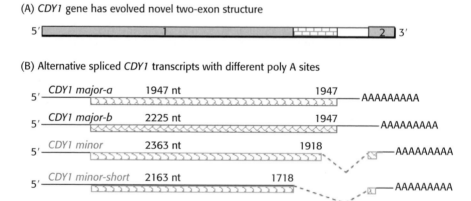

Figure 9.3   Schematic view of *CDY1* locus in AZFc. The transcription of this *CDY* gene copy in human testis produces at least four alternative spliced mRNAs published with the following GenBank accession numbers: *CDY1* major-a (AF080597), *CDY1* major-b (BC033041), *CDY1* minor (NM004680) and *CDY1* minor-short. The last variant was identified by Kleiman *et al.* (2001) and is not deposited in the GenBank. Both minor variants spliced out an intron sequence from the CDY1 exon at two different 5′ splicing sites but with identical 3′ splicing sites. This results in an alternative two-exon structure of the *CDY1* gene with an variable 5′ intron part (A) and the translation of 3 protein isoforms. The extensions of their coding frames are given in numbers of nucleotides without the poly(A) tail (B). This figure is presented also in Vogt (2005a) and used here with permission from the editor: Reproductive Healthcare Ltd

that of the CDY protein (Lahn *et al.*, 2002). This suggests that the Y gene copies in human have been evolutionarily adapted for a specific spermatogenic function (neo-functionalisation) and that both genes probably diverged before primate evolution. In this context it is interesting to note that a second autosomal *CDYL* gene, isolated in mouse and human (*CDYL2; Cdyl2*), both with a similar exon structure as the *CDYL/Cdyl* gene pair, were also divergent from each other in their amino acid sequences like found for the *CDYL* and *CDY* genes (Dorus *et al.*, 2003). The *CDY*-related gene family offers thus another informative example of how duplicated genes can evolve towards divergent functionality with a tendency to transfer genes with a spermatogenic function to the Y chromosome.

A functional difference between genes mapped in proximal and distal AZFc, respectively, might be indicated by the work of Fernandes *et al.* (2002), who found deletions of the *DAZ1/DAZ2* gene doublet only in some men with severe oligozoospermia, but *DAZ3* and *DAZ4* deletions also in men with normal fertility.

However, recently it has been indicated that the *AZFc* gene content now published for the GenBank Y sequence and deposited in different databases (GenBank: http://www.ncbi.gov; ENSEMBL: http://www.ensembl.org/Homo_sapiens/mapview? chr=Y) can be variable and is probably different in distinct Y-chromosomal haplogroup (Jobling and Tyler-Smith, 2003; Vogt 2005b). The male-specific region (MSY) of the Y sequence published by Skaletsky *et al.* (2003) belongs to a Y-chromosome of Y-haplogroup R* (Fernandes *et al.*, 2004; Vogt 2005b). Different copy numbers of the AZFb/c multi-copy genes were already found in the four main Y-branches D2b, F(xH,K), I and N (Fernandes *et al.*, 2004; Machev *et al.*, 2004; Repping *et al.*, 2003, 2004). Consequently, it might be possible that the number of amplicons and palindromes in the structure of the AZFb and AZFc regions as shown in Figure 9.2 is only associated with the Y-chromosomes of branch R*. This raises the question which Y genes in the polymorphic AZFb/c subintervals are really essential for spermatogenesis, that means which gene deletion is really a causative agent for the man's clinically observed testicular pathology and which gene deletion is neutral (polymorphic) because the gene is only balancing and shaping the reproductive fitness factor(s) of the male in the different human populations (see also Quintana-Murci *et al.*, 2001; Vogt, 2005b). Consequently, the R*-Y sequence now readable in the GenBank may reflect a genetic redundancy of AZFc gene copies, or also lack sequence regions which are present on the Y-chromosome from another Y lineage.

In summary, due to the generally high dynamic palindromic sequence structure in the ampliconic AZFb and AZFc sequence regions and the presence of similar albeit smaller repetitive sequence blocks along the whole sequence in Yq11 (Skaletsky *et al.*, 2003) multiple genomic rearrangements causing partial deletions in the 'complete'[1]

---

[1] Complete or 'classical' AZF deletions are those defined with their molecular extensions by Kamp *et al.* (2001); Kuroda-Kawaguchi *et al.* (2001), Repping *et al.* (2002); see also (Fig. 9.2).

AZF sequence regions are expected to occur frequently in the different lineages of the human Y-chromosome currently present in the global population of over three billion men. Methods that compare the age of the Y-lineage with a distinct variant of the R*-AZFb and -AZFc amplicon structure would then help to determine whether the structure identified is compatible with neutrality, that is fertility, or associated with some spermatogenic failure and whether the preference of multi-copy genes especially in the AZFb/c amplicon structures reflects some genetic redundancy or some functional constraints from the germ line, like for example creating a counterbalance for the unstable AZFb/c amplicon structures to reduce the risk of male infertility.

9.1.3 Single gene defects in infertile men

Besides the *AZF* genes in Yq11, it has been predicted from mouse knock-out models that numerous autosomal and X-chromosomal genes also expressed in the human male (and female) germ line can cause infertility (Cooke and Saunders, 2002; Matzuk and Lamb, 2002). However, although most of their human homologues are known, it is often unclear whether and how these genes are also functional in the human male germ line. Only the genes functioning for meiosis seem to be functionally conserved in the eukaryotic kingdom, whereas a rapid evolution of just reproductive proteins has been reported (Swanson and Vacquier, 2002; Wyckoff *et al.*, 2000). Indeed, when 2820 functionally equivalent rodent and human gene sequences were compared, many genes functional in the male germ line were found among the 10% most divergent sequences (Makalowski and Boguski, 1998). Functional human male fertility genes might therefore be revealed only by extensive mutation analyses of human genes known to be expressed in testis tissues.

The number of non-Y-chromosomal human single gene defects known to impair spermatogenesis is still small (Table 9.2). Most of them are also involved in the genetic control of male gonad development or some somatic development indicating a functional linkage with the germ line. Clinically, the best known are the cystic fibrosis (CF) locus located on the long arm of chromosome 7 (7q31.2), because CF mutations were abundantly found in patients with a congenital bilateral aplasia of the vas deferens (CBAVD), that is with obstructive azoospermia (Oates and Amos, 1994). Less frequent are mutations in the androgen receptor (*AR*) gene which causes different pathologies, summarised under the phrase: *Androgen Insensitivity Syndromes* (AIS: Testicular feminisation, Reifenstein, Infertile male syndrome) and mutations in the genes for the Follicle-Steroid- or Luteinising hormone receptors (*FSHR/LHR*) causing the *Idiopathic Hypo-* and hyper-gonadotropic *Hypogonadism* (IHH) syndrome and the *KAL-1* gene causing Kallmann syndrome (Table 9.2). Less known in the clinic are mutations in the *INSL3* and *LGR8-GREAT* genes that cause cryptorchidism and the (CAG)-variants of the mitochondrial DNA polymerase (*POLG*) locus proposed to be associated with male infertility (Rovio *et al.*, 2001).

Table 9.2. Clinical syndromes with possible impairment of male infertility[1]

Syndrome	Chromosomal position	Gene-locus	OMIM reference-number	
			Disease	Gene
Androgen Insensitivity syndromes (AIS: CAIS; PAIS; MAIS)	Xq11–12	AR	300068	313700
AZoospermia Factor (Y-linked)	Yq11	Multiple AZF genes	415000	14 protein genes[2]
Bardett–Biedl–syndrome (BBS2)	16q21	BBS2	209900	606151
Cystic Fibrosis (CF)	7q31.2	CFTR	219700	602421
Congenital bilateral aplasia of the vas deferens (CBAVD)			277180	602421
Cryptorchidism	19p13.2	INSL3	219050	146738
		LGR8-GREAT		606655
Dystrophia Myotonica (DM-1)	19q13.2–q13.3	DMPK	160900	605377
Fragile-X (FRAXA)	Xq27.3	FMR-1	309550	309550
Globozoospermia	6q21	CAL/GOPC	102530	606845
	6p13.3-2	CSNK2A2		115442
Gorlin-syndrome (PPS)	1q32	Not known	119500	Not known
Kallmann 1 (X-linked) Anosomia	Xp22.3	KAL-1	308700	308700
Kallmann 2 (dominant)	8p11–12	FGFR1	147950	136350
Kallmann 3 (recessive)	Not known	Not known	244200	Not known
Kartagener-Syndrome	5p15-p14	DNAH5	244400	603335
	7p21	DNAH11		603339
	9p21-p13	DNAH1		604366
McKusick–Kaufman (MKKS)	20p12	MKKS	236700	604896
Mitochondrial DNA breakage syndrome	15q25	POLG	157640	174763
Noonan-syndrome (NS1)	12q24.1	PTPN11	163950	176876
Prader–Willi–syndrome (PWS)	15q11–13	SNRPN	176270	182279
		Necidin	176270	602117
Rothmund–Thomson–syndrome (RTS)	8q24.3	RECQL4	268400	603780
Stein–Leventhal–syndrome (PCO)	15q23–24	CYP11A	184700	118485
Werner-syndrome (WRN)	8p12-p11.2	RECQL2	277700	604611
Wilms-Tumor; Denys–Drash–syndrome	11p13	WT1	194080	194080

[1] The clinical phenotypes of the male infertility syndromes listed are described in detail with their profiles of inheritance in Victor McKusicks's 'Mendelian Inheritance in Man (MIM)', respectively online (OMIM: http://www3.ncbi.nlm.nih.gov/omim/), under the given OMIM reference numbers.

[2] For more details see Table 9.1A.

A polygenic inheritance pattern has been proposed for the *Kartagener Syndrome* (KS) and Globozoospermia (GS). In this chapter a basic science perspective of these genes is presented with their description ranked according to the frequency of their mutation (for detailed description of their clinical significance see the chapter of P. Turek).

9.1.3.1 The CFTR-gene in 7q31.2

The *Cystic Fibrosis Transmembrane Conductance Regulator* (*CFTR*) gene locus is a single copy gene spanning ~250 kb of genomic DNA in region q31.2 on the long arm of chromosome 7 (Fig. 9.4). It is composed of 27 short exons numbered 1–24 (with a and b subdivisions for the exons 6, 14 and 17) that encode a messenger RNA of 6.5 kb and a protein with 1480 amino acids (molecular weight = 168 kDa). CFTR protein is functioning as a low-voltage, cyclic-AMP-regulated transmembrane channel for chloride ions in all epithelial cells analysed (Ellsworth *et al.*, 2000). It is a member of the *ATP-Binding Cassette* (ABC) family of transporter proteins, as it is characterised by two transmembrane domains (TM1, TM2), two nucleotide-binding domains (NBD1 and NBD2) and a cytoplasmic regulatory domain (R) containing many potential phosphorylation sites (Akabas, 2000). The TM domains define the structure of the CFTR chloride channel, the NPDs and R domains regulate its activity. Since the CFTR protein is subject to complex post-translational processing, including phosphorylation and glycosylation in the Golgi organelle, only 30% of the protein produced at the ribosomes is reaching its cellular membrane target (Gelman and Kopito, 2003). The cellular transport of CFTR protein is mediated by the *GO*lgi-associated *PDZ*- and *C*oiled-coil motif (GOPC) protein, also functionally involved in formation of a functional acrosome (Yao *et al.*, 2002). Therefore, GOPC is also called *CFTR Associated Ligand* (CAL) protein (Cheng *et al.*, 2004). It modulates CFTR plasma membrane expression by retaining CFTR within the cell and targeting it for degradation (see also Globozoospermia candidate genes below).

  CFTR gene defects cause cystic fibrosis (CF) and CBAVD. The molecular aetiology of the CBAVD condition was for a long time unknown until it was recognised that CF men were often childless after some years of marriage and that their infertility was caused by the absence of the vas deferens (Holsclaw *et al.*, 1971; Kaplan *et al.*, 1968). *CFTR* gene mutations are divided into six classes (I–VI) and two major categories (Estivill, 1996; Welsh and Smith, 1993). The first category includes those mutants where the *CFTR* protein is unable to accumulate at the cell surface, either because of impaired biosynthesis (Class I and V) or because of defective folding at the endoplasmic reticulum (Class II). Mutants that belong to the second category express the CFTR protein at the cell surface but its mutated structure fails to translocate chloride ions because of a defect in activation (Class IV). *CFTR* class VI mutants appear to be normal in their biosynthetic processing and macroscopic chloride channel function but the biological stability of the mature, complex glycosylated form

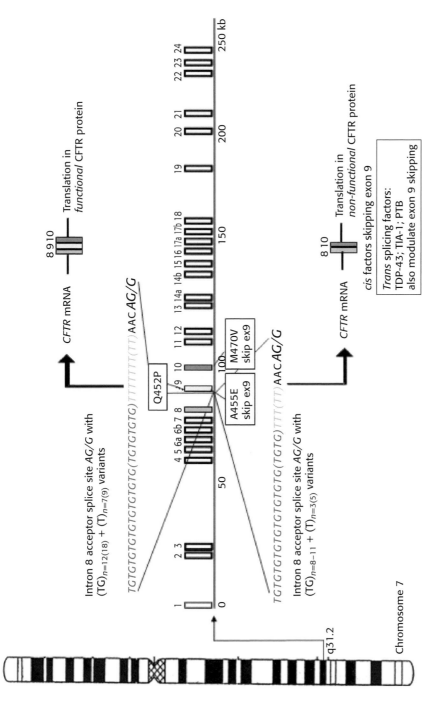

Figure 9.4   Schematic view on the exon structure of the human *CFTR* gene located on the long arm of chromosome 7 (7q31.2) along 250 kb. The variable number of TG + T nucleotides in intron 8 can result in skipping of exon 9 during the splicing process of *CFTR* primary transcripts as indicated. Exon variants which were shown to modulate this skipping process are given for exon 9 and 10. Additional *trans* splicing factors revealed by appropriate reporter CFTR minigene experiments (Niksic et al., 1999) are listed at the bottom of the figure. Translation of mRNAs without exon 9 results in a non-functional *CFTR* protein. For further details see text

is dramatically reduced (Haardt *et al.*, 1999). Most frequently found is a deletion of three nucleotides in exon 10 which results in the loss of a phenylalanine residue at position 508 of the putative *CFTR* protein (Bobadilla *et al.*, 2002). According to the *CFTR* online database (http://www.genet.sickkids.on.ca/CFTR) a surprisingly high number of 1005 pathological *CFTR* mutations and 208 variants are registered, most of them are rare and only present in single families. This suggests that the *CFTR* gene sequence can accommodate a degree of variability without loss of its basic chloride channel activity in the membranes of epithelial cells. Consequently, the severity of the CF pathology associated with a specific gene mutation is variable in different pedigrees (Estivill, 1996), ranging from severe pulmonary disease with pancreatic insufficiency to chronic bronchiectasis (Girodon *et al.*, 1997).

CFTR mutations causing a distinct somatic CF pathology most often cause CBAVD in male gonads. Other *CFTR* mutations only cause the CBAVD pathology (Oates and Amos, 1994). This suggests a different need for the *CFTR* protein in the different tissues. Indeed, it was found that the epithelial cells in the male genital tract appear to be more sensitive to a quantitative CFTR protein deficiency than the same cell type in other organs and also the processing of *CFTR* mutant transcripts seems to be different in the two cell types especially when changing the efficiency of the 3′splicing site of intron 8 (Kiesewetter *et al.*, 1993; Mak *et al.*, 1997). Consequently, the most frequent *CFTR* mutations not causing CF but CBAVD is based on the different sequence variants in this 3′splicing region (Fig. 9.4). Four different T alleles (3T, 5T, 7T, 9T) have been diagnosed in this *CFTR* sequence part. The reduction of the number of Ts results in reduction of the efficiency of splicing exon 9 in *CFTR* mRNA. In the presence of the 5T allele only 10–40% of *CFTR* mRNA contains exon 9. Exon 9 encodes part of the functionally important first nucleotide-binding domain (NBD1).

A remarkable number (60%) of heterozygous mutations in the *CFTR* gene form 'compound heterozygotes' in the CBAVD patient group, that is different mutations in each gene copy are analysed (Patrizio *et al.*, 1993). Compound heterozygotes of CBAVD patients with a 5T allele in one gene copy and an Arg117-to-His117 (R117H) mutation in exon 4 of the second gene copy also have a severe CF phenotype, whereas the 7T allele only results in CBAVD (Kiesewetter *et al.*, 1993).

The *CFTR* T alleles and their influence on the processing of exon 9 (skipping or inclusion in the *CFTR* mRNA) is linked to the extension of a polymorphic $(TG)_n$ dinucleotide ($n = 9$–13) flanking the T alleles in the intron 8 sequence and the presence of some exonic variants in exon 9 (Q452P; A455E) and exon10 (M470V) of the *CFTR* protein (Cuppens *et al.*, 1994, 1998; Fig. 9.4). These variants have no deleterious consequences for the production of *CFTR* mRNA but in combination with the 5T allele, the presence of these variants results in a different production of *CFTR* mRNA with and without exon 9 thereby causing the CBAVD pathology (for review see

Claustres, 2005). The higher proportion of *CFTR*-transcripts without exon 9 found in the vas deferens cells independent of the T_n genotype suggests a distinct processing efficiency of *CFTR* transcripts in the male germ line (Mak *et al.*, 1997; Teng *et al.*, 1997).

Using reporter *CFTR* minigenes, including the genomic sequence between exon 8 and exon 10, the dependence of the splicing efficiency for the exon 9 sequence on the presence of the different TG and T allele combinations (*cis* factors) was confirmed and it was also shown that additional specific nuclear proteins (TDP-43; TIA-1; PTB) were physically interacting with these target sequences (*trans*-factors), all involved in a tissue specific exon 9 splicing control (Buratti *et al.*, 2001; Niksic *et al.*, 1999; Zuccato *et al.*, 2004). Targeting mutations in the 5′ and 3′ splice site of the exon 9 sequence revealed that this exon already contains only natural suboptimal splicing conditions making it inherently vulnerable for skipping (Hefferon *et al.*, 2004). Interestingly, this vulnerability is absent in the mouse *CFTR* gene containing two strong splicing consensus sites and a very short and non-polymorphic polypyrimidine tract (Ellsworth *et al.*, 2000). Studies on the testis pathology of human CFTR mutations can therefore not be deduced from the mouse animal model.

9.1.3.2 The Kallmann 1 (KAL-1) gene locus

Kallmann syndrome is the most common X-linked male infertility disorder. Genetically, Kallmann syndrome is heterogenous, and genotype–phenotype correlations are difficult to settle (Quinton *et al.*, 1996). The patients can usually be successfully treated by hormone replacement therapy. The KAL-1 locus has been mapped to the X-chromosome (Xp22.3) (del Castillo *et al.*, 1992; Franco *et al.*, 1991; Legouis *et al.*, 1991). *KAL-1* expression escapes X inactivation, has a putative non-functional homologue on the Y-chromosome (Fig. 9.1) and shows an unusual pattern of conservation across species including Caenorhabditis elegans (Bulow *et al.*, 2002). The predicted protein anosmin-1 plays a key role in the migration of Gonadotropin Releasing Hormone (GnRH) neurons and olfactory nerves to the hypothalamus and has significant similarities with other proteins involved in neural cell adhesion and axonal pathfinding, as well as with protein kinases and phosphatases. This supports that the *KAL-1* gene could have a specific role in neuronal migration control (Hardelin, 2001) and that GnRH is a key regulator of reproduction and sexual behaviour.

KALl-1 mutations, for example intragenic deletions and point mutations (Bick *et al.*, 1992; Hardelin *et al.*, 1992), cause the pathology of Kallmann syndrome typically defined as an association between hypogonadotropic hypogonadism and anosmia, that is the inability to smell. Since it occurs more frequently in men (1 : 10,000) than in women (1 : 50,000) X-linked inheritance has been predicted (*KAL-1*) although examples of dominant (*KAL-2*) and autosomal recessive (*KAL-3*) inheritance have also been described (Table 9.2). Loss-of-function mutations in the fibroblast growth factor receptor 1 (*FGFR1*) gene located on the short arm of chromosome 8 (8p11–12) were identified recently as the molecular base of the dominant autosomal *KAL-2* locus (Dode *et al.*, 2003). The *KAL-1* and *FGFR1* genes were found to be co-expressed at different sites during embryonic development, a functional interaction between both proteins can therefore be proposed. This would also explain the higher prevalence of Kallmann syndrome in males.

9.1.3.3 The AR gene locus

The *AR* gene is a member of the large intracellular family of glucocorticoid receptors that are made inactive by inhibitors and the absence of their ligands. Upon ligand binding, they get activated, move to the nucleus and bind to DNA. For its full activity, a strong interaction between the N- and C-terminal peptide domain is essential. Ligands are the hormones testosterone (T) and dihydrotestosterone (DHT) that mediate a wide range of developmental and physiological responses in male sexual differentiation, pubertal maturation and the maintenance of spermatogenesis. They are therefore also called androgens. Production of testosterone (T) begins at the 8th week of pregnancy in foetal Leydig cells initiating the development of the male gonad from the Wolffian ducts. This includes formation of the epididymis, vas deferens, and seminal vesicles. Formation of the male external genitalia, that is penis, scrotum, requires the conversion of testosterone to dihydrotestosterone by the steroid 5α-reductase 2 (SRD5A2). The androgen receptor gene is not expressed in germ cells but at different phases in Sertoli cells (Suarez-Quian, 1999), supporting its role in male gonad and germ line development. After ligand binding the protein dimerizes and translocates to the cell nucleus where it binds to specific palindromic DNA elements (5′-TGTTCT-NNN-AGAACA-3′) defined as *Androgen Responsive Element* (ARE) sites. Binding to a number of nuclear co-activators (Heinlein and Chang, 2002), the dimerised AR protein promotes the transcription of multiple target genes. The AR interacting proteins are listed in a database (http://ww2.mcgill.ca/androgendb/ARinteract.pdf).

The androgen receptor gene is composed of eight exons along a genomic sequence region of ~90 kb at Xq11–12 (Fig. 9.5). The long N-terminal peptide domain (555 amino acids) encoded by exon 1 functions as a transactivation domain (TAD) by modulating the transcriptional activity of the AR-dependent downstream-genes. Exons 2–3 encode the DNA-binding peptide domain (DBD) (557–616 aa) and exons 4–8 encode the C-terminal peptide domain (664–915 aa), responsible for the protein's androgen-binding (ABD) activity. The DBD domain contains two zinc-fingers that are required to bind to the ARE of the DNA sequence. In addition to these principal functions, all three domains embody subsidiary functions that affect dimerisation, nuclear localisation and transcriptional regulation (Gobinet *et al.*, 2002).

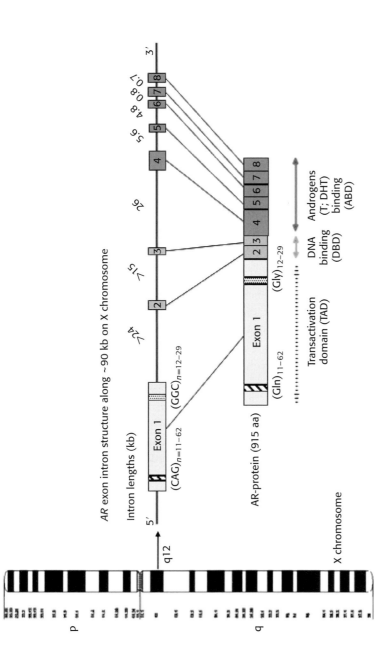

Figure 9.5   Schematic view on the exon structure of the human *Androgen Receptor* (*AR*) gene with its three functional domains distinguished by different grey tones. The *AR* gene is located on the long arm of the X chromosome along 90 kb as indicated. The first exon encodes the transactivation domain (TAD) forming the active gonad-specific transcription factor complex by binding with a series of other transcription factors. It has a polymorphic length due to two repetitive triplets $(CAG)_n$ and $(GGC)_n$ with variable n-values as indicated. Above the $n = 38$ for the CAG repeat, the androgen receptor becomes a causative agent for SBMA a severe neuro-degenerative disease. The DNA-binding region (DBD) of the AR protein has been mapped to exon 2 and 3. The androgens testosterone (T) and dihydrotestosterone (DHT) are the ligands binding to the androgen-binding region (ABD) encoded by exon 4–8. Specific point mutations associated with male infertility were found in the TAD and ABD region, respectively

The TAD region in exon 1 is variable in length encoding a repetitive tract of glutamines (coded by CAG_n; $n = 11–62$) and of glycins (coded by GGC_n; $n = 12–29$). This polymorphism quantitatively regulates AR promoter activity that is enhanced with lower and reduced with higher numbers of the CAG-repeat (Tut *et al.*, 1997). Whether lower AR transactivation values also impair the rate of spermatogenesis is still an open question (Casella *et al.*, 2003; Hiort and Holterhus, 2003; Patrizio *et al.*, 2001). In a large comparative study including 600 fertile and 674 infertile men from Europe, numbers of CAG-repeats in the fertile and infertile men were not statistically different (Rajpert-De Meyts *et al.*, 2002), and this was confirmed in other studies with 119 infertile men of Caucasoid origin (Dadze *et al.*, 2000) and 280 men from an Indian population (Thangaraj *et al.*, 2002). However, ethnical differences probably exist for the functional phenotype of the TAD peptide activating downstream spermatogenesis genes in some other human populations.

It this context it is interesting to note that CAG repeat length greater than $n = 38$ are usually not associated with male infertility but with the occurrence of a severe neurodegenerative disease, *Spinal Bulbar Muscular Atrophy* (SBMA: Kennedy syndrome: OMIM-ref: 313200). The SBMA CAG disease alleles range between $n = 38–62$ (La Spada *et al.*, 1991). Intracellular AR is essential for androgen action (T and DHT). Hence the AR is essential for normal primary sexual development before birth and for normal secondary male development at puberty (virilisation) including sperm maturation (Holdcraft and Braun, 2004). Therefore, the AR gene must also be involved in the regulative genetic network controlling spermatogenesis.

In the cell cytoplasm the function of the *AR* is inhibited by the binding of a number of heat-shock proteins (Hsps). They are released after androgen binding and phosphorylation has transformed the AR protein structure into a confirmation able to be translocated to the nucleus and to bind to the ARE sequence elements after dimerisation. After binding to a number of co-factors, including basal transcription factors and core promoter elements, the AR target genes are becoming transcriptional active (Gobinet *et al.*, 2002).

The general high grade of sequence variations in the *AR* gene (more than 300 point mutations in the AR-database: http://ww2.mcgill.ca/androgendb/AR23C.pdf) reflects a high structural flexibility of the dimeric AR-protein in its functional complex with the multiple co-activators, together resulting in a gonad-specific transcription factor. Consequently, no specific pathology is found for most *AR* gene mutations but more a variety of pathological phenotypes ranging from testicular feminisation with male infertility (CAIS: complete androgen insensitivity syndrome) to male infertility with mild androgen insensitivity (MAIS). This variability is the consequence of the quantitative gradient of the T/DHT binding efficiency in the ABD region of the AR protein (Gottlieb *et al.*, 2005). Mutation analysis of the *AR* gene should therefore be offered to all patients where male infertility is associated with a mild androgen resistance syndrome like Rosewater-Syndrome and Reifenstein-Syndrome (OMIM-ref. 312100, 312300).

9.1.3.4 Follicle-steroid hormone/luteinizing hormone receptor (FSHR/LHR) locus

The receptors for the gonadotropins follicle-stimulating hormone (FSH) and luteinizing hormone (LH) belong to the family of G-protein-coupled receptors. These receptors are characterised by a large extracellular domain that specifically binds the LH or FSH heterodimers. The α-helical transmembrane domain is linked to the intracellular domain, which is coupled to the cellular G-protein signal pathway converting ATP to c-AMP via the adenylcyclase enzyme complex. Upon FSH or LH binding, a conformational change of the intracellular receptor protein domain leads to the binding of G-proteins (Aittomaki, 1998). This structural relationship indicates a common origin and functional relationship of both genes (designated as *FSHR* and *LHR*). Additional support comes from their clustered localisation on the short arm of chromosome 2 (2p21) and their related exon structures. The extracellular domain is encoded by exon 1–9 (*FSHR*) and exon 1–10 (*LHR*) respectively. The transmembrane, as well as the intracellular domain, are encoded for by the last long exon in both genes (1251 nt in *FSHR*; 1200 nt in *LHR*).

Surprisingly, a variable suppression of spermatogenesis and fertility was diagnosed in men homozygous for the inactivating A189V mutation in exon 7 of the *FSHR* gene (Tapanainen *et al.*, 1997). As a result, the essential role of FSH and *FSHR* expression for the initiation of spermatogenesis in human is questionable. Although FSH/FSHR action is required to increase testicular size, spermatogenesis can occur in the presence of severe FSH resistance as long as there is a normal testosterone production. These observations have been confirmed recently in *FSHR* and *FSH* gene-knockout mice (Abel *et al.*, 2000). Three single nucleotide polymorphisms (SNP) of the *FSHR* gene, one in the promoter region and two in exon 10 had no influence on male fertility despite a significant correlation between these polymorphisms and the basal FSH levels diagnosed in females (Simoni *et al.*, 2002).

Mutations in the *LHR* gene leads to hypogonadal phenotypes (Leydig cell hypoplasia, LCH) due to a delay in foetal and pre-pubertal male development (male pseudo-hermaphroditism, MPH). MPH can be caused by different genetic anomalies. Among them are anomalies of Leydig cell differentiation, causing hypoplasia or even absence of Leydig cells (LCH). A number of mutations in the *LHR* gene resulting in complete or partial resistance to LH and associated with variable pathologies of the male gonad have been reported (Sultan and Lumbroso, 1998). Male infertility then occurs because of male gonad dysgenesis including micropenis and hypospadias.

Familial male-limited precocious puberty (FMPP) has been diagnosed in patients with a constitutive activation of the LH transduction pathway (Sultan and Lumbroso, 1998). It is a dominant disorder that is caused by two *LHR* mutations (D578G and

M571I) located in the sixth transmembrane domain (Kremer *et al.*, 1993). The most severe phenotype, resulting from altered LH–LHR interaction, is characterised by an external female phenotype with a blind ending vagina and primary amenorrhoea. In summary, the variance of pathological phenotypes associated with *LHR* gene mutations is similar, as has been found with mutations in the androgen receptor gene (see above).

FSH and LH are hetero-dimeric molecules that share a common α-subunit (also with chorionic gonadotropin, CG and thyroid-stimulating hormone, TSH) and have specific β-subunits. The single gene encoding the common α-subunit has been mapped to chromosome 6 (6q12–21). The FSH-β subunit encoding gene has been mapped to chromosome 11 (11p13) and the LH-β subunit encoding gene to chromosome 19 (19q13.32), where it is linked with six copies of the human CG gene. FSH is essential for Sertoli-cell proliferation and maintenance of sperm quality in the testis. The functional action of FSH might be different in the mouse and human germ line since males with *FSH-β* mutations present with azoospermia (Achermann *et al.*, 2001), whereas homozygous *FSH-β* knockout mice have small testes, are oligozoospermic but are fertile (Matzuk and Lamb, 2002). Only one *LH-β* gene mutation associated with male infertility has been reported (Acherman *et al.*, 2001).

9.1.3.5 INSL3 and LGR8-GREAT gene loci are functional for testis descent

INSL3/LGR8-GREAT are both functionally involved in the molecular mechanism of testis descent. Testicular descent from abdomen to scrotum occurs in two distinct phases: the trans-abdominal phase and the inguinal–scrotal phase. The gubernaculum connects the gonad to the inguinoscrotal region and is involved in testis descent. It rapidly develops in the male foetus, whereas development in the female foetus is lacking. Since absence of *Insl3* in male mice results in bilateral impairment of testis descent, that is cryptorchidism (Adham *et al.*, 2000; Nef and Parada, 1999), it has been proposed that mutations involving this gene may also be a cause of cryptorchidism in men. Cryptorchidism is one of the most frequent congenital abnormalities in humans, involving 2% of male births (OMIM ref.: 219050; Table 9.2). Cryptorchidism can result in infertility and an increased risk for development of germ-cell tumours. The aetiology of cryptorchidism is for the most part unknown and appears to be genetically heterogeneous. Other factors are involved in gubernaculum development, for example androgens and anti-Mullerian hormone (AMH).

In human, *INSL3* has been mapped on chromosome 19 (19p13.2). It is also known as relaxin-like factor (RLF) and Leydig insulin-like protein (LEY I-L) and a member of the insulin/relaxin hormone superfamily that is highly expressed in Leydig cells (Burkhardt *et al.*, 1994). The frequency of *INSL3/RLF* gene mutations as a cause of cryptorchidism appears to be low because only 2 of 145 (1.4%) formerly cryptorchid patients were found to have a *INSL3* mutation (Tomboc *et al.*,

2000). Mutation analysis of the coding regions of the *INSL3* gene was performed in 145 formerly cryptorchid patients and 36 adult male controls using single-strand conformational polymorphism (SSCP) analysis. Two mutations, R63X and P93L, and several polymorphisms were identified.

INSL3 is the ligand for LGR8, one of the recently identified G protein-coupled orphan receptors (LGR4–8) homologous to gonadotropin and thyrotropin receptors (Kumagai *et al.*, 2002). Transgenic mice missing the *LGR8* gene also display cryptorchidism. The same mouse gene, but designated as G-protein-coupled Receptor Affecting Testis descent (*GREAT*), because it was identified by a different research group (Gorlov *et al.*, 2002), was screened for some nucleotide variants in 61 cryptorchid human patients. Compared with the GREAT cDNA sequence, a unique missense mutation (T222P) was identified in the ectodomain of the GREAT receptor (Gorlov *et al.*, 2002). Two sequence variants in exon 12 (A/G transversions at nucleotide positions 957 and 993) were identified in 40 out of the 61 cryptorchid patients but were also identified in the normal control men displaying three different haplotypes (A957 and A993, A957 and G993, G957 and G993).

The low frequency of mutations found in the *INSL3* and *GREAT/LGR8* gene locus of patients with testicular maldescent suggests that this frequent occurring pathology must be caused by mutations in some other genes as well. Indeed, some candidate genes have already been suggested based on chromosome analyses and were found to be located, probably, on chromosome 1, 2, 8, 9, 22, X- and the Y-chromosome (Moreno-Garcia and Miranda, 2002).

9.1.3.6 DNA polymerase G (POLG) locus

The human *POLG* gene locus encoding the catalytic subunit of mitochondrial DNA polymerase has been mapped to the long arm of chromosome 15 (15q25) (Zullo *et al.*, 1997). *POLG* is the only DNA polymerase responsible for mitochondrial DNA replication. The protein contains a polyglutamine tract encoded for by a CAG repeat in the first *POLG* exon. This CAG repeat is polymorphic in length, as found for the *AR* gene, although with a much lower variability. The common $(CAG)_{n=10}$ repeat allele is found with a uniformly high frequency (0.88) in different ethnic populations and absent in only 1% of the individuals (Rovio *et al.*, 1999). This indicates that, in contrast to the *AR*–CAG repeat, a strong positive selection for one major $(CAG)_{10}$-allele exists.

Interestingly, in infertile men with moderate oligozoospermia this common CAG allele was found to be absent. The mutant genotype (*absence of the common CAG$_{10}$-allele, 'abs10' POLG-allele*) was found at an elevated frequency in this patient class in all populations studied (Rovio *et al.*, 2001). Using sperm DNA from men in whom azoospermia was excluded, 9 of 99 infertile males (9%) from Finland or England were found to be homozygous for the 'abs10' POLG-allele. In contrast, this allele was present in sperm DNA from all 98 fertile males studied. The frequent finding of the 'abs10/abs10' genotype in infertile men (9.1%) is therefore highly significant. However, in a similar study with a large number of Italian patients the 'abs10/abs10' genotype was not found (Krausz et al., 2004). Screening 195 individuals with some sort of sperm abnormalities including numbers and 190 fertile control samples with a normal sperm count from the same area *no* absence of the common $(CAG)_{10}$ allele could be registered in the infertile men population. The same conclusion was drawn from a multi-center study in France (Aknin-Seifer et al., 2005).

A higher frequency of heterozygosity for the 'abs10' allele in infertile males than in fertile males would suggest a causative influence of this *POLG* allele on the men's fertility. Given the many rounds of cell division during spermatogenesis and the functional necessity of mitochondrial DNA (mt-DNA) for sperm function, it seems plausible that a suboptimal mt-DNA polymerase would result in the accumulation of mt-DNA mutations and in failure to complete differentiation. Obviously, the 'abs10/abs10' *POLG* variant in infertile men was not found at an elevated frequency in all populations studied. This indicates only a weak impairment of the *POLG* gene in mitochondria of men with an increased or reduced length of the common CAG 10-repeat allele; probably being dependent on the ethnic background as found for the CAG-repeat alleles of the *AR* gene (Rajpert-De Meyts et al., 2002).

9.1.3.7 Gene defects causing Kartagener syndrome and Globozoospermia

Two prominent examples where defects of different genes are causing the same testicular pathology are the multiple genes causing Kartagener syndrome (KS) and Globozoospermia (Table 9.2). KS is also associated with immotile cilia syndrome, that is primary ciliary dyskinesia (PCD; OMIM no. 242650). The prevalence of PCD is estimated to be 1 in 20,000–60,000 but, like KS, it occurs more frequently (range between 1 in 8000–25,000). Spermatozoa from men with KS are immotile, like the cilia in their respiratory tract. Complete absence of dynein arms forming temporary cross bridges between adjacent ciliary filaments are causative factors. Dynein arms are believed to be responsible for generating movement in cilia and sperm tails. Although pedigree analysis mostly suggests an autosomal recessive inheritance pattern of KS, X-linked and autosomal dominant inheritance patterns were reported as well (Narayan et al., 1994). This points to genetic heterogeneity of KS, that is caused by mutation in multiple genes although of the same genetic network. A genome-wide linkage analysis has now confirmed the expected extensive locus heterogeneity for the PCD syndrome (Blouin et al., 2000) and the first three genes causing KS, if mutated, have been isolated: the gene encoding the dynein axonemal intermediate chain 1 (DNAH1) on the short arm of chromosome 9 (9p13–21) (Pennarum et al., 1999), the gene encoding the dynein axonemal heavy chain 5 (DNAH5) on the short arm of chromosome 5 (Olbrich et al., 2002), and the gene encoding dynein axonemal heavy chain 11 (DNAH11) on the short of chromosome 7 (7p21) (Bartoloni *et al.*, 2002). The axoneme is composed of about 250 distinct proteins (Dutcher, 1995). Therefore it can be expected that mutations in the other dynein axonemal arm genes will also cause a KS phenoytpe.

A polygenic inheritance pattern has also been discussed for round-headed spermatozoa phenotype (globozoopspermia), induced by malformations or absence of the acrosome (Florke-Gerloff *et al.*, 1984). The number of round-headed sperm in the ejaculate can vary between 14% and 71%. Two types of globozoospermia are distinguished: Type I is characterised by a complete lack of acrosome and acrosomal enzymes and by a spherical arrangement of the chromatin. These sperm are unable to penetrate the zona pellucida, causing infertility. Type II has some acrosomal activity covering a canonical nucleus surrounded by large cytoplasmic droplets (Singh, 1992). Elevated chromosome aneuplodies were found in round-headed sperm with FISH using probes for chromosomes 13, 15, 18, 21, X, and Y (Carrell *et al.*, 1999, 2001), although this could not be confirmed by other authors (Vicari *et al.*, 2002; Viville *et al.*, 2000). However, in all cases, an increased damage of the sperm chromatin structure has been reported, indicating a high mutational load in the paternal DNA structure of these patients. Globozoospermic sperm will therefore have an inherently low fertilisation rate even with intracytoplasmic sperm injection (ICSI), because an increased damage of sperm chromatin and DNA is generally decreasing the sperms fertilisation capacity and also impair early embryonic development (Sakkas *et al.*, 1998).

It has been found that the mouse gene encoding the protein kinase casein kinase II (Ck2) encodes a germ line-specific isoform (*Csnk2a2*) expressed in late stages of spermatogenesis and, if disrupted, cause globozoospermia (Xu *et al.*, 1999). Casein kinase II is a cyclic-AMP and calcium-independent serine-threonine kinase that is composed of two catalytic subunits (alpha and alpha′) and two regulatory beta-subunits. The highly conserved amino acid sequences of its subunits and their broad expression suggest that Ck2 may have a fundamental role in cell function. Ck2 has been implicated in DNA replication, regulation of basal and inducible transcription, translation and control of metabolism. The Ck2alpha and Ck2alpha′ isoforms (products of the genes *Csnk2a1* and *Csnk2a2*, respectively) are highly homologous, but the reason for their redundancy and evolutionary conservation is unknown. No mutations were yet found in the homologous human genes, *CSNK2A2* and *CSNK2B*, after screening six patients suffering from globozoospermia (Pirrello *et al.*, 2005).

A second mouse gene causing globozoospermia if disrupted (knock-out mutant) is the gene encoding the *GO*lgi-associated *PDZ*- and *Coiled*-coil motif- (GOPC) protein (Yao *et al.*, 2002). In these mice the acrosome in round-headed sperm is absent because of fragmentation in the early round spermatids. The GOPC protein is localised at the Golgi apparatus as well as the trans-Golgi network in spermatids.

It plays a role in the vesicular transport of other proteins from the Golgi apparatus to the plasma membrane. Interestingly, its human homologue has been isolated as CFTR *Associated Ligand* (CAL) protein that modulates CFTR plasma membrane expression by retaining CFTR within the cell and targeting it for degradation (Cheng *et al.*, 2004).

Multiple somatic genetic disorders cause male infertility pleiotropically (Table 9.2). That means that patients with mutations in, for example, the DM-1 gene causing myotonic dystrophy, are not always infertile. Considering different cell systems, the primary effect of a gene mutation is not identical and, only sometimes but not always, a second pathology occurs in an apparently remote cell system, that is pleiotropically. The over-all pattern of heterozygous mutations in the personal genome is therefore called 'individual specific heterozygosity' or 'genetic load factor'. According to these rules, it is often doubtful whether a given gene mutation with a recessive somatic gene defect may have a dominant inheritance pattern in the germ line, like that suggested for the CF/CBAVD locus (see above). It is therefore also not surprising when the same mutation in a given gene locus causes a variable pathology (see e.g. *AR, CFTR, FSHR*) or male infertility as a single pathology.

9.2 Male fertility marker genes

Mature mammalian spermatozoa require a post-testicular maturation process, including their exposure to the specific microenvironment provided by the epididymis. Therefore, ICSI fertilisation rates with testis-extracted spermatozoa (TESE) are usually lower then when mature spermatozoa isolated from the patient's ejaculates are used (Tournaye, 1999; but see also Bukulmez *et al.*, 2001). Also, a reduced implantation rate has been reported for ICSI cycles using testicular sperm compared with those using ejaculated sperm (Pasqualotto *et al.*, 2002; Ubaldi *et al.*, 1999). Thus, there is ample circumstantial evidence that epididymal function is essential for male fertility and that epididymal proteins are involved in this process (Kirchhoff, 1999). However, our understanding of how the individual proteins implement the acquisition of sperm fertilizing ability is still unclear. In order to better appreciate the role of the epididymis at a molecular level, a careful analysis of its specific pattern of gene expression needs to be elaborated (Kirchhoff, 2002). In any case, the diagnosis of the fertility potential of a semen sample is essential. Accurate molecular genetic diagnostic tests are needed to determine the sperm's fertility potential.

9.2.1.1 PHGPx expression in the male germ line

A prominent male fertility marker protein already expressed in spermatids and located as major structural protein in the midpiece of mature sperm tails is the mitochondrial capsule selenoprotein (MCS) encoded for by an isoform of the Gluthathione peroxidase gene GPX-4 (Ursini *et al.*, 1999), which is located on the short arm of chromosome 19 (19p13.3) (Kelner and Montoya, 1998). The GPX-4 isoform encodes the phospholipid hydroperoxide glutathione peroxidase (PHGPx) enzyme expressed in three different forms using alternative start codons. These target the enzyme to the cytosol, mitochondria, or to the nucleus, respectively. Preferential PHGPx gene transcription is observed in the late round spermatids, but ceases abruptly upon transition to elongated spermatids. The change in shape from round spermatids to the elongated form parallels, in time, the change of the chromosomal packaging proteins from histones to protamines. PHGPx activity in spermatids may therefore also functionally contribute to crosslinking of the protamine thiols, which is essential for stabilisation of the postmeiotic condensation of sperm chromatin.

In mature spermatozoa PHGPx activity is hardly detectable because it has been transformed to the oxidatively inactivated MCS protein (Ursini *et al.*, 1999). This switch in the redox status during late sperm maturation is explained by the disappearance of GSH, the usual PHGPx reductant. PHGPx, thus deprived of its usual GSH reduction, becomes cross-linked with itself and with other SH-proteins via seleno-disulphide bridges. In the midpiece of mature spermatozoa, the oxidised PHGPx protein represents at least 50 percent of the capsule material that embeds the helix of mitochondria. The mechanical instability of the mitochondrial midpiece that is observed after selenium deficiency also points to an essential role of PHGPx as a structural sperm tail protein.

The PHGPx protein content in sperm can be estimated after reductive solubilisation by measuring the rescued PHGPx activity (Foresta *et al.*, 2002). It was found that the rescued PHGPx activity in infertile men ranged significantly below that of controls (93.2 ± 60.1 units/mg sperm protein versus 187.5 ± 55.3 units/mg). It was particularly low in oligoasthenozoospermic specimens (61.93 ± 45.42 units/mg; $P < 0.001$) compared with asthenozoospermic samples and controls. In isolated motile sperm samples, motility decreased faster with decreasing PHGPx content. Obviously, irrespective of the cause of alteration, the content of PHGPx in spermatozoa is correlated with fertility-related parameters and their residual PHGPx protein activities can be used as a predictive marker for the fertilization capacity of the patients' sperm.

9.2.1.2 PRM-1/PRM-2 expression and sperm chromatin condensation

Male infertility can be also associated with abnormal sperm chromatin condensation due to a lack of protamines (Balhorn *et al.*, 1988). Protamines are the major DNA-binding proteins in the nucleus of sperms in most vertebrates, packaging the DNA in a volume less than 5% of a somatic cell nucleus. Many mammals have one protamine, but a few species, including humans and mice, have two. Mouse knock-out studies for both protamine genes have now shown that they are functional, not redundant, and that both protamines are essential for sperm chromatin condensation and that haploinsufficiency caused by a mutation in one allele of *Prm-1* or *Prm-2* prevents genetic transmission of both mutant and wild-type alleles (Cho *et al.*, 2001). It has now been shown experimentally in mice that protamines are essential for compaction of the sperm nucleus, and COMET assays have demonstrated that there is a direct correlation between the fraction of sperm with haploinsufficiency of Prm-2 and the frequency of sperm with damaged DNA (Cho *et al.*, 2003). As expected, ultrastructural analysis revealed reduced compaction of the sperm chromatin. ICSI with Prm-2-deficient sperms result in activation of most metaphase II-arrested mouse eggs, but only few were able to develop to the blastocyst stage. These findings suggest that the integrity of sperm DNA is also important for early embryonic development, which fails if there is increased sperm DNA damage. Prm-2 protein is therefore one of the crucial gene products for maintaining the integrity of sperm chromatin.

Acknowledgements

I like to thank all my friends and colleagues, especially, Martin Bergmann, Paul Burgoyne, Ann Chandley, Ilpo Huhtaniemi, Franklin Kieswetter, Martin Matzuk and Ewa Rajpert-De Meyts, who have contributed significantly with their discussions and materials to my understanding of the basic genetic aspects of the human male fertility genes presented in this chapter. I am undebted to Mrs. Christine Mahrla for her help in preparing the final version of this manuscript. Prof. Thomas Strowitzki, the director of my University department is thanked for his valuable and continuous support of my research on the human male fertility genes. My studies on the AZF locus in Yq11 are supported by grants from the Deutsche Forschungsgemeinschaft (DFG: Vo403/10-2; 11-5).

REFERENCES

Abel MH, Wootton AN, Wilkins V *et al.* (2000) The effect of a null mutation in the follicle stimulating hormone receptor gene on mouse reproduction. *Endocrinology* 141, 1795–1803.

Achermann JC, Weiss J, Lee EJ *et al.* (2001) Inherited disorders of the gonadotropin hormones. *Mol Cell Endocrinol* 179, 89–96.

Adham IM, Emmen JM and Engel W (2000) The role of the testicular factor INSL3 in establishing the gonadal position. *Mol Cell Endocrinol* 160, 11–16.

Aittomaki K (1998) FSH receptor defects and reproduction. In: *Fertility and Reproductive Medicine 1998*; eds RD Kempers, J Cohen, AF Haney and JB Younger, Amsterdam: Elsevier Science BV, pp. 761–788.

Akabas MH (2000) Cystic fibrosis transmembrane conductance regulator. Structure and function of an epithelial chloride channel. *J Biol Chem* 275, 3729–3732.

Aknin-Seifer IE, Touraine RL, Lejeune H *et al.* (2005) Is the CAG repeat of mitochondrial DNA polymerase gamma (POLG) associated with male infertility? A multi-centre French study. *Human Reprod* 20, 736–740.

Balhorn R, Reed S and Tanphaichitr N (1988) Aberrant protamine 1/protamine 2 ratios in sperm of infertile human males. *Experientia* 44, 52–55.

Bartoloni L, Blouin J-L, Pan Y *et al.* (2002) Mutations in the DNAH11 (axonemal heavy chain dynein type 11) gene cause form of situs inversus totalis and most likely primary ciliary dyskinesia. *Proc Natl Acad Sci USA* 99, 10282–10286.

Bick D, Franco B, Sherins RJ *et al.* (1992) Brief report: intragenic deletion of the KALIG-1 gene in Kallmann's syndrome. *New Engl J Med* 326, 1752–1755.

Blouin JL, Meeks M, Radhakrishna U *et al.* (2000) Primary ciliary dyskinesia: a genome-wide linkage analysis reveals extensive locus heterogeneity. *Eur J Human Genet* 8, 109–118.

Bobadilla JL, Macek Jr., M, Fine JP *et al.* (2002) Cystic fibrosis: a worldwide analysis of CFTR mutations–correlation with incidence data and application to screening. *Human Mutat* 19, 575–606.

Bukulmez O, Yucel A, Yarali H *et al.* (2001) The origin of spermatozoa does not affect intracytoplasmic sperm injection outcome. *Eur J Obstet Gynecol Reprod Biol* 94, 250–255.

Bulow HE, Berry KL, Topper LH *et al.* (2002) Heparan sulfate proteoglycan-dependent induction of axon branching and axon misrouting by the Kallmann syndrome gene kal-1. *Proc Natl Acad Sci USA* 99, 6346–6351.

Buratti E, Dork T, Zuccato E *et al.* (2001) Nuclear factor TDP-43 and SR proteins promote *in vitro* and *in vivo* CFTR exon 9 skipping. *EMBO J* 20, 1774–1784.

Burkhardt E, Adham IM, Brosig B *et al.* (1994) Structural organization of the porcine and human genes coding for a Leydig cell-specific insulin-like peptide (LEY I-L) and chromosomal localization of the human gene (INSL3). *Genomics* 20, 13–19.

Carrell DT, Emery BR and Liu L (1999) Characterization of aneuploidy rates protamine levels ultrastructure and functional ability of round-headed sperm from two siblings and implications for intracytoplasmic sperm injection. *Fertil Steril* 71, 511–516.

Carrell DT, Wilcox AL, Udoff LC *et al.* (2001) Chromosome 15 aneuploidy in the sperm and conceptus of a sibling with variable familial expression of round-headed sperm syndrome. *Fertil Steril* 7, 1258–1260.

Casella R, Maduro MR, Misfud A *et al.* (2003) Androgen receptor gene polyglutamine length is associated with testicular histology in infertile patients. *J Urol* 169, 224–227.

Chandley AC (1989) Asymmetry in chromosome pairing: a major factor in de novo mutation and the production of genetic disease in man. *J Med Genet* 26, 546–552.

Cheng J, Wang H and Guggino WB (2004) Modulation of mature cystic fibrosis transmembrane regulator protein by the PDZ domain protein CAL. *J Biol Chem* 279, 1892–1898.

Cho C, Willis WD, Goulding EH *et al.* (2001) Haploinsufficiency of protamine-1 or -2 causes infertility in mice. *Nat Genet* 28, 82–86.

Cho C, Jung-Ha H, Willis WD *et al.* (2003) Protamine-2 deficiency leads to sperm DNA damage and embryo death in mice. *Biol Reprod* 69, 211–217.

Claustres M (2005) Molecular pathology of the CFTR locus in male infertility. *Reprod BioMed Online* 10, 14–41.

Cooke HJ and Saunders PT (2002) Mouse models of male infertility. *Nat Rev Genet* 3, 790–801.

Cuppens H, Teng H, Raeymaekers P, De Boeck C and Cassiman JJ (1994) CFTR haplotype backgrounds on normal and mutant CFTR genes. *Human Mol Genet* 3, 607–614.

Cuppens H, Lin W, Jaspers M *et al.* (1998) Polyvariant mutant cystic fibrosis transmembrane conductance regulator genes. *J Clin Invest* 101, 487–496.

Dadze S, Wieland C, Jakubiczka S *et al.* (2000) The size of the CAG repeat in exon 1 of the androgen receptor gene shows no significant relationship to impaired spermatogenesis in an infertile Caucasoid sample of German origin. *Mol Human Reprod* 6, 207–214.

Daniel A (1985) Y isochromosomes and rings. In: eds AA Sandberg *The Y Chromosome, Part B: Clinical Aspects of Y Chromosome Abnormalities*. Alan R. New York: Liss, Inc., pp. 105–135.

Ditton HJ, Zimmer J, Kamp C, Rajpert-De Meyts E and Vogt PH (2004) The AZFa gene DBY (DDX3Y) is widely transcribed but the protein is limited to the male germ cells by translation control. *Human Mol Genet* 13, 2333–2341.

Dode C, Levilliers J, Dupont JM *et al.* (2003) Loss-of-function mutations in FGFR1 cause autosomal dominant Kallmann syndrome. *Nat Genet* 33, 463–465.

Dorus S, Gilbert SL, Forster ML *et al.* (2003) The CDY-related gene family: coordinated evolution in copy number, expression profile and protein sequence. *Human Mol Genet* 12, 1643–1650.

Dutcher SK (1995) Flagellar assembly in two hundred and fifty easy-to-follow steps. *Trends* 11, 389–404.

Elliott DJ, Venables JP, Newton CS *et al.* (2000) An evolutionarily conserved germ cell-specific hnRNP is encoded by a retrotransposed gene. *Human Mol Genet* 9, 2117–2124.

Ellsworth RE, Jamison DC, Touchman JW *et al.* (2000) Comparative genomic sequence analysis of the human and mouse cystic fibrosis transmembrane conductance regulator genes. *Proc Natl Acad Sci USA* 97, 1172–1177.

Estivill X. (1996) Complexity in a monogenic disease. *Nat Genet* 12, 348–350.

Ferlin A, Moro E, Rossi A *et al.* (2003) The human Y chromosome's azoospermia factor b. (AZFb) region: sequence structure and deletion analysis in infertile men. *J Med Genet* 40, 18–24.

Fernandes S, Huellen K, Goncalves J *et al.* (2002) High frequency of DAZ1/DAZ2 gene deletions in patients with severe oligozoospermia. *Mol Human Reprod* 8, 286–298.

Fernandes S, Paracchini S, Meyer LH *et al.* (2004) A large AZFc deletion removes DAZ3/DAZ4 and nearby genes from men in Y haplogroup N. *Am J Human Genet* 74, 180–187.

Fernandez-Capetillo O, Mahadevaiah K, Celeste A *et al.* (2003) H2AX is required for chromatin remodelling and inactivation of sex chromosomes in male mouse meiosis. *Dev Cell* 4, 497–508.

Florke-Gerloff S, Topfer-Petersen E, Muller-Esterl W *et al.* (1984) Biochemical and genetic investigation of round-headed spermatozoa in infertile men including two brothers and their father. *Andrologia* 16, 187–202.

Force A, Lynch M, Pickett FB *et al.* (1999) Preservation of duplicate genes by complementary, degenerate mutations. *Genetics* 151, 1531–1545.

Foresta C, Flohé L, Garolla A *et al.* (2002) Male fertility is linked to the selenoprotein phospholipid hydroperoxide glutathione peroxidase. *Biol Reprod* 67, 967–971.

Foster JW and Graves JA (1994) An SRY-related sequence on the marsupial X chromosome: implications for the evolution of the mammalian testis-determining gene. *Proc Natl Acad Sci USA* 91, 1927–1931.

Foss GL and Lewis FJ (1971) A study of four cases with Klinefelter's syndrome showing motile spermatozoa in their ejaculates. *J Reprod Fertil* 25, 401–408.

Franco B, Guioli S, Pragliola A *et al.* (1991) A gene deleted in Kallmann's syndrome shares homology with neural cell adhesion and axonal path-finding molecules. *Nature* 353, 529–536.

Fryns P, Kleczkowska A and Van den Berghe H (1985) Clinical manifestation of Y/autosome translocations in man In: ed AA Sandberg. *The Y chromosome Part B: Clinical aspects of Y chromosome abnormalities.* New York: Alan R. Liss Inc., pp. 213–243.

Gelman MS and Kopito RR (2003) Cystic fibrosis: premature degradation of mutant proteins as a molecular disease mechanism. *Method Mol Biol* 232, 27–37.

Girodon E, Cazeneuve C, Lebargy F *et al.* (1997) CFTR gene mutations in adults with disseminated bronchiectasis. *Eur J Human Genet* 5, 149–155.

Gobinet J, Poujol N and Sultan Ch (2002) Molecular action of androgens. *Mol Cell Endocrinol* 198, 15–24.

Goldberg EH (1988) H-Y antigen and sex determination. *Philos Trans R Soc B Biol Sci* 322, 73–81.

Gorlov IP, Kamat A, Bogatcheva NV *et al.* (2002) Mutations of the GREAT gene cause cryptorchidism. *Human Mol Genet* 11, 2309–2318.

Gottlieb B, Lombroso R, Beitel LK *et al.* (2005) Molecular pathology of the androgen receptor in male (in)fertility. *Reprod Biomed Online* 10, 42–48.

Haardt M, Benharouga M, Lechardeur D *et al.* (1999) C-terminal truncations destabilize the cystic fibrosis transmembrane conductance regulator without impairing its biogenesis A novel class of mutation. *J Biol Chem* 274, 21873–21877.

Habermann B, Mi HF, Edelmann A *et al.* (1998) DAZ (Deleted in AZoospermia) genes encode proteins located in human late spermatids and in sperm tails. *Human Reprod* 13, 363–369.

Hackstein JH, Hochstenbach R and Pearson PL (2000) Towards an understanding of the genetics of human male infertility: lessons from flies. *Trend Genet* 16, 565–572.

Hardelin JP (2001) Kallmann syndrome: towards molecular pathogenesis. *Mol Cell Endocrinol* 179, 75–81.

Hardelin JP, Levilliers J, del Castillo I *et al.* (1992) X chromosome-linked Kallmann syndrome: stop mutations validate the candidate gene. *Proc Natl Acad Sci USA* 89, 8190–8194.

Hefferon TW, Groman JD, Yurk CE *et al.* (2004) A variable dinucleotide repeat in the CFTR gene contributes to phenotype diversity by forming RNA secondary structures that alter splicing. *Proc Natl Acad Sci USA* 101, 3504–3509.

Heinlein AA and Chang C (2002) Androgen receptor (AR) coregulators: an overview. *Endocr Rev* 23, 175–200.

Hiort O and Holterhus P-M (2003) Androgen insensitivity and male infertility. *Int J Androl* 26, 16–20.

Holdcraft RW and Braun RE (2004) Androgen receptor function is required in Sertoli cells for the terminal differentiation of haploid spermatids. *Development* 131, 459–467.

Holsclaw DS, Perlmutter AD, Jockin H *et al.* (1971) Genital abnormalities in male patients with cystic fibrosis. *J Urol* 106, 568–574.

Hughes AL (1994) The evolution of functionally novel proteins after gene duplication. *Proc Roy Soc London B Biol Sci* 256, 119–124.

Jobling MA and Tyler-Smith C (2003) The human Y chromosome: an evolutionary marker comes of age. *Nat Rev Genet* 4, 598–612.

Kamp C, Huellen K, Fernandes S, Sousa M, Schlegel PN, Mielnik A, Kleiman S, Yavetz H, Krause W, Kupker W *et al.* (2001) High deletion frequency of the complete AZFa sequence in men with Sertoli-cell-only syndrome. *Mol Human Reprod* 7, 987–994.

Kaplan E, Shwachman H, Perlmutter AD *et al.* (1968) Reproductive failure in males with cystic fibrosis. *New Engl J Med* 279, 63–69.

Kelner MJ and Montoya MA (1998) Structural organization of the human selenium-dependent phospholipid hydroperoxide glutathione peroxidase gene (GPX4): chromosomal localization to 19p133. *Biochem Biophys Res Commun* 249, 53–55.

Kiesewetter S, Macek Jr., M, Davis C *et al.* (1993) A mutation in CFTR produces different phenotypes depending on chromosomal background. *Nat Genet* 5, 274–278.

Kim Y-S, Lee S-G, Park SH *et al.* (2001) Gene structure of the human DDX3 and chromosome mapping of its related sequences. *Mol Cells* 12, 206–214.

Kirchhoff C (1999) Gene expression in the epididymis. *Int Rev Cytol* 188, 133–202.

Kirchhoff C (2002) The dog as a model to study human epididymal function at a molecular level. *Mol Human Reprod* 8, 695–701.

Kirsch S, Keil R, Edelmann A *et al.* (1996) Molecular analysis of the genomic structure of the human Y chromosome in the euchromatic part of its long arm (Yq11). *Cytogen Cell Gene* 75, 197–206.

Kjessler B (1965) Karyotypes of 130 childless men. *Lancet* 10, 493–494.

Kleiman SE, Lagziel A, Yogev L, Botchan A, Paz G and Yavetz H (2001) Expression of *CDY1* may identify complete spermatogenesis. *Fertil Steril* 75, 166–173.

Krausz C, Forti G and McElreavey K (2003) The Y chromosome and male fertility and infertility. *Int J Androl* 26, 70–75.

Krausz C, Guarducci E, Becherini L *et al.* (2004) The clinical significance of the POLG gene polymorphism in male infertility. *J Clin Endocrinol Metab* 89, 4292–4297.

Kremer H, Mariman E, Otten BJ *et al.* (1993) Cosegregation of missense mutations of the luteinizing hormone receptor gene with familial male-limited precocious puberty. *Human Mol Genet* 2, 1779–1783.

Kumagai J, Hsu SY, Matsumi H *et al.* (2002) INSL3/Leydig insulin-like peptide activates the LGR8 receptor important in testis descent *J Biol Chem* 277, 31283–31286.

Kuroda-Kawaguchi T, Skaletzsky H, Brown LG *et al.* (2001) The AZFc region of the Y chromosome features massive palindromes and uniform recurrent deletions in infertile men. *Nat Genet* 29, 279–286.

La Spada AR, Wilson EM, Lubahn DB *et al.* (1991) Androgen receptor gene mutations in X-linked spinal and bulbar muscular atrophy. *Nature* 352, 77–79.

Lahn BT and Page DC (1997) Functional coherence of the human Y chromosome. *Science* 278, 675–679.

Lahn BT and Page DC (1999) Retroposition of autosomal mRNA yielded testis-specific gene family on human Y chromosome. *Nat Genet* 21, 429–433.

Lahn BT, Tang ZL, Zhou J et al. (2002) Previously uncharacterized histone acetyltransferases implicated in mammalian spermatogenesis. *Proc Natl Acad Sci USA* 99, 8707–8712.

Legouis R, Hardelin JP, Levilliers J et al. (1991) The candidate gene for the X-linked Kallmann syndrome encodes a protein related to adhesion molecules. *Cell* 67, 423–435.

Leroy P, Alzari P, Sassoon D et al. (1989) The protein encoded by a murine male germ cell-specific transcript is a putative ATP-dependent RNA helicase. *Cell* 57, 549–559.

Luetjens CM, Xu EY, Rejio Pera RA et al. (2004) Association of meiotic arrest with lack of BOULE protein expression in infertile men. *J Clin Endocrinol Metab* 89, 1926–1933.

McMillan DR, Christians E, Forster M et al. (2002) Heat shock transcription factor 2 is not essential for embryonic development, fertility, or adult cognitive and psychomotor function in mice. *Mol Cell Biol* 22, 8005–8014.

Machev N, Saut N, Longepied G et al. (2004) Sequence family variant loss from the AZFc interval of the human Y chromosome, but not gene copy loss, is strongly associated with male infertility. *J Med Genet* 41, 814–825.

Mahadevaiah SK, Odorisio T, Elliott DJ et al. (1998) Mouse homologues of the human AZF candidate gene RBM are expressed in spermatogonia and spermatids and map to a Y chromosome deletion interval associated with a high incidence of sperm abnormalities. *Human Mol Genet* 7, 715–727.

Mak V, Jarvi KA, Zielenski J et al. (1997) Higher proportion of intact exon 9 CFTR mRNA in nasal epithelium compared with vas deferens. *Human Mol Genet* 6, 2099–2107.

Makalowski W and Boguski MS (1998) Evolutionary parameters of the transcribed mammalian genome: an analysis of 2820 orthologous rodent and human sequences. *Proc Natl Acad Sci USA* 95, 9407–9412.

Marshall Graves JA (2000) Human Y chromosome, sex determination, and spermatogenesis – a feminist view. *Biol Reprod* 63, 667–676.

Marshall Graves JA (2002) The rise and fall of SRY. *Trends Genet* 18, 259–264.

Matzuk MM and Lamb DJ (2002) Genetic dissection of mammalian fertility pathways. *Nat Cell Biol* 4 (Suppl.) s41–49.

Mazeyrat S, Saut N, Grigoriev V et al. (2001) A Y-encoded subunit of the translation initiation factor *Eif2* is essential for mouse spermatogenesis. *Nat Genet* 29, 49–53.

Meadows L, Wang W, den Haan JM et al. (1997) The HLA-A*0201-restricted H-Y antigen contains a posttranslationally modified cysteine that significantly affects T cell recognition. *Immunity* 6, 273–281.

MHC sequencing consortium (1999) Complete sequence and gene map of a human major histocompatibility complex. *Nature* 401, 921–923.

Moore FL, Jaruzelska J, Fox MS et al. (2003) Human Pumilio-2 is expressed in embryonic stem cells and germ cells and interacts with DAZ (Deleted in AZoospermia) and DAZ-like proteins. *Proc Nat Acad Sci USA* 100, 538–543.

Moreno-Garcia M and Miranda EB (2002) Chromosomal anomalies in cryptorchidism and hypospadias. *J Urol* 168, 2170–2172.

Mroz K, Hassold TJ and Hunt PA (1999) Meiotic aneuploidy in the XXY mouse: evidence that a compromised testicular environment increases in incidence meiotic errors. *Human Reprod* 14, 1151–1156.

Murphy WJ, Sun S, Chen ZQ *et al.* (1999) Extensive conservation of sex chromosome organization between cat and human revealed by parallel radiation hybrid mapping. *Genome Res* 9, 1223–1230.

Narayan D, Krishnan SN, Upender M *et al.* (1994) Unusual inheritance of primary ciliary dyskinesia (Kartagener's syndrome). *J Med Genet* 31, 493–496.

Nef S and Parada LF (1999) Cryptorchidism in mice mutant for Insl3. *Nat Genet* 22, 295–299.

Neu RL, Matthew MS, Barlow Jr., MD *et al.* (1973) A 46,XYq-male with aspermia. *Fertil Steril* 24, 811–813.

Niksic M, Romano M, Buratti E *et al.* (1999) Functional analysis of cis-acting elements regulating the alternative splicing of human CFTR exon 9. *Human Mol Genet* 8, 2339–2349.

Oates RD and Amos JA (1994) The genetic basis of congenital bilateral absence of the vas deferens and cystic fibrosis. *J Androl* 15, 1–8.

Ohno S, Nagai Y, Ciccarese S *et al.* (1979) Testis-organizing H-Y antigen and the primary sex-determining mechanism of mammals. *Recent Prog Horm Res* 35, 449–476.

Olbrich H, Haffner K, Kispert A *et al.* (2002) Mutations in DNAH5 cause primary ciliary dyskinesia and randomization of left-right asymmetry. *Nat Genet* 30, 143–144.

O'Reilly AJ, Affara NA, Simpson E *et al.* (1992) A molecular deletion map of the Y chromosome long arm defining X and autosomal homologous regions and the localisation of the HYA locus to the proximal region of the Yq euchromatin. *Human Mol Genet* 1, 379–385.

Pasqualotto FF, Rossi-Ferragut LM, Rocha CC *et al.* (2002) Outcome of *in vitro* fertilization and intracytoplasmic injection of epididymal and testicular sperm obtained from patients with obstructive and nonobstructive azoospermia. *J Urol* 167, 1753–1756.

Patrizio P, Asch RH, Handelin B *et al.* (1993) Aetiology of congenital absence of vas deferens: genetic study of three generations. *Human Reprod* 8, 215–220.

Patrizio P, Leonard DG, Chen KL *et al.* (2001) Larger trinucleotide repeat size in the androgen receptor gene of infertile men with extremely severe oligozoospermia. *J Androl* 22, 444–448.

Quintana-Murci L, Krausz C, Heyer E *et al.* (2001) The relationship between Y chromosome DNA haplotypes and Y chromosome deletions leading to male infertility. *Human Genet* 108, 55–58.

Quinton R, Duke VM, de Zoysa PA *et al.* (1996) The neuroradiology of Kallmann's syndrome: a genotypic and phenotypic analysis. *J Clin Endocrinol Metab* 81, 3010–3017.

Rajpert-De Meyts E, Leffers H, Petersen JH *et al.* (2002) CAG repeat length in androgen-receptor gene and reproductive variables in fertile and infertile men. *Lancet* 5, 44–46.

Reijo RA, Dorfman DM, Slee R *et al.* (2000) DAZ family proteins exist throughout male germ cell development and transit from nucleus to cytoplasm at meiosis in humans and mice. *Biol Reprod* 63, 1490–1496.

Repping S, Skaletsky H, Lange J *et al.* (2002) Recombination between palindromes P5 and P1 on the human Y chromosome causes massive deletions and spermatogenic failure. *Am J Human Genet* 71, 906–922.

Repping S, Skaletsky H, Brown L *et al.* (2003) Polymorphism for a 1.6-Mb deletion of the human Y chromosome persists through balance between recurrent mutation and haploid selection. *Nat Genet* 35, 247–251.

Repping S, van Daalen SK, Korver CM *et al.* (2004) A family of human Y chromosomes has dispersed throughout northern Eurasia despite a 1.8-Mb deletion in the azoospermia factor c region. *Genomics* 83, 1046–1052.

Rovio A, Tiranti V, Bednarz AL *et al.* (1999) Analysis of the trinucleotide CAG repeat from the human mitochondrial DNA polymerase gene in healthy and diseased individuals. *Eur J Human Genet* 7, 140–146.

Rovio AT, Marchington DR, Donat S *et al.* (2001) Mutations at the mitochondrial DNA polymerase. (POLG) locus associated with male infertility. *Nat Genet* 29, 261–262.

Rozen S, Skaletsky H, Marszalek JD *et al.* (2003) Abundant gene conversion between arms of palindromes in human and ape Y chromosomes. *Nature* 423, 873–876.

Sakkas D, Urner F, Bizzaro D *et al.* (1998) Sperm nuclear DNA damage and altered chromatin structure: effect on fertilization and embryo development. *Human Reprod* 13 (Suppl. 4), 11–19.

Saxena R, de Vries JW, Repping S *et al.* (2000) Four DAZ genes in two clusters found in the AZFc region of the human Y chromosome. *Genomics* 67, 256–267.

Seboun E, Barbaux S, Bourgeron T *et al.* (1997) Gene sequence localization and evolutionary conservation of DAZLA a candidate male sterility gene. *Genomics* 41, 227–235.

Session DR, Lee GS and Wolgemuth DJ (2001) Characterization of D1Pas1, a mouse autosomal homologue of the human AZFa region DBY, as a nuclear protein in spermatogenic cells. *Fertil Steril* 76, 804–811.

Shan Z, Hirschmann P, Seebacher T *et al.* (1996) A SPGY copy homologous to the mouse gene Dazla and the Drosophila gene boule is autosomal and expressed only in the human male gonad. *Human Mol Genet* 5, 2005–2011.

Shinka T, Sato Y, Chen G *et al.* (2004) Molecular characterization of heart shock-like factor encoded on the human Y chromosome, and implications for male infertility. *Biol Reprod* 71, 297–306.

Simoni M, Nieschlag E and Gromoll J (2002) Isoforms and single nucleotide polymorphisms of the FSH receptor gene: implications for human reproduction. *Human Reprod Update* 8, 413–421.

Singh G (1992) Ultrastructural features of round-headed human spermatozoa. *Int J Fertil* 37, 99–102.

Skaletsky H, Kuroda-Kawaguchi T, Minx PJ *et al.* (2003) The male-specific region of the human Y chromosome is a mosaic of discrete sequence classes. *Nature* 423, 825–837.

Soudek D, Langmuir V and Stewart DJ (1973) Variation in the nonfluorescent segment of long Y chromosome. *Humangenetik* 18, 285–290.

Speed RM, Vogt P, Kohler MR *et al.* (1993). Chromatin condensation behaviour of the Y chromosome in the human testis I Evidence for decondensation of distal Yq in germ cells prior to puberty with a switch to Sertoli cells in adults. *Chromosoma* 102, 421–427.

Stouffs K, Lissens W, Van Landuyt L *et al.* (2001) Characterization of the genomic organization, localization and expression of four PRY genes (PRY1, PRY2, PRY3 and PRY4). *Mol Human Reprod* 7, 603–610.

Stouffs K, Lissens W, Verheyen G *et al.* (2004a) Expression pattern of the Y-linked PRY gene suggests a function in apoptosis but not in spermatogenesis. *Mol Human Reprod* 10, 15–21.

Stouffs K, Lissens W, Tournaye H *et al.* (2005) Possible role of USP26 in patients with severely impaired spermatogenesis. *Eur J Human Genet* 13, 336–340.

Suarez-Quian CA, Martinez-Garcia F, Nistal M *et al.* (1999) Androgen receptor distribution in adult human testis. *J Clin Endocrinol Metab* 84, 350–358.

Sultan C and Lumbroso S (1998) LH receptor defects. In: *Fertility and Reproductive Medicine*, eds RD Kempers, J Cohen, AF Haney and JB Younger, Amsterdam: Elsevier Science BV, pp. 769–782.

Swanson WJ and Vacquier VD (2002) The rapid evolution of reproductive proteins. *Nat Rev Genet* 3, 137–144.

Tapanainen JS, Aittomaki K, Min J *et al.* (1997) Men homozygous for an inactivating mutation of the follicle-stimulating hormone (FSH) receptor gene present variable suppression of spermatogenesis and fertility. *Nat Genet* 15, 205–206.

Teng H, Jorissen M, Van Poppel H *et al.* (1997) Increased proportion of exon 9 alternatively spliced CFTR transcripts in vas deferens compared with nasal epithelial cells. *Human Mol Genet* 6, 85–90.

Tessari A, Salata E, Ferlin A *et al.* (2004) Characterization of HSFY, a novel AZFb gene on the Y chromosome with a possible role in human spermatogenesis. *Mol Human Reprod* 10, 253–258.

Thangaraj K, Joshi MB, Reddy AG *et al.* (2002) CAG repeat expansion in the androgen receptor gene is not associated with male infertility in Indian populations. *J Androl* 23, 815–818.

Tiepolo L and Zuffardi O (1976) Localization of factors controlling spermatogenesis in the non-fluorescent portion of the human Y chromosome long arm. Localization of factors controlling spermatogenesis in the nonfluorescent portion of the human Y chromosome long arm. *Human Genet* 34, 119–124.

Tomboc M, Lee PA, Mitwally MF *et al.* (2000) Insulin-like 3/relaxin-like factor gene mutations are associated with cryptorchidism. *J Clin Endocrinol Metab* 85, 4013–4018.

Tournaye H (1999) Surgical sperm recovery for intracytoplasmatic sperm injection which method is to be preferred? *Human Reprod* 14 (Suppl. 1), 71–81.

Tournaye H, Staessen C, Liebaers I *et al.* (1996) Testicular sperm recovery in nine 47XXY Klinefelter patients. *Human Reprod* 11, 1644–1649.

Tut TG, Ghadessy FJ, Trifiro MA *et al.* (1997) Long polyglutamine tracts in the androgen receptor are associated with reduced trans-activation impaired sperm production and male infertility. *J Clin Endocrinol Metab* 82, 3777–3782.

Ubaldi F, Nagy ZP, Rienzi L *et al.* (1999) Reproductive capacity of spermatozoa from men with testicular failure. *Human Reprod* 14, 2796–2800.

Unnérus V, Fellmann J and De La Chapelle A (1967) The length of the human Y chromosome. *Cytogenet* 6, 213–227.

Ursini F, Heim S, Kiess M *et al.* (1999) Dual function of the selenoprotein PHGPx during sperm maturation. *Science* 285, 1393–1396.

Van Assche E, Bonduelle M, Tournaye H *et al.* (1996) Cytogenetics of infertile men. *Human Reprod* 11, 1–24.

Vera Y, Dai T, Hikim AP *et al.* (2002) Deleted in azoospermia associated protein 1 shuttles between nucleus and cytoplasm during normal germ cell maturation. *J Androl* 23, 622–628.

Vicari E, Perdichizzi A, De Palma A *et al.* (2002) Globozoospermia is associated with chromatin structure abnormalities: case report. *Human Reprod* 17, 2128–2133.

Viville S, Mollard R, Bach ML *et al.* (2000) Do morphological anomalies reflect chromosomal aneuploidies?: Case report. *Human Reprod* 15, 2563–2566.

Vogt PH (1997) Molecular basis of male (in)fertility. *Int J Androl* 20 (Suppl. 3), 2–10.

Vogt PH (2005a) Azoospermia factor (AZF) in Yq11: towards a molecular understanding of its function for human male fertility and spermatogenesis. *Reprod BioMed Online* 10, 81–93.

Vogt PH (2005b) AZF deletions in Y-chromosonal haplogroups: history and update based on sequence. *Hum Reprod. Update* 11, 319–336.

Vogt MH, de Paus RA, Vogt PJ *et al.* (2000a) DFFRY codes for a new human male-specific minor transplantation antigen involved in bone marrow graft rejection. *Blood* 95, 1100–1105.

Vogt MHJ, Goulmy E, Kloosterboer FM *et al.* (2000b) UTY gene codes for an HLA-B60-restricted human male-specific minor histocompatibility antigen involved in stem cell graft rejection: characterization of the critical polymorphic amino acid residues for T-cell recognition. *Blood* 96, 3126–3132.

Vogt MH, van den Muijsenberg JW, Goulmy E *et al.* (2002) The DBY gene codes for an HLA-DQ5-restricted human male-specific minor histocompatibility antigen involved in graft-versus-host disease. *Blood* 99, 3027–3032.

Vogt PH, Edelmann A, Hirschmann P *et al.* (1995) The azoospermia factor (AZF) of the human Y chromosome in Yq11: function and analysis in spermatogenesis. *Reprod Fertil Dev* 7, 685–693.

Vogt PH, Edelmann A, Kirsch S *et al.* (1996) Human Y chromosome azoospermia factors (AZF) mapped to different subregions in Yq11. *Human Mol Genet* 5, 933–943.

Vogt PH, Affara N, Davey P *et al.* (1997) Report on the third international workshop on Y chromosome mapping 1997. *Cytogen Cell Genet* 79, 1–20.

Wang PJ, McCarrey JR, Yang F *et al.* (2001) An abundance of X-linked genes expressed in spermatogonia. *Nat Genet* 27, 422–426.

Wang PJ (2004) X chromosomes, retrogenes and their role in male reproduction. *Trend Endocrinol Metab* 15, 79–83.

Wang W, Meadows LR, den Haan JM *et al.* (1995) Human H-Y: a male-specific histocompatibility antigen derived from the SMCY protein. *Science* 269, 1588–1590.

Warren EH, Gavin MA, Simpson E *et al.* (2000) The human UTY gene encodes a novel HLA-B8-restricted H-Y antigen. *J Immunol* 164, 2807–2814.

Welsh MJ and Smith AE (1993) Molecular mechanisms of CFTR chloride channel dysfunction in cystic fibrosis. *Cell* 73, 1251–1254.

Westerveld GH, Gianotten J, Leschot NJ *et al.* (2004) Heterogeneous nuclear ribonucleoprotein G-T (HNRNP G-T) mutations in men with impaired spermatogenesis. *Mol Human Reprod* 10, 265–269.

Wong EY, Tse JY, Yao KM *et al.* (2003) Identification and characterization of human VCY2-interacting protein: VCY2IP-1, a microtubule-associated protein-like protein. *Biol Reprod* 70, 775–784.

Wyckoff GJ, Wang W and Wu CI (2000) Rapid evolution of male reproduction genes in the descent of man. *Nature* 403, 304–309.

Xu X, Toselli PA, Russell LD *et al.* (1999) Globozoospermia in mice lacking the casein kinase II alpha' catalytic subunit. *Nat Genet* 23, 118–121.

Xu EY, Moore FL and Pera RA (2001) A gene family required for human germ cell development evolved from an ancient meiotic gene conserved in metazoans. *Proc Natl Acad Sci USA* 98, 7414–7419.

Xu J, Burgoyne S and Arnold AP (2002) Sex differences in sex chromosome gene expression in mouse brain. *Human Mol Genet* 11, 1409–1419.

Yao R, Ito C, Natsume Y *et al.* (2002) Lack of acrosome formation in mice lacking a Golgi protein, GOPC. *Proc Natl Acad Sci USA* 99, 11211–11216.

Yen PH (2004) Putative biological functions of the DAZ family. *Int J Androl* 27, 125–129.

Zuccato E, Buratti E, Stuani C *et al.* (2004) An intronic polypyrimidine-rich element downstream of the donor site modulates cystic fibrosis transmembrane conductance regulator exon 9 alternative splicing. *J Biol Chem* 279, 16980–16988.

Zullo SJ, Butler L, Zahorchak RJ *et al.* (1997) Localization by fluorescence *in situ* hybridization (FISH) of human mitochondrial polymerase gamma. (POLG) to human chromosome band 15q24 —>q26 and of mouse mitochondrial polymerase gamma. (Polg) to mouse chromosome band 7E with confirmation by direct sequence analysis of bacterial artificial chromosomes (BACs). *Cytogenet Cell Genet* 78, 281–284.

Sex chromosome abnormalities and male infertility: a clinical perspective

Shai Shefi and Paul J. Turek

Department of Urology, University of California San Francisco, San Francisco CA, USA

10.1 Introduction

Although abnormalities of the Y chromosome have been associated with male infertility since 1976 (Tiepolo and Zuffardi, 1976), it was only in the last decade that the Y chromosome was shown to have regions and genes that govern spermatogenesis. More recently, it has become clear that the X chromosome may be just as important as the Y chromosome in determining male fertility potential. This chapter will review our current understanding of the genotype–phenotype relationships that underlie abnormalities of both the X and Y chromosomes, and discuss recognized syndromes of the gonosomes that are known to cause male infertility.

10.2 Y chromosome

Over the last 10 years, there has been significant progress both in analyzing the molecular structure of the Y chromosome and understanding the relationship of Y chromosome mutations to infertility phenotypes. Before its firm association with male fertility, the Y chromosome was widely considered a genetic black hole, a chromosome that evolved as a broken remnant of the X chromosome. It was clear that the Y harbored the male sex-determining region (testis-determining region or *sex-determining region Y (SRY)*), but it was also home to gene regions that govern stature, tooth enamel and hairy ears as well as 'junk' gene regions. Now that the genome of the human Y is known, we realize that this chromosome is structurally unique as a fertility chromosome.

10.2.1 Azoospermia factor

The postulation that deletions in the long arm of the Y chromosome cause azoospermia was made 30 years ago (Tiepolo and Zuffardi, 1976). Based on cytogenetic analysis, this theoretical region was termed the Azoospermia Factor (AZF). Currently, the positional patterns of deletions (termed 'microdeletions') in the

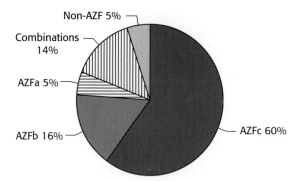

Figure 10.1   Relative frequency of specific AZF deletions in men (*n* = 5000) with Yq microdeletions (Foresta *et al.*, 2001a)

AZF region are used to subdivide this region into AZFa, AZFb, AZFc subregions (Vogt *et al.*, 1996). Regional deletions of the Y chromosome, termed Yq microdeletions occur in 6–8% of severely oligospermic men and in 3–15% of azoospermic men (Reijo *et al.*, 1996). Taken together, such deletions are the most commonly defined molecular cause of male infertility (Kostiner *et al.*, 1998). The relative frequency of individual AZF deletions among 5000 infertile men with Yq microdeletions is shown in Figure 10.1 (Foresta *et al.*, 2001a).

10.2.2 Mutations in Y chromosome genes that cause infertility

Although a handful of individual genes have been mapped to the AZF regions on Yq, very few reports define precise mutations within a gene that are associated with male infertility. The best example is a *de novo* point mutation described in an azoospermic male that included four base pairs in the Yq gene *USPY* in the AZFa region (Sun *et al.*, 1999). Another patient was found to have a deletion in the *DEAD box Y* (*DBY*) gene in the AZFa region, but the effect of the deletion on gene function was not fully analyzed (Foresta *et al.*, 2000).

10.2.3 Limitations of Y chromosome testing

Yq analysis is generally performed with polymerase chain reaction (PCR) technology on peripheral blood lymphocytes. There is wide variability among testing centers in primer number and types (sequence-tagged sites (STS)) used for analysis that often leads to incomplete descriptions of the extent and position of deletions (i.e. complete or partial deletion of region), and makes comparison of data from different centers very hard. Undoubtedly, this is hampering our ability to accurately define genotype–phenotype correlations (Ferlin *et al.*, 2004; Kleiman *et al.*, 2001). In addition, the euchromatic Yq consists of massive, nearly identical ampliconic repeats and palindromes that makes identification of AZF borders that much more difficult. Furthermore, genetic descriptions of 'microdeleted' regions of Yq do not necessarily correlate with actual deletions in specific genes, a problem that can also confound interpretation. Finally, it is also possible that some patients might be mosaic when comparing Yq deletions in leukocytes and sperm (Ferlin *et al.*, 1999). These variables pose significant barriers to a complete understanding of genotype–phenotype correlations in Yq-deleted patients. Despite these caveats, an attempt will be made to summarize currently understood genotype–phenotype correlations regarding Yq microdeletions.

10.2.4 Prognosis for AZF deletions: ejaculated sperm

There is considerable controversy regarding the prognostic value of specific AZF deletions. This is especially true regarding deletions in the AZFa and AZFb regions, as there are currently too few affected patients upon which to make unequivocal statements regarding genotype–phenotype correlations. In contrast to partial and complete AZFc deletion patients, in whom sperm can be found on semen analysis, the chance of finding ejaculated sperm in men with complete AZFa or AZFb deletions is highly unlikely (Hopps *et al.*, 2003). However, since fewer than 100 patients with isolated AZFa or AZFb deletions have been reported, more patients are needed to confirm these preliminary statements. Indeed, sperm have been detected in ejaculates of men with presumed and confirmed partial AZFa and AZFb deletions (Foresta *et al.*, 2001b). Similarly, ejaculated sperm in men with AZFa + b, and AZFb + c deletions (presumably partial deletions) has also been reported, but the finding of AZFa–c deletions has been associated with azoospermia.

10.2.5 Prognosis for AZF deletions: testis histological findings

When analyzing the testis histology associated with Yq microdeletions, it appears that several general patterns exist (Vogt *et al.*, 1996). Complete AZFa deletions are associated with germ cell aplasia or Sertoli cell-only histology (Type I). Complete AZFb deletions are generally associated with maturation arrest at the primary spermatocyte (early) or spermatid (late) stages. As might be expected, partial AZFa or AZFb deletions have a mixed testis phenotype. AZFc deletions are associated with hypospermatogenesis or a Sertoli cell-only Type II (better chance of finding foci of spermatogenesis than Type I) phenotype. Combined deletions of two or more regions that include AZFb are associated with Sertoli cell-only or maturation arrest phenotype. An important consideration for fertility treatment in these patients is the observation that there may be a time-dependent decline in sperm production in AZFc-deleted patients (Simoni *et al.*, 1997).

10.2.6 Prognosis for AZF deletions: testis sperm retrieval and intra-cytoplasmic sperm injection results

Patients with AZFc deletions carry the best prognosis for finding sperm during testicular sperm retrieval procedures performed for intra-cytoplasmic sperm injection (ICSI). Although results vary by center experience and retrieval method, approximately 50–55% of AZFc deleted men will have testis sperm available for ICSI (Hopps *et al.*, 2003; Krausz *et al.*, 1999). In patients with complete AZFa or AZFb microdeletions, a negative prognosis for sperm retrieval is the expectation, but this is based on a very limited number of cases to date (Hopps *et al.*, 2003; Krausz *et al.*, 1999). Deletions involving one or more regions that include AZFa or AZFb have met with a similar poor prognosis. The ability to find testicular sperm in patients with partial deletions of AZFa or AZFb regions is not well described. One critical variable in this analysis is the technique and expertise of the reporting center, as a sperm retrieval that involves a single or few testis biopsies may not have the same sperm 'yield' as a testicular microdissection or be as informative as a systematic fine needle aspiration 'map' in this cohort of patients (Turek *et al.*, 2000).

Four studies have assessed *in vitro* fertilization (IVF)–ICSI outcomes in men with AZF deletions (Table 10.1), presumably to assess whether such deletions may affect embryogenesis in addition to spermatogenesis. In one study, normal oocyte fertilization rates and embryo quality were poorer than contemporary, non-AZF-deleted controls (van Golde *et al.*, 2004). In the other studies, no discernable or significant differences were noted in fertilization or pregnancy rates (Choi *et al.*, 2004; Kihaile *et al.*, 2004; Oates *et al.*, 2002). However, these studies constitute small

Table 10.1. Summary of studies that address IVF-ICSI outcomes in Yq deleted couples

Author	No of patients	Yq deletions	Normal fertilization rate		Pregnancy/cycle	
			Controls (%)	AZF (%)	Controls (%)	AZF (%)
Mulhall *et al.* (1997)	3	AZFc	45 (*n* = 25 cycles)	36 (*n* = 6 cycles)	–	–
van Golde *et al.* (2004)	8	AZFc with oligozoospermia	71 (*n* = 107 patients)	55	25	16
Oates *et al.* (2002)	26	AZFc	–	47	–	27
Choi *et al.* (2004)	17	AZFb and c with azoospermia and oligozoospermia	58 (*n* = 53 patients)	49	43	33

numbers of patients and are subject to Type II statistical errors that may render it difficult to detect small but real differences in outcomes.

10.2.7 Prognosis for AZF deletions: offspring

It has been shown that men with AZF deletions who conceive with IVF–ICSI will pass on the Yq deletion to male offspring (Mulhall *et al.*, 1997, Oates *et al.*, 2002). Thus far, children conceived with an affected father are somatically healthy. However, male offspring would be expected to show similar spermatogenic deficiencies that currently exist in Yq-deleted men. Given that genetic mutations can remain stable or increase in extent as a species evolves, it is likely that male offspring of Yq-deleted men could possess a more severe phenotype than their fathers. In this scenario, a father with non-obstructive azoospermia and isolated foci of spermatogenesis and a Yq microdeletion phenotype might bear a son who is completely sterile.

Another important consideration mentioned earlier is the observation that there may be a time-dependent decline in sperm production in AZFc-deleted patients. This finding demonstrates the importance of genetic counseling, since a male offspring of an AZFc-deleted male should consider cryopreservation in early adulthood (Krausz *et al.*, 1999).

10.3 X chromosome

10.3.1 Structural abnormalities of the X chromosome associated with male infertility

Although its role as a sex-determining chromosome is well recognized, an early suggestion that the X chromosome may harbor genes controlling male fertility arose from case reports of X chromosome translocations, partial deletions and inversions that resulted in severe infertility and azoospermia (Cantu *et al.*, 1985; Lee *et al.*, 2003; Madan, 1983; Mark *et al.*, 1999; Mattei *et al.*, 1982; Nameth *et al.*, 2002) (Table 10.2). Infertility from structural abnormalities has been postulated to occur through direct interruption of a gene at breakpoint regions or as a consequence of 'position effect,' in which an uninterrupted gene does not function normally because of its changed chromosomal environment, but not necessarily due to disruption of the X-inactivation gene on Xq13 (Nemeth *et al.*, 2002). As a consequence, the X chromosome garnered suspicion as an important chromosome for the determination of male as well as female fertility.

10.3.2 Studies on the mouse X chromosome

In 2001, Wang *et al.* began a systematic search for the genes expressed exclusively in mouse spermatogonia (Wang *et al.*, 2001). Of 25 genes identified by complementary DNA (cDNA) subtraction, 3 localized to the Y chromosome, 12 to autosomes and 10 (9 novel) were found on the X chromosome. Verifying the value of the

Table 10.2. Abnormalities of the human X chromosome associated with an infertile male phenotype

Region	Genetic locus	Genes or function	Pathology	Phenotype	Reference
Xp	?	?	Deletion	Klinefelter	Mark *et al.* (1999)
Xq	Xq12–25	?	Paracentric inversion	Klinefelter	Nemeth *et al.* (2002)
Xp22	Xp22;8q11	?*TEX13A, B*	X-autosomal translocation	Azoospermia	Lee *et al.* (2003)
Xq22	Xq22;19q13.3	?*FTHL17* ?*TCTE1L*		Azoospermia	
Xq26	Xq26;3q13.2	?	X-autosomal translocation	Azoospermia	Cantu *et al.* (1985)

Note: Reports with mosaicism or Y chromosome involvement were not included in this analysis.
? = currently unknown.

Table 10.3. Human germ cell specific X-linked genes expressed in spermatogonia (10)

Mouse gene	Mouse chromosome	Human ortholog	Human chromosome	Comments
Fthl17	X	*FTHL17*	X	Ferritin, iron metabolism
Usp26	X	*USP26*	X	Ubiquitin specific protease 26
Tex11	X	*TEX11*	X	Testis expressed gene 11
Tafq2	X	*TAF2Q*	X	TBP-associated factor; RNA polymerase II
Nxf2	X	*NXF2*	X	Nuclear RNA export factor
Tex13	X	*TEX13A, 13B*	X	Testis expressed gene 13
mUtp14b	X	*UTP14*	X	Juvenile spermatogonia depletion (jsd) phenotype

cDNA subtraction, these experiments recovered the mouse homologs of 3 well-described human Y chromosome genes: *ubiquitin specific protease 9 Y* (*USP9Y*), *RNA binding motif Y-linked* (*RBMY*), and *deleted in azoospermia* (*DAZ*). The strong and quite unexpected predilection of genes solely expressed in spermatogonia to the X chromosome, indicating a 15-fold enrichment relative to chance, led the investigators to conclude that the X chromosome has a predominant role in pre-meiotic stages of mammalian spermatogenesis. Interestingly, many of the protein products of these genes were found to have a role in transcriptional or post-transcriptional regulation of gene expression. In addition, human homologues of 6 of the 9 novel mouse X chromosome genes were identified and mapped to chromosomal regions of known conserved synteny between mouse and human genomes (Table 10.3). Thus, similar to genes on the Y chromosome, it is possible

Table 10.4. Clinical studies of X-linked genes in male infertility

Human gene	Study patients	Mutations detected	Clinical phenotype	Reference
SOX3	56	3 nucleotide substitutions, no mutations	Oligozoospermia	Raverot *et al.* (2004)
FATE	144	4 polymorphisms 2 mutations (1.4%)	Random, infertile men	Olesen *et al.* (2003)

that these X chromosome genes may also prove to be sites of mutation in human spermatogenic failure.

10.3.3 Clinical studies of human X-linked genes and infertility

Few studies have examined mutations in X-linked genes in male infertility patients (Table 10.4). In a study of 56 infertile men with low or no sperm counts, Raverot *et al.* observed mutations in the *SOX3* gene (sex-determining region Y box 3) (Raverot *et al.*, 2004). The mouse homolog of this gene is found in the developing gonad and brain and, when disrupted, causes hypogonadism with loss of germ cells. Mutations in the human *fetal and adult testis-expressed* (*FATE*) gene (Xp28) have also been studied in infertile men (Olesen *et al.*, 2003). This gene encodes a polypeptide of 21 kDa that is not related to any known proteins. The *FATE* message is testis specific in fetal life soon after sex-determination and is co-expressed with *SRY* in the 7-week-old testis. Among 144 random chosen infertile men and 100 proven fertile men, a study of the *FATE* gene revealed 6 nucleotide substitutions, 4 of which were not amino acid altering, and 2 mutations. Each mutation was found only once in the experimental group, and neither was found in the controls. Neither affected patient had a karyotype abnormality nor a Y chromosome microdeletion. However, in one affected patient, a maternal uncle also carried the mutation and was fertile. The authors concluded that *FATE* gene mutations may be contributory but not necessarily common or important causes of male infertility.

There is also speculation that the *ZFX* gene in humans, a zinc finger protein located on the X chromosome that appears to be a transcriptional activator, may function in sex differentiation or spermatogenesis (Mardon and Page, 1989). To study this hypothesis, Luoh *et al.* used a reverse genetic strategy, mutagenized the mouse homolog *ZFX* and noted organismal effects that might suggest a role of this gene in reproductive development or function (Luoh *et al.*, 1997). The *ZFX* mutant had an impressive decrease in primordial germ cell number during the embryonic period before testicular differentiation. After birth, the mutant mice were smaller, had smaller testes and epididymides, and had sperm counts reduced by one half compared to wild type mice.

10.3.4 Why does the X chromosome have a role in male fertility?

It is interesting that, at least in mice, a disproportionate number of male-specific genes are located on the X chromosome. Two theories have been offered to explain this phenomenon: meiotic drive and sexually antagonistic genes (Wang *et al.*, 2001). Compared to the autosomes, the sex chromosomes are thought to be more susceptible to meiotic drive, in which there is preferential transmission of certain alleles to gametes and offspring rather than its homolog, in contradiction with Mendelian patterns. This process could skew transmission of X over Y chromosomes, perhaps driven by X-linked genes critical for spermatogenesis. Alternatively, the theory of sexually antagonistic genes, often invoked to explain why the Y chromosome is laden with spermatogenesis genes, could also be used to account for an abundance of X chromosome genes. Sexually antagonistic genes might enhance the reproductive strength in one sex and diminish it in the other and there is reason to believe that such genes might accumulate on the gonosomes. If recessive mutations existed that enhanced male reproductive fitness, they would be much more likely to have immediate benefit for males if located on the X chromosome rather than an autosome, thus increasing the chance that the allele would permeate the population. Once permeated, female 'fitness' might decrease and adaptive pressures would serve to limit the gene expression to males, thus augmenting the number of critical spermatogenesis genes on the X chromosomes (Wang *et al.*, 2001).

This scenario gets even more complicated when we consider that spermatogenesis genes also exist on autosomes. One theory presupposes that autosomal fertility genes arose as 'retrogenes' transposed from the X chromosome (Wang, 2004). Silencing of the X chromosome during male meiosis could have created a driving force for the shift of X-linked genes to autosomes to preserve expression of critical housekeeping genes required for developing germ cells during meiosis. Interestingly, it appears that many such 'retrogenes,' that lack introns in contrast with their progenitors, originated from X-linked progenitor genes and are specifically expressed in the testis (Wang, 2004). The evolution of autosomal, testis-specific retrogenes, by the compensation hypothesis, can be viewed as important in that they compensate for the transcriptionally silenced X chromosome genes that participate in spermatogenesis. Corroborating this hypothesis, several retrogenes have recently been identified that are autosomally located, testis-specific, with an origin from intron-containing X chromosome progenitor genes. The X-derived retrogene *juvenile spermatogonial depletion* (*Jsd*) is an excellent example of this phenomenon. This gene causes spermatogonial depletion in mice, which follows a single postnatal wave of spermatogenesis. The homolog retrogene in humans has been identified and is expressed only in the testis (Rohozinski and Bishop 2004). Both as 'rescue' genes that explain the widely variable phenotype observed in men with AZF deletions, or primary effectors of currently unexplained genetic infertility, X-derived retrogenes are likely important for normal human spermatogenesis.

10.4 Syndromes involving the sex chromosomes

Many well-established clinical syndromes involve abnormalities of the X or Y chromosome, generally taking the form of aneuploidy. The clinical phenotypes associated with the most common syndromes are described here.

10.4.1 Klinefelter syndrome (incidence 1 : 500)

This disorder is the most common genetic cause of azoospermia, accounting for 14% of cases. It is classically associated with a triad of findings: small, firm testes, azoospermia and gynecomastia. Other features of the syndrome are increased height, decreased intelligence, varicosities, obesity, diabetes, leukemia, increased likelihood of extragonadal germ cell tumors and breast cancer (20 $\times$ higher than normal). Most affected individuals, however, do not exhibit the classic clinical phenotype. This is an abnormality of chromosomal number in which 90% of men carry an extra X chromosome (47 XXY) and 10% are mosaic with a combination of XXY/XY chromosomes. It is thought that approximately half of XXY cases are paternally derived and recent evidence suggests that its occurrence may correlate with advanced paternal age (Lowe et al., 2001). Testis biopsies show sclerosis and hyalinization. Hormonal evaluation usually demonstrates a low testosterone and frankly elevated luteinizing hormone (LH) and follicle stimulating hormone (FSH). Natural paternity with this syndrome is possible, but almost exclusively with the mosaic (milder) form of the disease. Biological paternity in cases of non-mosaic XXY males is now possible using ICSI with sperm retrieval rates ranging from 27% to 45% in such cases (Denschlag et al., 2004; Palermo et al., 1998).

Interestingly, despite an abnormal somatic genotype, 80–100% of mature sperm from 47, XXY patients harbor a normal haploid sex chromosome complement (X or Y) (Shi and Martin, 2000, 2001; Blanco et al., 2001; Bergere et al., 2002). The lack of significant gonosomal aneuploidy in the presence of somatic aneuploidy suggests that abnormal germ cell lines may arrest at a meiotic checkpoint within the testis or that somatic–germ line mosaicism is more common than previously thought. Recent investigation into autosomal recombination events in Klinefelter testes that contain pachytene spermatocytes did not reveal any variation from normal fertile controls, suggesting that this quality control meiotic pathway remains intact in Klinefelter patients (Gonsalves et al., 2005). However, sex chromosomal recombination events have not yet been assessed in these patients.

10.4.2 XYY syndrome (1 : 1000)

An XYY chromosomal constitution can also result in infertility. Typically, men with 47, XYY are tall, may show decreased intelligence, could have a higher risk of leukemia, and may exhibit aggressive, often anti-social behavior (Palanduz *et al.*, 1998; Walzer and Gerald, 1975). Hormone evaluation reveals an elevated FSH and normal testosterone and LH. Semen analyses show either severe oligozoospermia or azoospermia. In azoospermic men, testis biopsies demonstrate maturation arrest or Sertoli cell-only syndrome.

Studies that have focused on the chromosomal complements in mature sperm from XYY men show findings similar to Klinefelter patients: very few sperm (<1%) harbor sex chromosomal disomy (YY, XX, XY) (Han *et al.*, 1994; Shi and Martin 2000; Wang *et al.*, 2000). This supports the hypothesis that the extra Y chromosome is eliminated at meiotic checkpoints during spermatogenesis.

10.4.3 Kallman syndrome (1 : 30,000)

Idiopathic hypogonadotropic hypogonadism (IHH) or Kallman syndrome is characterized by hypogonadism. Most patients experience a delay in puberty although those with less severe defects may present with only infertility. Other findings include anosmia, small testes and occasionally renal agenesis, bimanual synkinesia, cleft lip and dental agenesis. When anosmia is not present, the condition is termed IHH. Testicular biopsies display a wide range of findings from germ cell aplasia to focal areas of complete spermatogenesis (Patrizio and Broomfield, 1999). The condition is inherited as a familial disorder in one-third of cases. Both X-linked and autosomal inheritance patterns have been described (Bhasin *et al.*, 1998; Layman *et al.*, 1998). In the X-linked recessive form, deletions occur in *Kalig-1* (*kall*man-*interval* 1 or *KAL1*), a gene responsible for the migration of gonadotropin releasing hormone (GnRH) neurons to the pre-optic area of the hypothalamus during development (Bick *et al.*, 1992). The *KAL1* gene shares homology with other cell adhesion and axonal pathfinding molecules, further supporting the notion that a molecular defect in the gene causes the neuronal migration defect. The KAL protein is a secreted, diffusible molecule that easily incorporates into the extracellular matrix and is termed anosmin-1. Once incorporated into the extracellular matrix of the olfactory bulb, the KAL protein might promote the migration and target recognition of olfactory axons. As a consequence of mutations in this gene, there is failure of testicular stimulation by the anterior pituitary and hypothalamus and thus testis failure. Mutations in other genes have also been associated with the development of IHH including *double-dose associated sex-reversal* (*DAX1*) on the X chromosome (associated with congenital adrenal hyperplasia) (Guo *et al.*, 1995), the GnRH receptor (Layman *et al.*, 1998) and *phosphatidylcholine* (*PC1*) (associated with diabetes and obesity) (Jackson *et al.*, 1997). In addition to the X-linked form,

Table 10.5. Recognized forms of Kallman syndrome

Descriptor	Inheritance	Gene identified
KAL1	X-linked	KALIG-1 (Xp22.3)
KAL2	Autosomal dominant	FGFR1 (8p11–12)
KAL3	Autosomal recessive	None

autosomal dominant (*KAL2*) and recessive (*KAL3*) transmission of Kallman syndrome has also been reported (Dode *et al.*, 2003; Oliveira *et al.*, 2001) (Table 10.5).

Phenotypically, Kallman patients with documented *KAL1* mutations have apulsatile LH secretion, indicating complete lack of neuronal migration. In contrast, men with autosomal inheritance are more variably affected, generally with weakened but present LHRH-induced LH pulses. Although mental or intellectual disturbance was described in the original report of Kallman syndrome, more current analyses show that Kallman syndrome patients with mental disorders have large deletions on Xp that extend well beyond the *KAL1* locus. Infertility can be treated with gonadotropin (LH and FSH) replacement over 12–18 months, which stimulates spermatogenesis and the presence of sperm in the ejaculate in 80% of men (Buchter *et al.*, 1998). The clinical diagnosis of Kallman syndrome is confirmed by blood tests revealing a low total testosterone associated with low LH and low FSH levels in combination with normal prolactin.

10.4.4 XX male syndrome (1 : 20,000)

This structural and numerical chromosomal condition presents as either a male with gynecomastia at puberty or with azoospermia (Schweikert *et al.*, 1982). Typically, there are normal male external and internal genitalia. Hormone evaluation reveals elevated FSH and LH and low or normal testosterone. Testis biopsy demonstrates an absence of spermatogenesis with hyalinization, fibrosis and clumps of Leydig cells. The most obvious explanation for the disease is that *SRY* is translocated from the Y to the X chromosome so that testis differentiation is present. However, the AZF regions on the Y chromosome are not similarly translocated, resulting in azoospermia. This mechanism has been suggested because of the high degree of homology (98.7%) that exists between the short arm of the X and Y chromosomes (van der Auwera *et al.*, 1992).

10.4.5 Mixed gonadal dysgenesis (rare)

This heterogeneous condition is characterized by male or females with a unilateral testis on one side and a streak gonad on the opposite side. Genotypically, patients are usually 46, XY/45, X/46, XY, both of which are associated with impaired gonadal development. Interestingly, mutations in the *SRY* gene have not been detected in most patients (80% have normal *SRY*), suggesting that the gonadal dysgenesis may be due to cytogenetic mosaicism or to mutations in testis-organizing genes downstream from *SRY*. Suspect genes include the upstream *Wilms tumor suppressor gene (WT1)* and the downstream *DAX1* gene. Another gene may include the testatin gene (20p11.2), a putative cathepsin inhibitor that is expressed very early in testis development, just after *SRY* expression. Affected patients may present with ambiguous external genitalia, but the vast majority will have intra-abdominal testes. Scrotal testes may be associated with inguinal hernias and almost uniformly reveal seminiferous tubules with Sertoli cells only and normal Leydig cells (Wegner *et al.*, 1994). The dysgenetic gonad is predisposed to malignant degeneration (25% incidence) to gonadoblastoma or dysgerminoma, typically before puberty.

10.4.6 *SRY* Gene Defects (rare)

Located on the short arm of the Y chromosome (Yp11.3) is the *SRY* gene, important for determining 'maleness' (Berta *et al.*, 1990). Both 46XX *SRY* (+) males and 46XY *SRY* (−) females have been described in the literature and constitute a rare form of phenotypic sex reversal (Jager *et al.*, 1990; Mittwoch 1992). The *SRY* gene encodes a protein that harbors a high-mobility group box (HMG) sequence, a highly conserved DNA-binding motif that helps kink DNA (Sinclair *et al.*, 1990). This DNA-bending effect may alter the ability of target genes to be transcribed.

Interestingly, *SRY* mutations are not always detected in 46, XY phenotypic females, suggesting that genes other than *SRY* and in locations other than on the Y chromosome are important for complete male gonadal differentiation. Indeed, a locus termed dosage sensitive sex reversal (DSS) has been identified on Xp21 that may contain a Wolffian inhibitory gene to suppress male differentiation. Within this locus it is known that the 'anti-testis gene' *DAX1* (Xp21.3–p21.1), a member of the nuclear hormone receptor family, can alter *SRY* activity during development by suppressing downstream genes that induce testis differentiation (Fig. 10.2). *DAX1* over-expression may account for some X-linked cases of 46, XY female phenotype because of direct inhibition of *SRY* activity, or indirectly through affecting the ability of *SRY* to upregulate *SOX9* and *anti-Mullerian hormone (AMH)* gene expression (Yu *et al.*, 1998). Another gene, largely confined to the adult ovary, may serve as an anti-testis gene during male development. A *wingless-type MMTV integration site 4 (WNT4)* (1p34) deletion has been associated with XY female sex reversal in a patient with 1p31–35 duplication (Hughes, 2002). In the male, *SRY* defects are generally detected by cytogenetic analysis showing a shortened or absent Y chromosome. Analysis with fluorescence *in situ* hybridization (FISH) can locate the *SRY* gene within the existing chromosomal complement. With mutations or

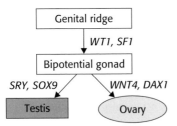

Figure 10.2   Putative genes involved with male sex differentiation

translocations of *SRY*, genes on Yq that control spermatogenesis are also usually affected resulting in infertility.

10.4.7 Androgen receptor gene mutations (1 : 60,000)

In this condition, the androgen receptor (AR) is absent or functionally altered such that testosterone or its more bioactive derivative, dihydrotestosterone, cannot activate target genes. Thus, androgens have little to no effect on tissues; as such the development of both internal and external genitalia are affected. Depending on the severity of the AR defect, serum testosterone levels can be low, normal or high. The androgen balance in each individual depends on the functional integrity of AR within the pituitary and hypothalamus. The clinical picture of infertility is also variable (nomenclature includes Reifenstein, Lub and Rosewater syndromes) and ranges from apparent females with testes (complete androgen insensitivity) to normal but infertile males (Shkolny *et al.*, 1999).

Over 300 distinct (mainly point) mutations and have been found in the AR, a large steroid receptor gene on the X chromosome (Xq11–q12) (Bhasin *et al.*, 1998). Given the widely variable phenotype and numerous mutations noted in the AR gene, it has been proposed that as many as 40% of men with low or no sperm counts may have subtle AR abnormalities as an underlying cause (Aiman *et al.*, 1979). It is not clear whether the infertility in the milder forms of this disorder is truly treatable despite a case report of success with exogenous testosterone supplementation (Yong *et al.*, 1994).

10.4.8 Kennedy disease (rare)

This disorder, also termed spinal and bulbar muscular atrophy, is a debilitating, neurodegenerative condition that begins by age 30 and consists of muscle cramping and atrophy as well as testicular atrophy. The genetic basis for the disease is not exactly a mutation but a variation in the length of the AR gene in a specific region (transcriptional activation domain) that results in decreased androgen-binding ability. The AR gene on Xq has eight exons and it is clear that a critical region of CAG-nucleotide repeats, usually 15–30 in number, exists in exon 1. Elongation of

the number of CAG repeats in this region to more than 50 generally results in clinically apparent disease (Kupker *et al.*, 1999). The clinical infertility resembles that
due to mild androgen insensitivity and may include gynecomastia in addition to
testis atrophy. Interestingly, some affected patients may have only mild oligozoospermia and as such may be able to conceive naturally or with ICSI. Men, fertile at an early age, may actually experience a significant reduction in their sperm
counts with advancing age and disease progression. Importantly, affected couples
should be counseled about the phenomenon of genetic 'anticipation' that occurs
with this disorder, in which offspring may inherent an even larger number of CAG-
nucleotide repeats than that of the parent. Clinically, this translates into a more
severe disease phenotype that is manifest earlier in life. Specialized laboratories
offer exon 1 CAG-nucleotide repeat analysis of the AR gene.

10.4.9 Persistent Mullerian duct syndrome (rare)

This disorder involves altered male sexual differentiation with an abnormal persistence of Mullerian duct structures. It is a familial X-linked or an autosomal
dominant condition in which there is absence or impaired action of AMH (AMH,
Mullerian inhibiting substance, testis-secreted H-Y antigen, maps to 19p13.3)
during development (Cohen-Haguenauer *et al.*, 1987). This disorder can be caused
by either: (a) failure of Sertoli cells to elaborate AMH, (b) failure of end-organ
response to AMH (AMH receptor, mapped to 12q13) or (c) defects in the timing
of AMH release (Imbeaud *et al.*, 1994, 1995).

Affected males have normal male external and internal genitalia, but also a
fully developed uterus and fallopian tubes as a result of incomplete involution
of Mullerian derivatives. Persistent Mullerian duct syndrome presents clinically
as a hernia that contains a uterus and fallopian tubes (hernia uteri inguinalis)
or cryptorchidism. Cryptorchidism may be secondary to the tethering of the testes
to the Mullerian structure and inhibition of normal descent. During hernia
repair, all efforts should be made to preserve the integrity of the vas deferens and
epididymis. The fertility and cancer risk of cryptorchid patients with this syndrome is similar to other cryptorchid individuals. Patients with scrotal testes can
be fertile.

10.5 Conclusions

The human sex chromosomes play a significant role in sex determination and
reproductive function. Our knowledge of the relationship between Y chromosome
genetics and various infertility phenotypes is well known and advancing rapidly.
However, equally impressive and promising is discovering the potential that the
X chromosome has in controlling genetic male infertility.

REFERENCES

Aiman J, Griffin JE, Gazak JM *et al.* (1979) Androgen insensitivity as a cause of infertility in otherwise normal men. *New Engl J Med* 300, 223–227.

Bergere M, Wainer R, Nataf V *et al.* (2002) Biopsied testis cells of four 47, XXY patients: fluorescence *in-situ* hybridization and ICSI results. *Human Reprod* 17, 32–37.

Berta P, Hawkins JR, Sinclair AH *et al.* (1990) Genetic evidence equating SRY and the testis-determining factor. *Nature* 348, 448–450.

Bhasin S, Ma K, Sinha I *et al.* (1998) The genetic basis of male infertility. *Endocrinol Metab Clin North Am* 27, 783–805.

Bick D, Franco B, Sherins RJ *et al.* (1992) Brief report: intragenic deletion of the Kalig-1 gene in Kallmann's syndrome. *N Engl J Med* 326, 1752–1755.

Blanco J, Egozcue J and Vidal F (2001) Meiotic behaviour of the sex chromosomes in three patients with sex chromosome anomalies (47, XXY, mosaic 46, XY/47, XXY and 47, XYY) assessed by fluorescence *in-situ* hybrization. *Human Reprod* 16, 887–892.

Buchter D, Behre HM, Kliesch S *et al.* (1998) Pulsatile GnRH or human chorionic gonadotropin/human menopausal gonadotropin as effective treatment for men with hypogonadotropic hypogonadism: a review of 42 cases. *Eur J Endocrinol* 139, 298–303.

Cantu JM, Diaz M, Moller M *et al.* (1985) Azoospermia and duplication 3qter as distinct consequences of a familial t(X;3)(q26;q13.2). *Am J Med Genet* 20, 677–684.

Choi JM, Chung P, Veeck L *et al.* (2004) AZF microdeletions of the Y chromosome and *in vitro* fertilization outcome. *Fertil Steril* 81, 337–341.

Cohen-Haguenauer O, Picard JY, Mattei MG *et al.* (1987) Mapping of the gene for anti-mullerian hormone to the short arm of human chromosome 19. *Cytogenet Cell Genet* 44, 2–6.

Denschlag D, Tempfer C, Kunze M *et al.* (2004) Assisted reproductive techniques in patients with Klinefelter syndrome: a critical review. *Fertil Steril* 82, 775–779.

Dode C, Levilliers J, Dupont JM *et al.* (2003) Loss-of-function mutations in FGFR1 cause autosomal dominant Kallmann syndrome. *Nat Genet* 33, 463–465.

Ferlin A, Moro E, Onisto M *et al.* (1999) Absence of testicular DAZ gene expression in idiopathic severe testiculopathies. *Human Reprod* 14, 2286–2292.

Foresta C, Ferlin A and Moro E (2000) Deletion and expression analysis of AZFa genes on the human Y chromosome revealed a major role for DBY in male infertility. *Human Mol Genet* 9, 1161–1169.

Foresta C, Moro E and Ferlin A (2001a) Y chromosome microdeletions and alterations of spermatogenesis. *Endocr Rev* 22, 226–239.

Foresta C, Moro E and Ferlin A (2001b) Prognostic value of Y deletion analysis. The role of current methods. *Human Reprod* 16, 1543–1547.

Gonsalves J, Turek PJ, Schlegel PN, Hopps CV and Reijo Pera RA (2005) Recombination in men with Klinefelter Syndrome. *Reproduction* 130, 223–229.

Guo W, Burris TP and McCabe ER (1995) Expression of DAX-1, the gene responsible for X-linked adrenal hypoplasia congenita and hypogonadotropic hypongonadism, in the hypothalamic-pituitary-adrenal/gonadal axis. *Biochem Mol Med* 56, 8–13.

Han TH, Ford JH, Flaherty SP *et al.* (1994) A fluorescent *in situ* hybridization analysis of the chromosomal constitution of ejaculated sperm in a 47, XYY male. *Clin Genet* 45, 67–70.

Hopps CV, Mielnik A, Goldstein M *et al.* (2003) Detection of sperm in men with Y chromosome microdeletions of the AZFa, AZFb and AZFc regions. *Human Reprod* 18, 1660–1665.

Imbeaud S, Carre-Eusebe D, Rey R *et al.* (1994) Molecular genetics of the persistent Mullerian duct syndrome: a study of 19 families. *Human Mol Genet* 3, 125–131.

Imbeaud S, Faure E, Lamarre I *et al.* (1995) Insensitivity to anti-Mullerian hormone due to a mutation in the human anti-Mullerian hormone receptor. *Nat Genet* 11, 382–388.

Jackson RS, Creemers JW, Ohagi S *et al.* (1997) Obesity and impaired prohormone processing associated with mutations in the human prohormone convertase 1 gene. *Nat Genet* 16, 303–306.

Jager RJ, Anvret M, Hall K *et al.* (1990) A human XY female with a frame shift mutation in the candidate testis-determining gene SRY. *Nature* 348, 452–454.

Kihaile PE, Kisanga RE, Aoki K *et al.* (2004) Embryo outcome in Y-chromosome microdeleted infertile males after ICSI. *Mol Reprod Dev* 68, 176–181.

Kleiman SE, Bar-Shira Maymon B, Yogev L *et al.* (2001) The prognostic role of the extent of Y microdeletion on spermatogenesis and maturity of Sertoli cells. *Human Reprod* 16, 399–402.

Kostiner DR, Turek PJ and Reijo RA (1998) Male infertility: analysis of the markers and genes on the human Y chromosome. *Human Reprod* 13, 3032–3038.

Krausz C, Bussani-Mastellone C, Granchi S *et al.* (1999) Screening for microdeletions of Y chromosome genes in patients undergoing intracytoplasmic sperm injection. *Human Reprod* 14, 1717–1721.

Kupker W, Schwinger E, Hiort O *et al.* (1999) Genetics of male subfertility: consequences for the clinical work-up. *Human Reprod* 14 (Suppl 1), 24–37.

Layman LC, Cohen DP, Jin M *et al.* (1998) Mutations in gonadotropin-releasing hormone receptor gene cause hypogonadotropic hypogonadism (letter). *Nat Genet* 18, 14–15.

Lee S, Lee SH, Chung TG *et al.* (2003) Molecular and cytogenetic characterization of two azoospermic patients with X-autosome translocation. *J Assist Reprod Genet* 20, 385–389.

Lowe X, Eskanazi B, Nelson DO *et al.* (2001) Frequency of XY sperm increases with age in fathers of boys with Klinefelter syndrome. *Am J Human Genet* 69, 1046–1054.

Luoh SW, Bain PA, Polakiewicz RD *et al.* (1997) Zfx mutation results in small animal size and reduced germ cell number in male and female mice. *Development* 124, 2275–2284.

Madan K (1983) Balanced structural changes involving the human X: effect on sexual phenotype. *Human Genet* 63, 216–221.

Mardon G and Page DC (1989) The sex-determining region of the mouse Y chromosome encodes a protein with a highly acidic domain and 13 zinc fingers. *Cell* 56, 765–770.

Mark HF, Feldman D and Sigman M (1999) Conventional and molecular cytogenetic identification of a variant klinefelter syndrome patient with a deleted X chromosome. *Pathobiology* 67, 55–58.

Mattei MG, Mattei JF, Ayme S *et al.* (1982) X-autosome translocations: cytogenetic characteristics and their consequences. *Human Genet* 61, 295–309.

Mittwoch U (1992) Sex determination and sex reversal: genotype, phenotype, dogma and semantics. *Human Genet* 89, 467–479.

Mulhall JP, Reijo R, Alagappan R *et al.* (1997) Azoospermic men with deletion of the DAZ gene cluster are capable of completing spermatogenesis: fertilization, normal embryonic development and pregnancy occur when retrieved testicular spermatozoa are used for intracytoplasmic sperm injection. *Human Reprod* 12, 503–508.

Nemeth AH, Gallen IW, Crocker M *et al.* (2002) Klinefelter-like phenotype and primary infertility in a male with a paracentric Xq inversion. *J Med Genet* 39, E28.

Oates RD, Silber S, Brown LG *et al.* (2002) Clinical characterization of 42 oligospermic or azoospermic men with microdeletion of the AZFc region of the Y chromosome, and of 18 children conceived via ICSI. *Human Reprod* 17, 2813–2824.

Olesen C, Silber J, Eiberg H *et al.* (2003) Mutational analysis of the human FATE gene in 144 infertile men. *Human Genet* 113, 195–201.

Oliveira LM, Seminara SB, Beranova M *et al.* (2001) The importance of autosomal genes in Kallmann syndrome: genotype–phenotype correlations and neuroendocrine characteristics. *J Clin Endocrinol Metab* 86, 1532–1538.

Palanduz S, Aktan M, Ozturk S *et al.* (1998) 47, XYY karyotype in acute myeloid leukemia. *Cancer Genet Cytogenet* 106, 76–77.

Palermo GD, Schlegel PN, Sills ES *et al.* (1998) Births after intracytoplasmic injection of sperm obtained by testicular extraction from men with non-mosaic Klinefelter's syndrome. *New Engl J Med* 338, 588–590.

Patrizio P and Broomfield D (1999) The genetic basis of male infertility. In: Male Fertility and Infertility, eds TD Glover and CLR Barratt. Cambridge, UK: Cambridge University Press, pp. 162–179.

Raverot G, Lejeune H, Kotlar T *et al.* (2004) X-linked sex-determining region Y box 3 (SOX3) gene mutations are uncommon in men with idiopathic oligoazoospermic infertility. *J Clin Endocrinol Metab* 89, 4146–4148.

Reijo R, Alagappan RK, Patrizio P *et al.* (1996) Severe oligozoospermia resulting from deletions of azoospermia factor gene on Y chromosome. *Lancet* 347, 1290–1293.

Rohozinski J and Bishop CE (2004) The mouse juvenile spermatogonial depletion (jsd) phenotype is due to a mutation in the X-derived retrogene, mUtp14b. *Proc Natl Acad Sci USA* 101, 11695–11700.

Schweikert HU, Weissbach L, Leyendecker G *et al.* (1982) Clinical, endocrinological, and cytological characterization of two 46, XX males. *J Clin Endocrinol Metab* 54, 745–752.

Shi Q and Martin RH (2000) Multicolor fluorescence *in situ* hybridization analysis of meiotic chromosome segregation in a 47, XYY male and a review of the literature. *Am J Med Genet* 93, 40–46.

Shi Q and Martin RH (2001) Aneuploidy in human spermatozoa: FISH analysis in men with constitutional chromosomal abnormalities, and in infertile men. *Reproduction* 121, 655–666.

Sinclair AH, Berta P, Palmer MS *et al.* (1990) A gene from the human sex-determining region encodes a protein with homology to a conserved DNA-binding motif. *Nature* 346, 240–242.

Shkolny DL, Beitel LK, Ginsberg J *et al.* (1999) Discordant measures of androgen-binding kinetics in two mutant androgen receptors causing mild or partial androgen insensitivity, respectively. *J Clin Endocrinol Metab* 84, 805–810.

Simoni M, Gromoll J, Dworniczak B *et al.* (1997) Screening for deletions of the Y chromosome involving the DAZ (Deleted in Azoospermia) gene in azoospermia and severe oligospermia. *Fertil Steril* 67, 542–547.

Sun C, Skaletsky H, Birren B *et al.* (1999) An azoospermic man with a *de novo* point mutation in the Y-chromosomal gene USP9Y. *Nat Genet* 23, 429–432.

Tiepolo L and Zuffardi O (1976) Localization of factors controlling spermatogenesis in the non-fluorescent portion of the human Y chromosome long arm. *Human Genet* 34, 119–124.

Turek PJ, Cha I, Ljung B-M and Conaghan J (2000) Diagnostic findings from testis fine needle aspiration mapping in obstructed and non-obstructed azoospermic men. *J Urol* 163, 1709–1716.

van Golde RJ, van der Avoort IA, Tuerlings JH *et al.* (2004) Phenotypic characteristics of male subfertility and its familial occurrence. *J Androl* 25, 819–823.

Van der Auwera B, Van Roy N, De Paepe A *et al.* (1992) Molecular cytogenetic analysis of XX males using Y-specific DNA sequences, including SRY. *Human Genet* 89, 23–28.

Vogt PH, Edelmann A, Kirsch S *et al.* (1996) Human Y chromosome azoospermia factors (AZF) mapped to different subregions in Yq11. *Human Mol Genet* 5, 933–943.

Walzer S and Gerald PS (1975) Social class and frequency of XYY and XXY. *Science* 190, 1228–1229.

Wang JY, Samura O, Zhen DK *et al.* (2000) Fluorescence *in-situ* hybridization analysis of chromosomal constitution in spermatozoa from a mosaic 47, XYY/46, XY male. *Mol Human Reprod* 6, 665–668.

Wang PJ (2004) X chromosomes, retrogenes and their role in male reproduction. *Trends Endocrinol Metab* 15, 79–83.

Wang PJ, McCarrey JR, Yang F *et al.* (2001) An abundance of X-linked genes expressed in spermatogonia. *Nat Genet* 27, 422–426.

Wegner HE, Ferszt AN, Wegner AD *et al.* (1994) Mixed gonadal dysgenesis: a rare cause of primary infertility. Report of two cases and a review of the literature. *Urologe* 33, 342–346.

Yong EL, Ng SC, Roy AC, Yun G and Ratnam SS (1994) Pregnancy after hormonal correction of severe spermatogenic defect due to mutation in androgen receptor gene. *Lancet* 344, 826–827.

Young D (1970) Surgical treatment of male infertility. *J Reprod Fertil* (Abst) 23, 541.

Yu RN, Masafumi I, Saunders TL *et al.* (1998) Role of Ahch in gonadal development and gametogenesis. *Nat Genet* 20, 353–357.

11

Epigenetic patterning in male germ cells: importance of DNA methylation to progeny outcome

Sophie La Salle[1] and Jacquetta M. Trasler[1,2,3]

[1] Departments of Pharmacology and Therapeutics, [2] Pediatrics and [3] Human Genetics, McGill University and the Montreal Children's Hospital Research Institute, Montreal, QC, Canada

Epigenetics refers to non-sequence based mechanisms that control gene expression and has been described as the next 'frontier' in genetics. This chapter focuses on DNA methylation, one of the best-characterized DNA modifications associated with the modulation of gene activity. In humans, DNA methylation abnormalities have been linked to infertility, imprinting disorders in children and cancer. Recent studies have suggested that assisted reproductive technologies (ARTs) may be associated with an increased incidence of epigenetic defects in children and it is unclear whether the etiology is related to infertility with an underlying epigenetic cause or the specific techniques used. Gametes may be particularly vulnerable to epigenetic defects since genome-wide epigenetic methylation patterns are first initiated in the male and female germ lines; the acquisition of gametic methylation patterns is subsequently essential for normal embryonic development. Here, recent progress in our understanding of when and how methylation patterns are established in the male germ line, as well as the enzymes involved in this process, will be discussed. We will also review the factors involved in modulating DNA methylation and the disorders associated with DNA methylation abnormalities in the germ line. Although we will emphasize human studies where they exist, mouse studies will be included since much of our understanding of DNA methylation pattern establishment and propagation comes from studies done in mice.

11.1 Epigenetics and gene expression

Epigenetic alterations lead to heritable changes in gene expression without altering the underlying DNA sequence. To date three main mechanisms, RNA-associated silencing, histone modifications and DNA methylation, have been associated with epigenetic silencing of gene expression. Recent advances made in our understanding of the relationships between these systems have illustrated how they interact and stabilize each other, emphasizing how disrupting one or more of these interacting systems could lead to inappropriate expression or silencing of genes, resulting in 'epigenetic diseases'. Imprinting diseases, molar pregnancies and childhood cancers are some of the human disorders associated with epigenetic abnormalities.

Post-translational modification of histone tails, including acetylation, phosphorylation and methylation of specific amino acid residues, are associated with changes in transcriptional competence (Geiman and Robertson, 2002; Rice and Allis, 2001). Heterochromatic silencing is also mediated by antisense transcripts, non-coding RNAs and RNA interference (Lippman and Martienssen, 2004; Panning and Jaenisch, 1998; Rougeulle and Heard, 2002). Links between histone modifications and DNA methylation have been established in mammals (Lehnertz et al., 2003) and more recently, between DNA methylation and RNA interference in human cells (Kawasaki and Taira, 2004; Morris et al., 2004). Conservation of epigenetic mechanisms across higher eukaryotes, including humans, suggests they act in concert to regulate higher order chromatin and, ultimately, genome integrity (Grewal and Moazed, 2003).

The best-characterized modification of DNA associated with modulation of gene expression is methylation of cytosine residues by DNA methyltransferases (DNMTs); it takes place at approximately 30 million CpG sites throughout the genome following DNA replication and is both reversible and heritable (Bestor and Tycko, 1996). Unmethylated CpGs are found in CpG islands, short sequences relatively rich in G + C (>55%) and associated with the promoter region of genes (Goll and Bestor, 2004). DNA methylation is commonly associated with transcriptional repression as well as genome organization and stabilization, and more specifically with a number of specialized biochemical processes, such as allele-specific gene expression (genomic imprinting), X-chromosome inactivation and heritable transcriptional silencing of parasitic sequence elements (Goll and Bestor, 2004). Several mechanisms are associated with the regulation of gene expression through DNA methylation. Accessibility of target sequences can be directly blocked by cytosine methylation, preventing binding of transcription regulatory factors. Gene expression can also be repressed through several methyl-CpG-binding proteins that recognize and 'read' methylation patterns. For instance, transcription can be repressed in a methylation-dependent manner via formation of a complex between the methyl-binding protein MeCP2, histone deacetylases (HDACs) and a co-repressor protein, Sin3a (Jones et al., 1998; Nan et al., 1998). MBD2, another methyl-CpG-binding protein, forms a complex with NuRD, a multi-subunit complex containing an ATP-dependent chromatin-remodeling protein, Mi-2, and HDACs (Wade et al., 1999; Zhang et al., 1999); the MBD2–NuRD complex, formerly known as MeCP1, represses transcription and remodels methylated chromatin with high efficiency (Feng and Zhang, 2001; Ng *et al.*, 1999). Finally, DNMTs have also been shown to directly interact with HDACs and are able to repress transcription through this association (reviewed by Burgers *et al.*, 2002).

Genomic methylation patterns are initially acquired during gametogenesis in a sex- and sequence-specific manner and are further consolidated following birth (Bestor, 2000; Reik *et al.*, 2001). Early studies identified the sperm genome as being more highly methylated than that of the oocyte (Monk *et al.*, 1987; Sanford *et al.*, 1987); more recent work has begun to determine the precise mechanisms governing differential methylation of the paternal and maternal genomes. The most striking modulations in methylation are observed for imprinted genes and repetitive sequence elements (Bestor, 2000; Reik *et al.*, 2001). Imprinted genes are expressed exclusively from one of the parental alleles and DNA methylation is the best-studied epigenetic mark known to distinguish the maternal and paternal alleles. In many cases, imprinted genes have been shown to contain sequences that are differentially methylated between gametes, with the two parental alleles showing different levels of methylation constrained within an area called a differentially methylated domain (DMD) (Spahn and Barlow, 2003; Tycko and Morison, 2002). Stable propagation of DNA methylation patterns after DNA replication ensures maintenance of monoallelic gene expression throughout life. The majority of CpGs in the genome are found in repetitive DNA sequences such as endogenous retroviruses (like intracisternal A particles or IAPs), long interspersed nuclear elements (LINEs) and satellite sequences (O'Neill *et al.*, 1998; Smit, 1996; Viegas-Pequignot and Dutrillaux, 1976; Xu *et al.*, 1999; Yoder *et al.*, 1997). It has been proposed that retrotransposons are maintained in a predominantly methylated state to prevent their random retrotransposition and protect the integrity of the genome.

Over the last decade, technical progress has permitted a more precise assessment of the developmental timing of methylation pattern acquisition in the germ line and the embryo. Purified populations of prenatal germ cells can be isolated by means of germ cell surface or green fluorescent protein (GFP) markers (Davis *et al.*, 2000; Hajkova *et al.*, 2002; Lane *et al.*, 2003; Szabo *et al.*, 2002; Yamazaki *et al.*, 2003). Several techniques (reviewed in Oakeley, 1999; Shiraishi *et al.*, 2002) are available to assess DNA methylation at an overall genomic level (e.g. thin layer chromatography or 5-methyl cytosine antibody staining), at CpG islands (e.g. restriction landmark genomic scanning), or at specific sequences (e.g. methylation-sensitive restriction enzyme digestion followed by Southern blotting or polymerase chain reaction, PCR). A significant advance has been the introduction of bisulfite genomic sequencing, a sensitive method for the detection of methylated cytosine residues in any gene, in small numbers of cells and on individual maternal and paternal alleles (Clark *et al.*, 1994; Frommer *et al.*, 1992).

11.2 Genomic methylation reprogramming in the germ line: dynamics and timing

Experimental evidence in mice suggests that genomic methylation patterns inherited from the parental gametes are erased upon entry into the reproductive cycle, reestablished in immature germ cells according to their fate as either male or female gametes and further consolidated and maintained during early embryonic development, giving rise to methylation profiles that will be preserved throughout adulthood (Fig. 11.1, Color plate 9).

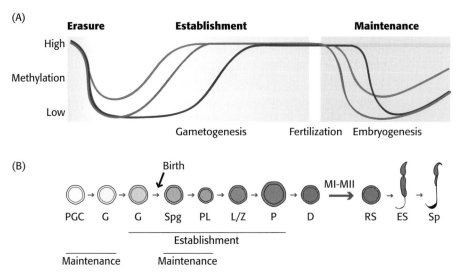

Figure 11.1 Methylation dynamics during germ cell and preimplantation embryo development.
(A) Methylation dynamics of maternal (red) and paternal (blue) genomes. During
gametogenesis, non-imprinted genes acquire their methylation similarly to imprinted
genes, however, after fertilization, both the maternal and paternal genomes become
demethylated while imprinted genes retain their methylation status, as shown by the
paler red and blue lines. Some repeat sequences (dark gray) appear to escape complete
demethylation during gametogenesis and retain a high proportion of their initial
methylation marking during preimplantation development. Methylation levels are not to
scale. (B) Progression of genomic methylation pattern acquisition during male germ cell
development, as represented by the intensity of the blue shading. *De novo* and
maintenance methylation events are indicated under the appropriate germ cell types.
PGC: primordial germ cell; G: gonocyte; Spg: spermatogonia; PL: preleptotene; L/Z:
leptotene/zygotene; P: pachytene; D: diplotene; RS: round spermatid; ES: elongating
spermatid; Sp: sperm; MI–MII: meiosis I–II. Model based on mouse data and adapted
from Lucifero *et al.* (2004b) (see Color plate 9)

11.2.1 Mouse studies

11.2.1.1 Erasure of methylation patterns in the germ line

Founding cells of the germ line, the primordial germ cells (PGCs), are thought to carry full complements of parental methylation profiles when they begin migrating towards the genital ridge. Upon their entry into the genital ridge, around 10.5 days of gestation, they undergo extensive genome-wide demethylation. Early studies employing methylation-sensitive restriction enzymes and Southern blot and PCR approaches indicated that PGCs have completely demethylated genomes by 13.5 days of gestation (Brandeis *et al.*, 1993; Chaillet *et al.*, 1991; Kafri *et al.*, 1992; Monk *et al.*, 1987). Recent work done using bisulfite sequencing to examine the methylation status of imprinted genes and repetitive sequences has helped better define the timing and sequence specificity of these early epigenetic events in PGCs. A number of imprinted genes, including *Peg3*, *Kcnq1ot1* (also known as *Lit1*), *Snrpn*, *H19*, *Rasgrf1* and *Gtl2*, as well as non-imprinted genes such as *α-actin*, were shown to become demethylated between 10.5 and 13.5 days of gestation (Hajkova *et al.*, 2002; Li *et al.*, 2004). However, certain sequences (at least some repetitive elements) appear to be treated differently: IAP, LINE-1 and minor satellite sequences are only subject to partial demethylation, whereas most imprinted and single-copy genes become demethylated (Hajkova *et al.*, 2002; Lane *et al.*, 2003; Lees-Murdock *et al.*, 2003; Szabo *et al.*, 2002).

Assessing the expression of imprinted genes has also been used by investigators to ascertain the state of epigenetic reprogramming of germ cells. Monoallelic expression would be expected prior to erasure of epigenetic marks on imprinted genes in PGCs, while biallelic expression would be an indication of ongoing or complete erasure of these marks. Using this approach, Szabo and colleagues (2002) found monoallelic expression of the four imprinted genes examined, including *H19* and *Snrpn*, in PGCs at 9.5 days of gestation. In contrast, *Snrpn* was biallelically expressed at day 10.5 as were the other genes examined by day 11.5. Consistent with the DNA methylation data this expression study points to the time of entry into the genital ridge as the period when demethylation of imprinted genes takes place in PGCs. Another approach used to examine epigenetic reprogramming in the early germ line has been analysis of embryos derived from somatic cell nuclear transfer (SCNT) using PGC nuclei (Lee *et al.*, 2002; Yamazaki *et al.*, 2003). Although no viable offspring were obtained when PGC nuclei were used for cloning experiments, careful examination of these embryos indicated that methylation imprints were being erased between 10.5 and 12.5 days of gestation (Lee *et al.*, 2002; Yamazaki *et al.*, 2003).

Overall, it appears that rapid and possibly active genome-wide erasure of methylation patterns takes place between 10.5–12.5 days of gestation, leaving PGCs of both sexes in an equivalent epigenetic state by embryonic day 13.5 (Hajkova *et al.*,

2002; Kato *et al.*, 1999; Lee *et al.*, 2002; Li *et al.*, 2004; Szabo and Mann, 1995; Szabo *et al.*, 2002).

11.2.1.2 Differential timing of methylation pattern acquisition between germ lines

Following demethylation in PGCs, male and female gametes acquire sex- and sequence-specific genomic methylation patterns (Reik *et al.*, 2001). For non-imprinted genes and repeat sequences, DNA methylation can be assessed directly. For imprinted genes, determination of DNA methylation status and assessment of mono- or biallelic expression of the genes of interest in the resulting embryos are used. Nuclear transplantation and cloning experiments using germ cell nuclei at different stages have also been used to study the timing of acquisition of methylation on imprinted genes by assessing postimplantation embryos for monoallelic expression of the genes of interest (Bao *et al.*, 2000; Obata and Kono; 2002; Obata *et al.*, 1998).

The timing of acquisition of methylation patterns differs greatly between the two germ lines. In the male, techniques like Southern blotting and bisulfite genomic sequencing have shown that acquisition of DNA methylation patterns begins before birth, in prospermatogonia, and is completed for most of the sequences after birth, before the end of the pachytene phase of meiosis (Davis *et al.*, 1999, 2000; Kafri *et al.*, 1992; Lees-Murdock *et al.*, 2003; Li *et al.*, 2004; Ueda *et al.*, 2000; Walsh *et al.*, 1998). Initial acquisition of methylation occurs between 15.5 and 18.5 days of gestation; at this time germ cells begin to stain positively with an antibody directed against methylated cytosine, indicating increases in overall genomic methylation (Coffigny *et al.*, 1999). *H19*, a maternally expressed gene that becomes methylated in the male germ line (and remains unmethylated in oocytes) has been extensively characterized (Bartolomei *et al.*, 1991, 1993; Davis *et al.*, 1999; Ferguson-Smith *et al.*, 1993; Tremblay *et al.*, 1995; Ueda *et al.*, 2000). A DMD spanning a 2 kb region roughly 2–4 kb from the transcription start site of the gene begins to acquire its methylation between days 15.5 and 18.5 of gestation in prenatal male germ cells; methylation is completed postnatally by pachynema, persisting in sperm (Davis *et al.*, 1999, 2000; Ueda *et al.*, 2000). Additional experiments demonstrated that the paternal alleles of *H19* become methylated prior to the maternally inherited alleles in male germ cells, suggesting that paternal alleles may 'remember' their origin as methylated alleles (Davis *et al.*, 1999, 2000).

Two additional imprinted genes in the mouse, *Gtl2* (Takada *et al.*, 2002) and *Rasgrf1* (Yoon *et al.*, 2002), have also been reported to be methylated on the paternally inherited allele. Their respective DMDs become progressively methylated between 12.5 and 17.5 days of gestation, but not to the extent seen in mature sperm (i.e. fully methylated), suggesting ongoing postnatal *de novo* methylation as seen for *H19* (Li *et al.*, 2004). Other types of sequences are also known to become methylated in prospermatogonia: repetitive DNA elements such as LINE-1, IAP and minor satellite sequences are fully methylated by 17.5 days of gestation (Lees-Murdock *et al.*, 2003; Walsh *et al.*, 1998). Further proof that male germ cells have completely acquired their methylation prior to the haploid phase of spermatogenesis comes from studies using intracytoplasmic round spermatid and sperm injections (Shamanski *et al.*, 1999); expression of imprinted genes is similar in embryos derived from round spermatids as compared to embryos derived from epididymal spermatozoa.

In contrast to the male, female germ cells only begin to acquire their gametic DNA methylation postnatally, following the pachytene phase of meiosis (Brandeis *et al.*, 1993; Chaillet *et al.*, 1991; Kono *et al.*, 1996; Lucifero *et al.*, 2002, 2004a; Obata and Kono, 2002; Stoger *et al.*, 1993; Ueda *et al.*, 1992; Walsh *et al.*, 1998). DNA methylation analysis of imprinted genes and nuclear transplantation studies have both pointed to the oocyte growth phase as the time when functional imprints are acquired in the female (Bao *et al.*, 2000; Lucifero *et al.*, 2002, 2004a; Obata and Kono, 2002).

11.2.1.3 DNA methylation and testis-specific gene expression

That DNA methylation could be an important mechanism for the regulation of tissue-specific gene expression was proposed a number of years ago (Holliday and Pugh, 1975; Riggs, 1975). The role of DNA methylation in the regulation of testis-specific gene expression has been the subject of a number of studies. In examples of early mouse studies, genes including transition protein 1, phosphoglycerate kinase-2, apolipoprotein A1, Oct-3/4 and lactate dehydrogenase C, were methylated in non-expressing tissues and became demethylated at some CpG sites prior to their expression in the testis (Ariel *et al.*, 1994; Bonny and Goldberg, 1995; Kroft *et al.*, 2001; Trasler *et al.*, 1990). For a few testis-specific genes, increases in methylation precede expression. For example, a few CpG sites in the coding region of mouse protamine 1 and the 5′ upstream region of mouse protamine 2, increases in methylation in meiotic prophase prior to expression in spermatids (Choi *et al.*, 1997; Trasler *et al.*, 1990). More recently, careful developmental time-course studies using bisulfite genomic sequencing on isolated germ cells have shown that a decrease in the methylation of the promoter region of phosphoglycerate kinase-2 is one of the earliest events, taking place before changes in chromatin structure, DNase I hypersensitivity, tissue-specific binding of factors to the enhancer region and transcriptional activation in meiotic male germ cells (Geyer *et al.*, 2004). Interestingly, phosphoglycerate kinase-2 is remethylated during transit through the epididymis; it is currently the only gene whose methylation status has been examined for change between testicular and cauda epididymal sperm (Geyer *et al.*, 2004). The purpose of a remethylation event occurring in the epididymis is unclear at present since most DNA methylation patterns (except those at imprinted genes and retro-transposons) are removed from the paternal genome shortly after fertilization. Although more epididymal DNA methylation studies need to be done on other genes, it has been postulated that non-specific genome-wide alterations in DNA methylation might occur in the epididymis to prepare the sperm genome for post-fertilization and early developmental epigenetic events (Geyer *et al.*, 2004).

Although there are a number of examples of testis-specific genes that show a correlation between hypomethylation and germ cell expression, it is presently unresolved whether the alterations in DNA methylation associated with germ cell-specific expression of genes are a cause or consequence of expression or events (other than DNA methylation) leading to expression (for review see MacLean and Wilkinson, 2005). The same issue has arisen and has been discussed with respect to the role of DNA methylation in time- or cell-specific expression in other organs (Goll and Bestor, 2004).

11.2.1.4 Maintenance of DNA methylation patterns in early embryos

A second genome-wide demethylation occurs in the early embryo. Marks established on imprinted genes and some repeat sequences must be faithfully maintained during preimplantation development at a time when the methylation of non-imprinted sequences is lost (Fig. 11.1). The male pronucleus faces a rapid, presumably active demethylation process within about 4 h of fertilization (Mayer *et al.*, 2000; Oswald *et al.*, 2000; Santos *et al.*, 2002), while the maternal genome becomes demethylated more slowly, presumably through a passive process whereby maintenance methylation does not take place following cell division (Howlett and Reik, 1991; Rougier *et al.*, 1998). Preservation of methylation at imprinted loci during the wave of preimplantation demethylation is postulated to be important for subsequent postimplantation embryo development, allowing for appropriate allele-specific, monoallelic expression of genes required for embryonic development (Hanel and Wevrick, 2001; Olek and Walter, 1997; Reik and Walter, 2001; Tremblay *et al.*, 1997). The overall methylation level of non-imprinted genes reaches a minimum at the blastocyst stage of preimplantation development, following which initiation of genome-wide *de novo* methylation takes place, coincident with the time of the first differentiation event after the fifth cell cycle (Santos and Dean, 2004).

11.2.2 Human studies

11.2.2.1 Erasure, establishment and maintenance of genomic methylation

Indirect evidence concerning the timing of DNA methylation pattern erasure in human PGCs has been acquired through studies on embryonic germ (EG) cell lines. While embryonic stem (ES) cells are derived from the inner cell mass of blastocyst-stage embryos, EG cells are derived from PGCs from the developing gonadal ridges of human fetuses. Monoallelic expression of *H19*, *SNRPN*, *IGF2* and *TSSC5*, as well as the methylation status of *H19* were found to be normal in differentiated EG lines derived from 5-, 6- and 11-week-old human fetuses (Onyango *et al.*, 2002). More studies need to be done, however, these results appear to contrast with the situation seen in the mouse, where methylation patterns are erased upon entry into the gonadal ridge, suggesting that the timing of epigenetic resetting differs between human and mouse. On the contrary, a number of studies support conservation of various key aspects of the dynamics of methylation acquisition and maintenance between mouse and human, even if little information is available on the methylation status of imprinted genes during gametogenesis or embryogenesis in humans. For instance, the paternally inherited methylation imprint on *H19* is conserved in both human and mouse sperm (Hamatani *et al.*, 2001; Kerjean *et al.*, 2000; Marques *et al.*, 2004). The *H19* DMD is unmethylated in human fetal gonocytes while a methylated imprint is acquired and maintained in adult spermatogonia and other stages of male germ cell development, including mature sperm (Kerjean *et al.*, 2000). Jinno and colleagues (1996) have also observed conservation of the paternal methylation imprint on *H19* in preimplantation embryos as has been reported in the mouse. An initial study conducted on a small number of human oocytes suggested that the methylation imprint at the *SNURF–SNRPN* locus is absent in fully grown human oocytes and that this imprint must be acquired during or following fertilization in humans (El Maarri *et al.*, 2001). However, in keeping with the mouse data, another study performed on oocytes at different developmental stages found *SNRPN* to be methylated in human oocytes, an imprint being present by the germinal vesicle stage and maintained in metaphase I and II oocytes (Geuns *et al.*, 2003). Certainly, a stable parental allele-specific mark must be established before the four-cell stage as monoallelic expression of *SNRPN* is initiated in four-cell human embryos (Huntriss *et al.*, 1998).

With regard to the role for DNA methylation in the control of testis-specific gene expression, to our knowledge, there have been no studies examining possible links between abnormalities in DNA methylation of testis-specific genes and infertility in humans.

11.3 The mammalian DNMTs

A number of different enzymes have been postulated to be involved in either erasing or establishing distinguishable epigenetic marks, including DNA demethylases and histone-modifying enzymes, but to date, DNMTs remain the best-characterized group of enzymes involved in epigenetic programming. Methylation of cytosine residues involves the transfer of a methyl group donated by the cofactor

S-adenosylmethionine (SAM) to the 5′-carbon of the cytosine pyrimidine ring to create 5-methylcytosine, a reaction catalyzed by DNMTs. In mammals, three families of DNMTs have been described and are classified according to similarities found in their C-terminal catalytic domains (Goll and Bestor, 2004). The predominant mammalian DNMT is DNMT1, although four other enzymes, including DNMT2 (Yoder and Bestor, 1998), DNMT3a, DNMT3b (Okano *et al.*, 1998) and more recently DNMT3L (DNA methyltransferase 3-like) (Aapola *et al.*, 2001; Bourc'his *et al.*, 2001), have been characterized. Of these, only DNMT1, DNMT3a and DNMT3b are thought to be capable of methylating DNA *in vivo*; nonetheless, recent reports suggest that DNMT2 might have residual methylation activity (Hermann *et al.*, 2003).

Three types of enzymatic activities are required to erase, establish and perpetuate DNA methylation patterns: demethylation, *de novo* methylation and maintenance methylation (Fig. 11.2). Demethylation can occur passively if methylation is not maintained at the time of replication, or it can come about actively by some as yet unidentified mechanism *in vivo*. The methylation states of early germ cells and

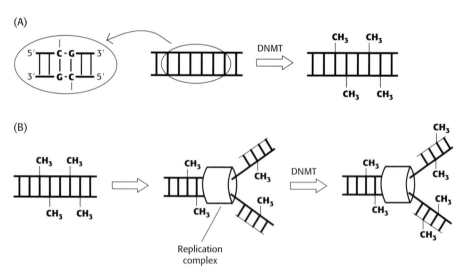

Figure 11.2   Schematic representation of *de novo* and maintenance methylation events. Two types of methylation activity are required in cells. (A) *De novo* methylation refers to the addition of methyl groups by DNMTs on an unmethylated substrate; this occurs mainly within CpG dinucleotides (i.e. the 3′ carbon atom of the cytosine is linked by a phosphodiester bond to the 5′ carbon atom of the guanine – left inset). (B) Following DNA replication, DNMTs performing maintenance methylation are responsible for adding methyl groups to the newly synthesized daughter strands at positions opposite to the methyl groups present on the parent strand, ensuring stable transmission of DNA methylation patterns following cell division

preimplantation stage embryos are established by DNMTs with *de novo* methyl-transferase activity, whereas differentiated cells present very little propensity to *de novo* methylation (Lei *et al.*, 1996). DNMTs with maintenance activity are required to ensure the accurate propagation of DNA methylation patterns at the time of cell division by faithfully copying the methylation status of the mother strand onto the daughter strand after replication.

All of the known mammalian DNMTs share similarities in their C-terminal catalytic domain, characterized by the 10 conserved amino acid motifs implicated in their catalytic function (reviewed by Bestor, 2000; Goll and Bestor, 2004; Hermann *et al.*, 2004). In addition, DNMT1, DNMT3a and DNMT3b contain large N-terminal regulatory domains (Fig. 11.3, Color plate 10). The mammalian DNMTs show little evidence of specificity for selected DNA sequences and thus how and why certain sequences become methylated has been a longstanding question in the field (for review, see Goll and Bestor, 2004). An equally important question is what prevents certain sequences from becoming methylated at different times. Recent results suggest that methylation of DNA at specific sites is the result of multiple inputs including the presence of repeat sequence elements in the DNA, interactions between RNA and DNA and histone modifications; precisely how these different mechanisms interact in germ cells to target specific sequences for methylation is unknown and an important area for future studies. Mouse gene-targeting studies have been particularly useful in shedding light on the biological functions of the different DNMTs. In

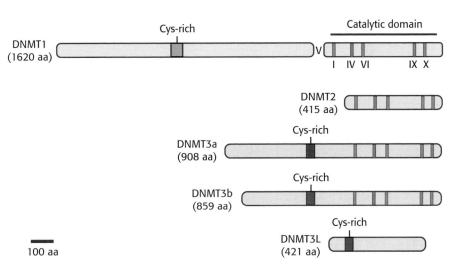

Figure 11.3 Organization of known mammalian DNMTs. Specific motifs are represented by boxes; five of the important amino acid motifs involved in catalysis are illustrated to demonstrate homology in the catalytic domain. Sizes in amino acids (aa) are those of the murine proteins (see Color plate 10)

the following section, current knowledge on the DNMTs from mouse, bovine and human studies will be reviewed, including their expression in germ cells and early embryos, as well as the reproductive consequences of their disruption.

11.4 DNMT1

11.4.1 Mouse studies

The first identified and perhaps best-characterized mammalian DNMT, DNMT1, was purified and cloned from mouse cells in the late 1980s (Bestor *et al.*, 1988); to date, it remains the sole DNA methylating enzyme to have been identified by means of biochemical purification. Earlier studies showed DNMT1 to prefer hemimethylated DNA (Bestor, 1992; Yoder *et al.*, 1997), which caused it to be assigned a function in maintenance methylation. Although its activity on unmethylated DNA substrates is greater than that of DNMT3a and DNMT3b, the postulated *de novo* methyltransferases (Okano *et al.*, 1998), it remains unresolved whether DNMT1 has *de novo* methylation activity *in vivo*.

Expression of the mouse *Dnmt1* gene is controlled by the use of sex-specific exons and the use of alternative splicing to produce two major protein products, DNMT1 and DNMT1o, as well as an untranslated transcript, Dnmt1p (Mertineit *et al.*, 1998). The full-length somatic form originally characterized by Bestor and colleagues, DNMT1, is produced from exon 1s (Bestor *et al.*, 1988). Initiation of transcription through exon 1o results in a degradation-resistant form of DNMT1 only expressed in mouse oocytes (Carlson *et al.*, 1992; Mertineit *et al.*, 1998). This oocyte-specific form, DNMT1o, lacks the first 118 amino acids of the N-terminus of the somatic form and accumulates at very high levels in non-cycling oocytes and preimplantation embryos. In fact, DNMT1o is the only form of DNMT1 detected in oocytes following birth, coincident with their entry into the growth phase (Howell *et al.*, 2001; Mertineit *et al.*, 1998; Ratnam *et al.*, 2002). A tissue-dependent DMD (T-DMD) has recently been found in the region 5′ of exon 1o, but not in that of exons 1s/1p; the T-DMD is completely methylated in all tissues examined except for oocytes and early developing embryos (Ko *et al.*, 2005). Production of Dnmt1p, a non-translated mRNA transcript only expressed in pachytene spermatocytes, is initiated from exon 1p (Mertineit *et al.*, 1998; Trasler *et al.*, 1992). Monitoring of the translational status of this transcript as well as sequence analyses show that production of active DNMT1 is highly improbable and expression of this transcript correlates with the fall in DNMT1 content in maturing pachytene spermatocytes (Mertineit *et al.*, 1998; Trasler *et al.*, 1992).

DNMT1 is the major methyltransferase in all somatic tissues, but levels of *Dnmt1* mRNA are higher in the testis and the ovary than in any other adult tissue

(Trasler *et al.*, 1992). More so, DNMT1 expression is tightly regulated throughout both spermatogenesis and oogenesis (Benoit and Trasler, 1994; Howell *et al.*, 2001; Jue *et al.*, 1995a; La Salle *et al.*, 2004; Mertineit *et al.*, 1998; Ratnam *et al.*, 2002; Sakai *et al.*, 2001; Trasler *et al.*, 1992) and there are striking germ line-specific differences in DNMT1 expression pre- and perinatally (La Salle *et al.*, 2004). In the male, DNMT1 is clearly lacking in late prenatal gonocytes (days 15.5–18.5 in the mouse), the developmental time when methylation patterns are initially laid down, indicating that another DNMT must be responsible for *de novo* methylation at this time (La Salle *et al.*, 2004; Sakai *et al.*, 2001). In neonatal testes, expression of DNMT1 is first associated with resumption of mitosis in proliferating spermatogonia, where it can be found throughout the nucleoplasm (Jue *et al.*, 1995a; La Salle *et al.*, 2004). Entry into meiosis coincides with the formation of DNMT1 nuclear foci only detected in leptotene/zygotene spermatocytes, after which point the presence of DNMT1 gradually decreases to become completely absent at pachynema (Jue *et al.*, 1995a; Mertineit *et al.*, 1998). As mentioned previously, downregulation of DNMT1 protein is linked to the expression of Dnmt1p transcript in pachytene spermatocytes (Jue *et al.*, 1995a; Mertineit *et al.*, 1998; Trasler *et al.*, 1992). DNMT1 is predicted to play a role in maintaining DNA methylation patterns in the germ line; whether it plays other functional roles not directly linked to its DNMT activity, such as in early meiotic cells, is currently unknown.

The importance of DNA methylation in embryonic development was first demonstrated by gene targeting of *Dnmt1* (Li *et al.*, 1992). Homozygous targeted partial ($Dnmt^{n/n}$ and $Dnmt^{s/s}$) and complete ($Dnmt^{c/c}$) loss-of-function mutations in *Dnmt1* cause growth retardation and mid-gestational lethality; the $Dnmt^{c/c}$ mice display only ~5% of wild-type DNA methylation levels (Lei *et al.*, 1996; Li *et al.*, 1992). In addition, biallelic expression of imprinted genes (Li *et al.*, 1993), ectopic X-chromosome inactivation (Panning and Jaenisch, 1996), reactivation of normally silent IAP sequences (Walsh *et al.*, 1998) and increased levels of apoptosis (Li *et al.*, 1992) are all induced by *Dnmt1* deficiency in embryos. Based on the high levels of DNMT1 in the testis and evidence of tight regulation during male germ cell development, one could predict that *Dnmt1* inactivation would also affect spermatogenesis; because targeted disruption of *Dnmt1* is embryonic lethal, germ cell-specific inactivation of *Dnmt1* or knock-down approaches will be required to determine the precise role(s) of DNMT1 in male germ cells.

11.4.2 Expression of DNMT1 in the reproductive system of humans and other species

The *DNMT1* gene is conserved across deuterostomes (see Table 11.1 for mouse/ human sequence homologies; reviewed by Goll and Bestor, 2004). The use of alternative first exons to encode for distinct protein products most likely evolved after the divergence of mammals and amphibians but before the split between marsupials

Table 11.1. Dissecting the mammalian DNMTs

Gene	Function	Mouse mutant phenotype	Mouse/human homology DNA % (protein %)	Associated human disease	References
Dnmt1	Maintenance methylation	Genome-wide demethylation; developmental arrest at E8.5.	86.5 (86.4)	–	Li *et al.* (1992) Lei *et al.* (1996)
Dnmt2	Unknown	Normal	87.4 (85.5)	–	Yoder and Bestor (1998)
*Dnmt3a**[*]	*De novo* methylation	Spermatogenesis defects; die at ~4 weeks of age. *Germ cell-specific inactivation affects imprint establishment, perturbing both spermatogenesis and oogenesis.*	91.6 (96.8)	–	Okano *et al.* (1999) Kaneda *et al.* (2004)
*Dnmt3b**[*]	*De novo* methylation	Demethylation of minor satellite DNA; embryonic lethality at ~E14.5–E18.5. *Germ cell-specific inactivation does not affect spermatogenesis or oogenesis.*	88.4 (91.2)	ICF syndrome	Okano *et al.* (1999) Kaneda *et al.* (2004)
Dnmt3L	No catalytic activity; regulation of methylation	Failure to establish maternal imprints; no viable progeny obtained from *Dnmt3L*⁻/⁻ dams. Complete spermatogenic arrest (infertility); partial methylation of some paternally imprinted genes and complete absence of methylation of certain repeat sequences.	83.0 (69.8)	–	Bourc'his *et al.* (2001) Hata *et al.* (2002) Bourc'his and Bestor (2004) Webster *et al.* (2005)

E: embryonic day.

[*] Double mutant: failure to initiate *de novo* methylation after implantation; developmental arrest at E8.5 (Okano *et al.*, 1999).

and eutherian mammals (Ding *et al.*, 2003). Dnmt1o transcripts are detected in opossum (Ding *et al.*, 2003) and human oocytes (Hayward *et al.*, 2003; Huntriss *et al.*, 2004), but are undetectable in bovine oocytes (Golding and Westhusin, 2003). However, there is very little information available on the expression of *DNMT1* in the testis of non-murine species. Jue and colleagues (1995b) demonstrated that *Dnmt1* is also developmentally expressed in rat testes as it is in the mouse, but did not detect the presence of Dnmt1p in this model. There are also indications of *DNMT1* expression in human testis, as reported in the human transcriptome project (GEO profiles, NCBI). Some studies have identified a novel transcript variant of *DNMT1* that incorporates 48 nucleotides between exons 4 and 5 via alternative splicing (Hsu *et al.*, 1999). This variant, named DNMT1b, was demonstrated to be a functional DNMT expressed in many human cell lines but only at ∼2–5% of the levels of DNMT1 (Bonfils *et al.*, 2000). It remains to be determined whether DNMT1b is expressed in the testis. To date, mutation of the human *DNMT1* gene has not been associated with any common human disorders; mutations have only been reported in very rare incidences of colorectal cancers where a one-base deletion results in deletion of the whole catalytic domain (Kanai *et al.*, 2003).

11.5 DNMT3a and DNMT3b

The mammalian genome encodes two functional cytosine methyltransferases of the DNMT3 family, DNMT3a and DNMT3b, which are more closely related to multispecies DNMTs than to DNMT1 or DNMT2 (Bestor, 2000; Goll and Bestor, 2004). They are postulated to function primarily as *de novo* methyltransferases, without any sequence specificity beyond CpG dinucleotides (Okano *et al.*, 1998). DNMT3a and DNMT3b are encoded by two different essential genes and are highly expressed in undifferentiated ES cells but their expression is downregulated upon differentiation (Okano *et al.*, 1998, 1999); genetic evidence indicates that the functions of DNMT3a and DNMT3b are distinct (Okano *et al.*, 1999).

11.5.1 Mouse studies

Organization of the *Dnmt3a* and *Dnmt3b* genes is complex, as is the regulation of their expression (Chen *et al.*, 2002; Ishida *et al.*, 2003; Okano *et al.*, 1998; Weisenberger *et al.*, 2002). Originally, several tissue-specific transcripts of *Dnmt3a* were identified by northern blot analysis (Okano *et al.*, 1998), pointing to the possible existence of more than one protein product. It was later determined by Chen and colleagues (2002) that two distinct proteins originate from the *Dnmt3a* gene, DNMT3a and DNMT3a2. DNMT3a is the full-length protein initially characterized and shown to possess *de novo* methylation activity (Okano *et al.*, 1998), while

DNMT3a2 is encoded by a transcript initiating from a downstream intronic promoter and is a shorter protein product lacking the first 219 N-terminal amino acids residues of DNMT3a (Chen *et al.*, 2002). Although their cytosine methyltransferase activity is very similar *in vitro*, they display different subcellular localization patterns suggesting that while DNMT3a associates with heterochromatin, DNMT3a2 associates with euchromatin (Chen *et al.*, 2002).

Several different transcripts of the *Dnmt3b* gene, resulting from alternative splicing of exons 11, 22 and/or 23, have also been reported (Aoki *et al.*, 2001; Chen *et al.*, 2002; Okano *et al.*, 1998; Weisenberger *et al.*, 2004). In all, there are potentially eight different splicing variants, each producing a slightly different protein product. Only DNMT3b1 and DNMT3b2 are capable of methylating DNA and are presumably both *de novo* methyltransferases, whereas DNMT3b3 appears unable of transferring methyl groups, despite its ability to bind DNA (Aoki *et al.*, 2001; Okano *et al.*, 1998; Weisenberger *et al.*, 2004). The other isoforms are most likely inactive, as they lack some of the conserved motifs conferring catalytic activity, but their specific roles remain elusive (Chen *et al.*, 2002; Weisenberger *et al.*, 2004); some have been postulated to act as negative regulators of DNA methylation (Saito *et al.*, 2002).

Dnmt3a and *Dnmt3b* are highly expressed in undifferentiated ES cells and, to a lesser extent, in a range of adult tissues (Okano *et al.*, 1998). They are also expressed in a stage- and cell-specific manner during embryogenesis, possibly reflecting distinct functions during embryonic development (Okano *et al.*, 1998, 1999; Watanabe *et al.*, 2002). As seen for *Dnmt1*, striking sex-specific differences in the expression of these genes are also observed during gametogenesis, the most remarkable modulations detected in the male germ line (La Salle *et al.*, 2004). *Dnmt3a* is very highly expressed in prenatal testes, whereas *Dnmt3b* expression is minimal; however, a spike in expression is observed for *Dnmt3b* shortly after birth, whereas expression of *Dnmt3a* is sustained to similar levels as seen before birth. Levels of both transcripts gradually decrease as testis development takes place (La Salle *et al.*, 2004). Immunostaining studies indicate that DNMT3a2 is present in the nuclei of prenatal gonocytes at the time when methylation patterns are initially laid down in the male, whereas DNMT3a expression is restricted to the nuclei of Sertoli cells and surrounding tissues at all stages examined (Sakai *et al.*, 2004); postnatal expression of DNMT3a has also been detected but appears to be restricted to type B spermatogonia (Watanabe *et al.*, 2004). DNMT3b is expressed at low levels in prenatal gonocytes (Sakai *et al.*, 2004) and expressed at higher levels specifically in type A spermatogonia after birth (Watanabe *et al.*, 2004). Certain transcript variants of Dnmt3b have been reported to be expressed in the testis (Chen *et al.*, 2002; Watanabe *et al.*, 2004), but their specific nature or role is still unclear. As for *Dnmt1*, detailed developmental studies are needed to fully understand these enzymes in the context of male germ cell development.

Some of the key functions of DNMT3a and DNMT3b have been identified by gene-targeting experiments. DNMT3a-deficient mice survive to term but are underdeveloped, die 3–4 weeks after birth and have impaired spermatogenesis; their global methylation levels appear normal (Okano *et al.*, 1999). Inactivation of *Dnmt3b* has more deleterious consequences, resulting in a more severe, mid-gestation embryonic lethal phenotype with demethylation of minor satellite repeats (Okano *et al.*, 1999). Combination of DNMT3a and DNMT3b deficiencies act synergistically, where embryos fail to develop past gastrulation and show global demethylation of their genomes (Okano *et al.*, 1999). Conditional inactivation of *Dnmt3a* in germ cells has revealed the crucial role it plays in establishing *de novo* methylation patterns in male germ cells, more specifically at paternally imprinted loci (Kaneda *et al.*, 2004). Deletion of the *Dnmt3a* gene in male germ cells causes demethylation of the DMDs of *H19* and *Gtl2–Dlk1* but does not affect the methylation of *Rasgrf1* (Kaneda *et al.*, 2004). Whether the demethylation defect is restricted to the DMDs of imprinted genes or affects other regions of the genome is still unknown. Germ cell-specific inactivation of *Dnmt3b* does not produce any apparent phenotype; viable offspring are produced from these *Dnmt3b* conditional mutants and the methylation status of all analyzed sequences is not perturbed (Kaneda *et al.*, 2004). Based on the high levels of *Dnmt3b* transcripts detected in the testis (La Salle *et al.*, 2004), one would expect a more severe phenotype following germ cell-specific inactivation of this gene.

11.5.2 DNMT3A and DNMT3B in the reproductive system of humans and other species

The human equivalents of the mouse *Dnmt3* genes, *DNMT3A* and *DNMT3B*, are highly homologous to their murine counterparts (see Table 11.1 for mouse/human sequence homologies; Xie *et al.*, 1999), showing the same type of genomic organization as well as expressing similar transcript variants (Chen *et al.*, 2002; Weisenberger *et al.*, 2002; Xie *et al.*, 1999). *DNMT3A* is ubiquitously expressed, being detected in a variety of tissues, whereas lower levels of *DNMT3B* transcripts are detected in these same tissues; both genes are expressed in the ovary and the testis (Xie *et al.*, 1999). Work done on human oocytes has shown that *DNMT3A* and at least two splicing variants of *DNMT3B* are developmentally expressed during the oocyte growth phase, in addition to showing that at least four transcript variants of *DNMT3B* are expressed in human testis (Huntriss *et al.*, 2004). Golding and Westhusin (2003) have also shown *DNMT3A* and *DNMT3B* to be expressed in bovine fetal and adult testis and ovary.

To date, *DNMT3B* is currently the only DNMT shown to be mutated and result in a human disease. Various mutations in *DNMT3B* cause a human autosomal recessive genetic disorder characterized by immunodeficiency, centromeric instability and facial anomalies known as ICF syndrome (Xu *et al.*, 1999). Cytogenetic abnormalities affecting predominantly the pericentric regions of chromosomes 1, 9 and 16 are observed in ICF patients; these regions contain a type of satellite DNA that is normally methylated but is almost completely demethylated in the DNA of ICF patients (Jeanpierre et al., 1993). Demethylation of CpG islands on the inactive X has also been reported in ICF patients (Kondo et al., 2000). None of the patients reported are homozygous for null alleles of *DNMT3B*, suggesting that complete loss of function of DNMT3B is lethal, as is seen in the mouse model (Okano et al., 1999). A specialized role in methylation of certain repeated sequences and CpG islands on the inactive X chromosome can thus be ascribed to DNMT3B. Effects on fertility have not been reported in patients with ICF syndrome.

11.6 DNMT3L

DNMT3L is related to DNMT3a and DNMT3b in both N- and C-terminal domains but lacks some of the key amino acid residues conferring catalytic activity (Fig. 11.3; Aapola et al., 2000, 2001; Bourc'his et al., 2001; Hata et al., 2002). DNMT3L does not possess methyltransferase activity, but genetic studies have demonstrated its importance for the establishment of a subset of methylation patterns in both male and female germ cells (Bourc'his et al., 2001; Hata et al., 2002; Webster et al., 2005). *In vitro* and *in vivo* studies suggest that DNMT3L interacts with DNMT3a and/or DNMT3b to stimulate their methyltransferase activity, implying that DNMT3L could by a cofactor to both proteins and a stimulator of *de novo* methylation (Chedin et al., 2002; Hata et al., 2002; Margot et al., 2003; Suetake et al., 2004).

11.6.1 Mouse studies

The mouse *Dnmt3L* gene was identified *in silico* based on its homology with *Dnmt3a* and *Dnmt3b* (Aapola et al., 2001). Recent studies have described the promoter region of *Dnmt3L*, characterized by a TATA-less and CpG-rich minimal promoter (Aapola et al., 2004). This genomic organization is reminiscent of the human *DNMT3A* and *DNMT3B* genes, which were shown to contain several promoters that are either CpG-rich or CpG-poor and typically lacking TATA consensus sequences (Yanagisawa et al., 2002). Methylation analysis of the *Dnmt3L* promoter region showed that in a highly expressing tissue such as the testis, all CpG sites studied are fully unmethylated (Aapola et al., 2004).

Like other DNMT family members, *Dnmt3L* is highly expressed in ES cells, but its expression becomes restricted to a few tissues upon differentiation, namely the chorion of E7.5 and E8.5 embryos and the gonads (Aapola et al., 2001; Bourc'his et al., 2001; Hata et al., 2002). Reciprocal expression patterns are observed in the male and female germ lines; testicular levels of *Dnmt3L* are highest before birth and then decrease dramatically after birth, whereas in the female they are lowest in the prenatal stages of ovarian development and then increase drastically in the postnatal period (La Salle *et al.*, 2004). In both germ lines, peak expression correlates with the window of acquisition of methylation patterns (La Salle *et al.*, 2004) and DNMT3L protein is only detected in germ cells (Bourc'his *et al.*, 2001; Hata *et al.*, 2002; Webster *et al.*, 2005). Activity of a reporter gene controlled by the endogenous *Dnmt3L* promoter suggests DNMT3L is only present in pre- and perinatal prospermatogonia and that expression of DNMT3L in spermatogonia is for the most part extinguished by 6 days post partum (Bourc'his *et al.*, 2001; Bourc'his and Bestor, 2004; Webster *et al.*, 2005). Using a similar approach, Hata and colleagues (2002) also detected DNMT3L in differentiating spermatocytes of newborn and adult mice. Immunostaining studies will prove decisive in determining the exact endogenous expression and localization of DNMT3L in male germ cells.

The central role played by *Dnmt3L* in reproduction was clearly demonstrated by gene-targeting studies. While homozygous *Dnmt3L* null mice are viable, both males and females are sterile (Bourc'his *et al.*, 2001; Hata *et al.*, 2002). Homozygous oocytes can be fertilized but the resulting heterozygous progeny die at midgestation, showing demethylation of DMDs of maternally methylated imprinted genes and corresponding biallelic expression of normally paternally expressed imprinted genes (Bourc'his *et al.*, 2001; Hata *et al.*, 2002). The reproductive impact of DNMT3L deficiency is different in males, as they suffer from hypogonadism and are azoospermic (Bourc'his *et al.*, 2001; Hata *et al.*, 2002; Webster *et al.*, 2005). Seminiferous cords appear normal at 1 week of age postnatally but there are few differentiated spermatocytes in the testes of *Dnmt3L*-deficient mice by 4 weeks (Hata *et al.*, 2002; Webster *et al.*, 2005). Targeting of the *Dnmt3L* gene causes partial demethylation of the *H19* and *Rasgrf1* DMDs (Bourc'his and Bestor, 2004; Webster *et al.*, 2005), while it clearly prevents methylation of both LINE-1 and IAP elements, leading to their massive transcription in spermatogonia and spermatocytes (Bourc'his and Bestor, 2004). While DNMT3L is dispensable for female meiosis, abnormal synapsis accompanies DNMT3L deficiency in the male, triggering an apoptotic checkpoint that prevents spermatocytes from progressing to pachynema (Bourc'his and Bestor, 2004).

11.6.2 DNMT3L in the reproductive system of humans

The human *DNMT3L* gene was initially characterized before its murine homolog (see Table 11.1 for mouse/human sequence homologies) and its expression was detected in testis, ovary and thymus (Aapola *et al.*, 2000). Recent studies have reported the expression of *DNMT3L* in preimplantation embryos but failed to detect it in developing human oocytes (Huntriss *et al.*, 2004), suggesting that the mechanism of imprint acquisition might be different between mouse and human. Although expression of *DNMT3L* is highest in the testis, expression profiling studies in human male germ cells at different steps in their development are clearly lacking.

11.7 Germ line epigenetic inheritance: regulation and dysregulation

11.7.1 Mechanisms of epigenetic inheritance in genomic imprinting

The functional non-equivalence of the maternal and paternal genomes is underscored by the failure of uniparental embryos to develop normally, confirming the requirement of both parental genomes for normal development (reviewed by Reik and Walter, 2001). As previously mentioned, genomic imprinting regulates the expression of a subset of mammalian genes by restricting their expression to one of the parental alleles. Differential epigenetic marking of the parental alleles takes place during gametogenesis or in the first few divisions after fertilization; differential DNA methylation and chromatin structure, for example, histone modifications and hypersensitivity sites, and asynchronous replication timing are common features of the maternally and paternally inherited alleles of imprinted genes (reviewed by Bartolomei and Tilghman, 1997; Reik and Walter, 2001; Reik *et al.*, 2001). Extensive studies have unveiled some of the characteristic features shared by a subset of imprinted genes, namely genomic clustering, regulation by antisense transcripts and the presence of repeat elements near or within their differentially methylated domain (DMD). The clustering of imprinted genes into large imprinted domains raises the possibility that a common imprinting mechanism may regulate an entire imprinted area, allowing coordinated regulation of genes in a given chromosomal region. Supporting this concept is the discovery that *cis*-acting imprinting control elements or imprinting centers (IC) have been found in some clusters and shown to have an impact on genes many kilobases away (Spahn and Barlow, 2003).

11.7.1.1 The *H19* subdomain: a model for paternally inherited imprinting marks

A well-characterized imprinted cluster is found on human chromosome 11p15.5, spanning a region of 1 Mbase separated into two independent imprinting subdomains, the *H19* subdomain and the *KCNQ1OT1* subdomain (reviewed by Verona *et al.*, 2003); mouse distal chromosome 7 shows conserved genomic organization and imprinting of this cluster. The *H19* subdomain includes the *H19*, *IGF2* and *INS* genes; *H19* encodes a non-translated RNA with exclusive maternal expression while *IGF2* is reciprocally imprinted and paternally expressed. Both the mouse and human *H19* genes exhibit paternal-specific methylation of a region located 2 kb upstream of the *H19* promoter known as the DMD or the imprinting control

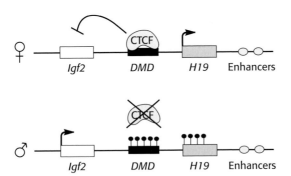

Figure 11.4 Imprinting regulation at the *H19* subdomain. On the maternal alleles, binding of the insulator protein CTCF to the unmethylated DMD (black box) prevents access of *Igf2* (white box) to downstream enhancer elements, allowing for maternal expression of *H19* (gray box). However, paternal-specific methylation (filled circles) of the DMD prevents binding of CTCF, silencing *H19* and allowing expression of *Igf2*. Black arrows indicate transcriptional activity of a given gene. Adapted from Verona *et al.* (2003)

region (ICR), and this DMD is thought to harbor the imprinting mark that distinguishes the parental alleles of *H19* (Bartolomei *et al.*, 1991; Frevel *et al.*, 1999; Tremblay *et al.*, 1995, 1997). In the mouse, studies suggest the *H19* DMD acts as a methylation-sensitive insulator element in regulating the imprinting of *Igf2* by blocking promoter–enhancer interactions through binding of the methylation-sensitive insulator factor CTCF (Bell and Felsenfeld, 2000; Hark *et al.*, 2000; Kanduri *et al.*, 2000). Together, these data have led to the elaboration of the following model to account for reciprocal imprinting of H19 and Igf2 (Fig. 11.4): on the maternal allele, binding of CTCF to the unmethylated DMD insulates the *Igf2* promoter from enhancer elements situated 3′ of *H19*, allowing *H19* exclusive access to these elements and ensuring maternal expression of *H19*. On the paternal allele, methylation of the DMD prevents binding of CTCF and formation of an insulator, resulting in paternal expression of *Igf2* by allowing access to downstream enhancers. Another imprinted cluster on human chromosome 14 and mouse chromosome 12 is reminiscent of this arrangement; the paternally expressed gene *Dlk* is flanked by a maternally expressed gene *Gtl2*, which is a non-coding RNA, and these genes contain DMDs that are reciprocally imprinted (Schmidt *et al.*, 2000; Takada *et al.*, 2000; Wylie *et al.*, 2000). The factors that regulate the establishment of parental imprints at these loci remain to be identified.

11.7.2 Sex chromosome inactivation during spermatogenesis

The process of spermatogenesis in mammals is a complex series of events leading to the formation of haploid cells starting from diploid precursors. Going through meiosis requires the pairing of homologous autosomal chromosomes, while the X- and Y-chromosomes pair only at their pseudoautosomal regions to form the sex (or XY) body (reviewed by Handel, 2004). Several genes on the X chromosome are subject to transcriptional repression during meiosis, beginning at pachytene with reactivation by the spermatid stage (McCarrey *et al.*, 1992, 2002); RNA polymerase II is excluded from the XY body at pachynema (Ayoub *et al.*, 1997; Fernandez-Capetillo *et al.*, 2003). In somatic cells, X inactivation is accompanied by DNA methylation. However, DNA methylation does not seem to be involved in transcriptional repression of genes on the X chromosome during spermatogenesis since the promoter region of a number of housekeeping genes on the X chromosome remains unmethylated throughout germ cell development in both humans and mice (Driscoll and Migeon, 1990; McCarrey *et al.*, 1992). *Xist* (X-inactive-specific transcript gene), which is associated with X inactivation in female cells, is transiently transcribed in pachytene spermatocytes and repressed again in spermatids but it is not essential to normal spermatogenesis and formation of the XY body, indicating that another mechanism must be responsible for transient X inactivation during spermatogenesis (Marahrens *et al.*, 1997; McCarrey and Dilworth, 1992; McCarrey *et al.*, 2002; Salido *et al.*, 1992; Turner *et al.*, 2002).

Recent reports in the literature suggest that histone modifications are involved in XY inactivation during spermatogenesis (Peters *et al.*, 2001). Using immuno-cytochemistry and *in situ* DNA hybridization, Khalil and colleagues (2004) demonstrated that histones of both the X and Y chromosomes undergo sequential modifications (both acetylation and methylation) beginning at the pachytene stage and that in spermatids, these modifications are reversed to their status in early spermatogenesis. At the pachytene stage, specific lysine residues on histone H4 become progressively underacetylated, while H3–K9 goes from an acetylated to a hypermethylated state. Coincident with enrichment in H3–K9 dimethylation is the exclusion of RNA polymerase II from the XY body at the pachytene stage. Some of these modifications persist through the first and second meiotic cell divisions, indicating that the chromatin of the X and Y chromosome is transcriptionally silent even when the chromosomes are physically separated. Together, these data provide evidence that some but not all histone modifications reflect the transient inactivation of sex chromosomes during spermatogenesis (Khalil *et al.*, 2004).

11.7.3 Errors in erasure, acquisition or maintenance of DNA methylation patterns

11.7.3.1 Single-site loss of DNA methylation

11.7.3.1.1 Imprinting disorders
Loss of function of a number of imprinted genes has been linked to human genetic diseases, progression of certain cancers and has also been implicated in a number

of neurological disorders. Some of the most extensively studied disorders involving imprinted genes are Prader–Willi syndrome (PWS), Angelman syndrome (AS), Beckwith–Wiedemann syndrome (BWS) and Russell–Silver syndrome; the clinical features as well as the specific molecular determinants associated with these imprinting disorders are reviewed elsewhere (Lucifero *et al.*, 2004b). Diverse molecular events can lead to phenotypic abnormalities involving imprinted genes (reviewed by Jiang *et al.*, 2004). Generally, uniparental disomy can result in overexpression or underexpression of imprinted genes implicated in the control of fetal growth and postnatal development. Another general mechanism involves the deletion of one or more genes or point mutations affecting a specific locus. Epigenetic defects can also give rise to imprinting disorders, in which case a chromosome of one parental origin has an abnormal epigenetic status (DNA methylation, chromatin structure and gene expression), often that of the opposite parental origin. Mutations or deletions in the IC can be associated with imprinting diseases, and this is particularly well characterized in the case of PWS and AS; these genetic events can have secondary epigenetic effects resulting in the *de novo* acquisition of epigenetic marks. Finally, imprinting defects can also be epigenetic in origin (gain or loss of imprinting at a specific locus) when no identifiable genetic defect is observed. Imprinting defects have the potential to arise at any step of epigenetic reprogramming and could result from problems with the enzymes responsible for erasing, establishing and maintaining imprints. Alternatively, the methylation status or chromatin structure may be affected by epigenetic insults leading to abnormal imprinted gene expression.

Of note, loss of imprinting is also involved in the progression of a number of cancers (Tycko and Morison, 2002). Tumors that show imprinting defects include Wilm's tumor, where loss of function of the maternal allele leading to the suppression of *H19* and biallelic expression of *IGF2* appears to be involved. Some imprinted genes act as tumor suppressor genes, the best characterized being *IGF2R* and *WT1*; in the case of imprinted tumor suppressor genes, inactivation of only one allele is required to cause loss of function, compared to non-imprinted tumor suppressor genes where loss of function requires mutation of both alleles.

11.7.3.1.2 *Male germ cell culture and assisted reproductive technologies: cause for concern*

Epigenetic marks, in particular DNA methylation patterns, tend to be unstable and amenable to modification by culture conditions and cellular manipulations. A number of animal studies have examined how different types of media or the addition of serum to culture media affect the methylation status and expression of imprinted genes of cultured preimplantation embryos (Doherty *et al.*, 2000; Khosla *et al.*, 2001); significant DNA methylation perturbations were found in both cases.

Introduction of intracytoplasmic sperm injection (ICSI) has greatly improved chances to conceive for couples with previous fertilization failures using *in vitro* fertilization (IVF). The success of ICSI with freshly ejaculated spermatozoa has been extended to epididymal spermatozoa, and even to elongating and round spermatids (reviewed by Tsai *et al.*, 2000). It is unlikely that ARTs themselves, involving the use of haploid gametes, interfere with either erasure or acquisition of genomic imprints, as both processes appear to be complete by the spermatid phase of spermatogenesis.

Nonetheless, there is cause for concern when abnormal or more immature gametes are used in ARTs to overcome male infertility. In mice, multiple approaches have been developed to overcome spermatogenic arrest, including injection of secondary and primary spermatocyte nuclei into oocytes (Kimura and Yanagimachi, 1995; Kimura *et al.*, 1998; Sasagawa *et al.*, 1998). Upon electrical activation of the oocyte, oocyte and spermatocyte chromosomes complete meiosis (producing two pronuclei and two polar bodies) and participate in embryogenesis; but it appears that mouse primary spermatocyte nuclei complete meiosis with less efficiency than secondary spermatocytes. A number of reasons could explain poor embryo outcome: suboptimal culture conditions, unsuccessful DNA repair or incomplete paternal genomic imprint acquisition. Nevertheless, *in vitro* culture of spermatocytes has been proposed to overcome spermatogenic arrest in humans (Tesarik *et al.*, 1998, 1999) and the first live births using both primary and secondary spermatocytes have been reported respectively in 1999 by Tesarik *et al.* and 1998 by Sofikitis *et al.* To date, there is only one report linking an imprinting defect to disruptive spermatogenesis. Marques *et al.* (2004) found that 17–30% of moderate to severe oligozoospermic (very low sperm counts) patients seeking an infertility diagnosis presented defective *H19* methylation, with most patients having normally methylated and hypomethylated alleles in the same semen sample; all patients presented complete erasure of the maternally methylated gene *MEST*. Since maternal imprints appear to be properly erased, abnormal genomic imprinting could indicate changes in DNMT activity or DNA methylation modulating factors. Recent studies suggest a possible link between the increased incidence of imprinting disorders and human ARTs (reviewed by Lucifero *et al.*, 2004b). However, it is unclear whether the imprinting disorders are due to underlying infertility (i.e. that there exist epigenetic causes for infertility) or the techniques being used. Interestingly, a recent study reported an increased prevalence of imprinting defects in patients with AS born to subfertile couples; the findings suggest that imprinting defects and subfertility may have a common cause (Ludwig *et al.*, 2005). In light of the apparent instability of epigenetic marks, studies are required to look for epigenetic causes of infertility and examine the effects of culture conditions on spermatogenic cell maturation. These studies should provide an understanding of male germ cell epigenetic plasticity, as well as the safety of procedures used in assisted reproduction.

11.7.3.1.3 Epimutations

As mentioned previously, epigenetic changes can also play a major role in the development of human cancer. For example, a high proportion of patients with sporadic colorectal cancers with microsatellite instability display abnormal methylation and silencing of the gene *MLH1* (Kane *et al.*, 1997). Germ line 'epimutations' in the *MLH1* gene have been proposed to predispose individuals carrying aberrant methylation patterns to multiple cancers (Gazzoli *et al.*, 2002; Suter *et al.*, 2004). In some patients, the epimutation is detected in normal somatic tissues derived from the three founding cell lineages (endoderm, buccal mucosa; mesoderm, blood; ectoderm, hair follicles), implying that the event occurred in the germ line (Suter *et al.*, 2004); more so, spermatozoa display the same promoter-associated methylation found in tumors, evidence that the epimutation can be transmitted through the germ line (Suter *et al.*, 2004). More examples of epimutations are likely to be reported in the future, some of which may be associated with infertility or subfertility.

11.7.3.2 Global loss of DNA methylation

11.7.3.2.1 Trophoblastic diseases and molar pregnancies

Complete hydatidiform moles (CHM) originate from the growth of cells with two identical parental genomes. Although most CHM have a uniparental etiology (with two paternal genomes), a small number of women have an autosomal recessive disorder causing recurrent CHM of biparental origin, in which a global loss of imprinting or maternal DNA methylation on imprinted genes has been implicated (Judson *et al.*, 2002). In this disorder, most of the imprinted loci spread across the maternal genome are unmethylated or acquire a paternal epigenotype, suggesting a defect in a *trans*-acting factor involved in the establishment of epigenetic marks at imprinted gene loci in the female germ line. Involvement of the known DNMTs seems unlikely since no mutations were detected in any of the human *DNMT* genes (Judson *et al.*, 2002). Moglabey and colleagues (1999) originally mapped a maternal locus responsible for biparental CHM to chromosome 19q13.4 but the gene coding for the putative factor involved in imprint establishment/maintenance has not been identified as of today. Whether a similar condition occurs in the human male (i.e. global loss of imprinting in the male germ line) is unknown; such a condition would be expected to result in teratomas (the result of two maternal genomes). In mice, one condition already mentioned above is similar to a global loss of imprinted gene methylation in the male germ line. DNMT3L deficiency in the male germ line results in a loss of methylation at some imprinted loci as well as

IAP; however, since the mutation is associated with infertility, the outcome in the offspring cannot be examined (Bourc'his and Bestor, 2004). It would be interesting to know if mutations in *DNMT3L* exist in infertile men.

11.8 Epigenetic modulators with potential reproductive implications

11.8.1 Chromatin modification and remodeling factors

Numerous types of chromatin modifying factors including histone modification enzymes have been described and are postulated to be involved in modulating transcription, X-chromosome inactivation, genome stability and chromosome events during meiosis (Goll and Bestor, 2002; Hendrich and Bickmore, 2001; Li, 2002). Chromatin modification and chromatin remodeling are the principal mechanisms by which global gene silencing and higher order chromatin structure are established and maintained. Discussed here are additional factors with chromatin remodeling or modifying activities that greatly influence genome stability and, perhaps, DNA methylation patterning during gametogenesis.

11.8.1.1 SWI2/SNF2 remodeling proteins

Lymphoid-specific helicase (LSH) is a member of the SNF2 family of chromatin remodelers and is involved in mammalian development and cellular proliferation (Geiman *et al.*, 2001; Raabe *et al.*, 2001). More specifically, LSH is required for genome-wide methylation, normal histone methylation and formation of heterochromatin (Dennis *et al.*, 2001; Yan *et al.*, 2003). Targeted deletion of *Lsh* results in perinatal lethality with substantial loss of methylation throughout the genome. Various sequences are affected by LSH deficiency, including repetitive elements such as satellite sequences, LINE-1s and IAPs, as well as single-copy genes, suggestive of a role for this enzyme in maintenance methylation during development (Dennis *et al.*, 2001). Recent studies indicate that LSH is specifically required to maintain the methylation status of the imprinted gene *Cdkn1c* but not of other imprinted genes such as *H19* or *Igf2r* during development, implying that LSH is only crucial to the maintenance of imprinting marks at specific loci (Fan *et al.*, 2005). So far, the only non-lymphoid tissue found to express *Lsh* at very high levels is the adult testis, both in mouse and human (Geiman *et al.*, 1998).

The α-thalassaemia/mental retardation syndrome, X-linked (ATRX) localizes to pericentromeric heterochromatin and to the short arms of human acrocentric chromosomes. It contains a PHD-like zinc-finger domain shared by the DNMT3 family members, and an SNF-like helicase domain, suggesting a role in transcriptional regulation (McDowell *et al.*, 1999). Mental retardation, facial dysmorphism and α-thalassaemia result from mutations in the human *ATRX* gene. Patients suffering from the ATRX syndrome present with specific changes in the pattern of methylation of several highly repeated sequences including hypomethylated rDNAs and hypermethylated Y-chromosome repeats (Gibbons *et al.*, 2000). More recently, ATRX was shown to be required for proper chromosome alignment and meiotic spindle organization in mouse metaphase II oocytes (De La Fuente *et al.*, 2004); it is currently unknown if this protein plays a similar role during spermatogenesis.

11.8.1.2 Histone modification enzymes

Modifications of histone tails by acetylation, phosphorylation and methylation have a fundamental role in gene regulation. Several classes of histone methyltransferases have been identified, one of which includes H3–K9 methyltransferases. Three members of this class are of particular interest: G9a, Suv39h1 (human homolog: *SUV39H1*) and Suv39h2. These histone methyltransferases appear to direct H3–K9 methylation to distinct chromatin domains: G9a targets euchromatin while Suv39h1 and Suv39h2 target heterochromatic regions of the genome (Rice *et al.*, 2003). Gene-targeting studies in mice have shown *G9a* to be essential to normal development, *G9a*-deficient embryos showing a drastic decrease in H3–K9 methylation and severe growth retardation leading to embryonic lethality (Tachibana *et al.*, 2002). More recently, studies using mouse *G9a*-deficient ES cells have shown that the maintenance of CpG methylation at the PWS IC requires the function of *G9a* (Xin *et al.*, 2003), while X inactivation is properly maintained in *G9a*-deficient embryos (Ohhata *et al.*, 2004). The *Suv39h* genes display overlapping expression profiles during mouse embryonic development, but *Suv39h2* expression becomes restricted to the testis of adult mice (O'Carroll *et al.*, 2000). Peters and colleagues (2001) demonstrated that the *Suv39h* histone methyltransferases regulate H3–K9 methylation of pericentromeric heterochromatin. Combined disruption of the *Suv39h* genes severely impairs viability, induces chromosomal instabilities and causes sterility in males; spermatogenic failure largely results from non-homologous chromosome pairing (Peters *et al.*, 2001). Interestingly, a recent report has directly linked *Suv39h*-associated H3–K9 methylation to DNMT3b-dependent DNA methylation at pericentric repeats (Lehnertz *et al.*, 2003). Together, these data demonstrate an evolutionarily conserved pathway between H3–K9 methylation and DNA methylation in mammals. Furthermore, they provide an attractive avenue to pursue to explain the role these proteins play during spermatogenesis.

11.8.2 Nutritional and genetic factors: folic acid and the folate pathway

The folate pathway is central to the production of methionine and to the synthesis of purines and pyrimidines, in addition to being integral to the production of methyl groups necessary for numerous methylation reactions, including DNA methylation. Briefly, two pathways are linked via methionine synthase: the reduction of 5-methyltetrahydrofolate to tetrahydrofolate and the subsequent remethylation of homocysteine to methionine. It is the conversion of homocysteine to methionine that provides the methyl group required for SAM, the universal methyl donor in numerous cellular reactions. One can hypothesize that disruption of one part of the folate pathway could alter the balance of SAM levels and perturb methylation reactions. Indeed, hypomethylation of DNA is observed when one of the folate pathway enzymes is mutated in mice (Chen *et al.*, 2001).

Few studies to date have characterized the effects of folate pathway enzyme deficiency on the testis or examined the consequences on DNA methylation pattern establishment in the germ line; the systemic effects that deficiency causes are a major obstacle in studying the effects on reproduction. One exception is for methylenetetrahydrofolate reductase (MTHFR), the enzyme that catalyses the conversion of 5, 10-methylenetetrahydrofolate to 5-methyltetrahydrofolate, a methyl donor serving in the remethylation of homocysteine to methionine, the precursor of SAM (Chen *et al.*, 2001). Inactivation of this enzyme results in reduced levels of 5-methyltetrahydrofolate, methionine and SAM, as well as decreased DNA methylation levels (Chen *et al.*, 2001). MTHFR activity is higher in the testis than in any other organ of the adult mouse (Chen *et al.*, 2001). *Mthfr* homozygous null male mice have smaller testes, histological evidence of abnormal germ cell development and are infertile (Kelly *et al.*, 2005). Interestingly, supplementation with betaine, an alternative methyl donor serving in the remethylation of homocysteine to methionine, benefits both testis histology and fertility (Kelly *et al.*, 2005). Together, these data suggest an important role for MTHFR in the testis and encourage further investigation.

11.8.2.1 Transgenerational epigenetic inheritance and early dietary influences

Phenotypic variation cannot always be accounted for by genetic or environmental heterogeneity. Studies on murine models of variable expressivity have suggested that this variability could be explained by the stochastic establishment of epigenetic modifications, such as DNA methylation (Rakyan *et al.*, 2001). Both the $Axin^{Fu}$ (axin-fused) allele and the A^{iapy}, A^{hvy} and A^{vy} alleles of the agouti locus have been subjected to insertion of an IAP retrotransposon; the methylation state of the inserted IAP element correlates with the variability of the phenotype (Morgan *et al.*, 1999; Rakyan *et al.*, 2003; Waterland and Jirtle, 2003). Recent evidence suggests that these epigenetic modifications are sometimes transmitted to the next generation (reviewed by Rakyan *et al.*, 2001). Transgenerational epigenetic inheritance could result from inefficient erasure of the epigenetic state of certain sequences (like IAPs) during gametogenesis, resulting in maternal or paternal transmission of variable phenotypes (Morgan *et al.*, 1999; Rakyan *et al.*, 2001, 2003).

Mammalian one-carbon metabolism, which ultimately provides the methyl groups for all methylation reactions, depends on dietary methyl donors and cofactors. Thus, early nutrition could greatly impact the establishment and the maintenance of DNA methylation patterns. An initial study conducted by Wolff *et al.* (1998) suggested that maternal methyl-donor supplementation affected the phenotype of the A^{vy}/a offspring. Recently, Waterland and Jirtle (2003) confirmed that maternal diet containing methyl donors could influence offspring phenotype and showed that this effect was mediated via increased A^{vy} methylation in the offspring of supplemented dams. Further studies are required to determine if other types of sequences are epigenetically labile to early nutrition in the mouse. By using animal models to better understand the mechanisms underlying epigenetic plasticity during early nutrition, we will be able to identify similar epigenetic targets amenable to metabolic imprinting in humans.

11.8.3 Drugs-targeting epigenetic modifications

The development of new drugs targeting epigenetic modifications has been motivated by the fact that many human diseases, including cancers, have an epigenetic etiology. Many agents capable of modifying DNA methylation patterns or histone modifications are currently being tested in clinical trials (reviewed by Egger *et al.*, 2004). The cytosine analogs 5-azacytidine and 5-aza-2′ deoxycytidine are amongst the most commonly used agents to inhibit DNA methylation: they incorporate into DNA during replication, but due to the presence of nitrogen at position C5, they cannot accept the methyl group and the DNMT enzyme remains bound to DNA as a covalent adduct (Gabbara and Bhagwat, 1995). Formation of this adduct is thought to cause indirect genomic hypomethylation through decreased activity of the DNMTs. In the rat and mouse, disruption of DNA methylation patterns in male germ cells using these agents has severe consequences for both germ cells and progeny outcome (Doerksen and Trasler, 1996; Doerksen *et al.*, 2000; Kelly *et al.*, 2003). Decreased sperm counts, decreased fertility, increased preimplantation loss and decreased sperm DNA methylation are all consequences of chronic exposure to 5-azacytidine and 5-aza-2′ deoxycytidine. A number of agents are also being developed to inhibit HDACs in the hope of inducing expression of genes silenced by histone deacetylation. Trichostatin-A (TSA), a non-specific HDAC inhibitor, induces cell cycle arrest through stimulation of transcription of genes that negatively regulate cell growth and survival. Chronic exposure of mice to TSA impairs spermatogenesis, causing an increase in pachytene–diplotene spermatocyte apoptosis, decreased numbers of spermatids with increasing doses of TSA and decreased fertility (Fenic *et al.*, 2004). Although the effects on spermatogenesis appear reversible, consequences of long-term exposure to TSA have not been evaluated on germ cell and progeny outcome. Recently, there has been renewed interest in using cytosine analogs and HDAC inhibitors to treat certain diseases. As the doses used in human clinical trials are similar to the doses used in the mouse studies, one can predict that there will be adverse effects of these drugs on human germ cells.

11.9 Perspectives and outlook

Epigenetic reprogramming of the genome during gametogenesis and the preimplantation period sets the developmental program for normal embryogenesis. The sex-specific functional non-equivalence of the parental genomes (genomic imprinting) established during gametogenesis emphasizes the importance of epigenetic reprogramming during this period and confirms the requirement of both parental genomes to normal development. Studies done on highly specialized biological processes such as genomic imprinting and X inactivation have begun to unravel how epigenetic reprogramming works. Some of the key aspects involve dynamic changes in DNA methylation, histone modifications and chromatin remodeling taking place in a timely fashion during male and female germ cell development. Many DNA- and histone-modifying enzymes as well as chromatin-remodeling factors have recently been identified and have contributed to our understanding of the mechanisms governing epigenetic reprogramming. Some of the challenges that we face during the next decade include understanding how these epigenetic factors assemble into regulatory networks, how they are targeted to specific genes or chromosomal domains, as well as the consequences of perturbations occurring during gametogenesis.

11.9.1 Studies required and implications for research

More basic research on animal and human gametes and early embryos is clearly required to better understand the timing and the mechanisms governing epigenetic reprogramming. Most of our current knowledge comes from studies done in the mouse, where the methylation status of a number of genes has been examined at different times during development. More global approaches looking at the methylation profiles of multiple genes simultaneously throughout germ cell and embryonic development are still required to fully understand the nature of the sequences targeted for methylation as well as the precise timing of the methylation events (i.e. erasure, establishment and maintenance) taking place at these different sequences. The dynamic changes in histone modifications and chromatin structure also need to be explored. As technological advances diminish the number of cells required to perform certain assays, techniques like chromatin immunoprecipitation (ChIP) will prove very valuable in identifying the proteins associated with methylated DNA, as well as the histone modifications present at these methylated loci during gametogenesis and early embryogenesis.

Efforts should be continued to study epigenetic events in human gametes and early embryos. A limited number of studies have provided some answers, but these studies were conducted on a small number of cells in most cases. Once it becomes technologically feasible, complete developmental studies using appropriate numbers of cells would be useful to delineate the epigenetic status of multiple genes and determine if the same enzymes identified in mouse are involved in epigenetic reprogramming during human gametogenesis and embryogenesis. This approach will also impact on our comprehension of human diseases with an epigenetic etiology and confirm the validity of animal models used to study epigenetics. Studies are required to determine whether there is an epigenetic basis for some cases of infertility in both males and females. Finally, recent studies suggesting connections between human ARTs and epigenetic defects in the offspring indicate that prospective studies of children conceived by ART should include monitoring for epigenetic abnormalities. More basic research on animal gametes and embryos is required to model procedures such as ICSI, superovulation and gamete and embryo culture. Although the mouse is an excellent model, other models where embryo development may be more similar to humans, such as bovine or non-human primates, should be examined.

Understanding epigenetic programming (i.e. the timing and mechanisms) has potentially important implications for human stem cell research (Sapienza, 2002). Two types of cells are potential sources of material for transplantation medicine: ES cells and EG cells. Both cell types can be cultured *in vitro* and their pluripotent nature makes them capable of differentiating into multiple cell types. While ES cells are derived from the inner cell mass of blastocysts, EG cells are derived from PGCs collected from developing gonads of human fetuses. It has been suggested that EG cells might be a preferable source to establish stable cell lines that could be used for transplantation medicine, since some studies have questioned the stability of epigenetic marks in ES cells (Dean *et al.*, 1998; Humpherys *et al.*, 2001). A better understanding of the mechanisms governing erasure and establishment of epigenetic marks in human PGCs will directly impact the use of EG cell lines destined for stem cell-derived therapies.

11.10 Conclusions

As further investigations tease apart the complex organization of epigenetic reprogramming in germ cells and early embryos, more light will be shed on the interrelated functions of epigenetic marks and the instructions they provide to support development. Various human diseases have been linked to alterations in DNA methylation or chromatin structure; the underlying cause of these diseases might be elucidated by studying epigenetic regulation of suspected gene(s) during development.

As our understanding of epigenetic reprogramming grows, new drugs targeting epigenetic regulators without affecting the reproductive system will be developed and prove useful in treating disorders caused by altered epigenetic states.

Acknowledgments

Dr. Jacquetta M. Trasler is a William Dawson Scholar of McGill University and a Scholar of the Fonds de la recherche en sante du Quebec; Sophie La Salle is the recipient of a Canadian Institutes of Health Research (CIHR) studentship. This work was supported by a grant from CIHR to J.M.T.

REFERENCES

Aapola U, Kawasaki K, Scott HS, Ollila J, Vihinen M, Heino M, Shintani A, Kawasaki K, Minoshima S, Krohn K et al. (2000) Isolation and initial characterization of a novel zinc finger gene, DNMT3L, on 21q22.3, related to the cytosine-5-methyltransferase 3 gene family. *Genomics* 65, 293–298.

Aapola U, Lyle R, Krohn K, Antonarakis SE and Peterson P (2001) Isolation and initial characterization of the mouse Dnmt3l gene. *Cytogenet Cell Genet* 92, 122–126.

Aapola U, Maenpaa K, Kaipia A and Peterson P (2004) Epigenetic modifications affect Dnmt3L expression. *Biochem J* 380, 705–713.

Aoki A, Suetake I, Miyagawa J, Fujio T, Chijiwa T, Sasaki H and Tajima S (2001) Enzymatic properties of *de novo*-type mouse DNA (cytosine-5) methyltransferases. *Nucleic Acids Res* 29, 3506–3512.

Ariel M, Cedar H and McCarrey J (1994) Developmental changes in methylation of spermatogenesis-specific genes include reprogramming in the epididymis. *Nat Genet* 7, 59–63.

Ayoub N, Richler C and Wahrman J (1997) Xist RNA is associated with the transcriptionally inactive XY body in mammalian male meiosis. *Chromosoma* 106, 1–10.

Bao S, Obata Y, Carroll J, Domeki I and Kono T (2000) Epigenetic modifications necessary for normal development are established during oocyte growth in mice. *Biol Reprod* 62, 616–621.

Bartolomei MS and Tilghman SM (1997) Genomic imprinting in mammals. *Annu Rev Genet* 31, 493–525.

Bartolomei MS, Zemel S and Tilghman SM (1991) Parental imprinting of the mouse H19 gene. *Nature* 351, 153–155.

Bartolomei MS, Webber AL, Brunkow ME and Tilghman SM (1993) Epigenetic mechanisms underlying the imprinting of the mouse H19 gene. *Genes Dev* 7, 1663–1673.

Bell AC and Felsenfeld G (2000) Methylation of a CTCF-dependent boundary controls imprinted expression of the Igf2 gene. *Nature* 405, 482–485.

Benoit G and Trasler JM (1994) Developmental expression of DNA methyltransferase messenger ribonucleic acid, protein, and enzyme activity in the mouse testis. *Biol Reprod* 50, 1312–1319.

Bestor TH (1992) Activation of mammalian DNA methyltransferase by cleavage of a Zn binding regulatory domain. *EMBO J* 11, 2611–2617.

Bestor TH (2000) The DNA methyltransferases of mammals. *Hum Mol Genet* 9, 2395–2402.

Bestor TH and Tycko B (1996) Creation of genomic methylation patterns. *Nat Genet* 12, 363–367.

Bestor T, Laudano A, Mattaliano R and Ingram V (1988) Cloning and sequencing of a cDNA encoding DNA methyltransferase of mouse cells. The carboxyl-terminal domain of the mammalian enzymes is related to bacterial restriction methyltransferases. *J Mol Biol* 203, 971–983.

Bonfils C, Beaulieu N, Chan E, Cotton-Montpetit J and MacLeod AR (2000) Characterization of the human DNA methyltransferase splice variant Dnmt1b. *J Biol Chem* 275, 10754–10760.

Bonny C and Goldberg E (1995) The CpG-rich promoter of human LDH-C is differentially methylated in expressing and nonexpressing tissues. *Dev Genet* 16, 210–217.

Bourc'his D and Bestor TH (2004) Meiotic catastrophe and retrotransposon reactivation in male germ cells lacking Dnmt3L. *Nature* 431, 96–99.

Bourc'his D, Xu GL, Lin CS, Bollman B and Bestor TH (2001) Dnmt3L and the establishment of maternal genomic imprints. *Science* 294, 2536–2539.

Brandeis M, Ariel M and Cedar H (1993) Dynamics of DNA methylation during development. *Bioessays* 15, 709–713.

Burgers WA, Fuks F and Kouzarides T (2002) DNA methyltransferases get connected to chromatin. *Trends Genet* 18, 275–277.

Carlson LL, Page AW and Bestor TH (1992) Properties and localization of DNA methyltransferase in preimplantation mouse embryos: implications for genomic imprinting. *Genes Dev* 6, 2536–2541.

Chaillet JR, Vogt TF, Beier DR and Leder P (1991) Parental-specific methylation of an imprinted transgene is established during gametogenesis and progressively changes during embryogenesis. *Cell* 66, 77–83.

Chedin F, Lieber MR and Hsieh CL (2002) The DNA methyltransferase-like protein DNMT3L stimulates *de novo* methylation by Dnmt3a. *Proc Natl Acad Sci USA* 99, 16916–16921.

Chen Z, Karaplis AC, Ackerman SL, Pogribny IP, Melnyk S, Lussier-Cacan S, Chen MF, Pai A, John SW, Smith RS *et al.* (2001) Mice deficient in methylenetetrahydrofolate reductase exhibit hyperhomocysteinemia and decreased methylation capacity, with neuropathology and aortic lipid deposition. *Hum Mol Genet* 10, 433–443.

Chen T, Ueda Y, Xie S and Li E (2002) A novel Dnmt3a isoform produced from an alternative promoter localizes to euchromatin and its expression correlates with active *de novo* methylation. *J Biol Chem* 277, 38746–38754.

Choi YC, Aizawa A and Hecht NB (1997) Genomic analysis of the mouse protamine 1, protamine 2, and transition protein 2 gene cluster reveals hypermethylation in expressing cells. *Mamm Genome* 8, 317–323.

Clark SJ, Harrison J, Paul CL and Frommer M (1994) High sensitivity mapping of methylated cytosines. *Nucleic Acids Res* 22, 2990–2997.

Coffigny H, Bourgeois C, Ricoul M, Bernardino J, Vilain A, Niveleau A, Malfoy B and Dutrillaux B (1999) Alterations of DNA methylation patterns in germ cells and Sertoli cells from developing mouse testis. *Cytogenet Cell Genet* 87, 175–181.

Davis TL, Trasler JM, Moss SB, Yang GJ and Bartolomei MS (1999) Acquisition of the H19 methylation imprint occurs differentially on the parental alleles during spermatogenesis. *Genomics* 58, 18–28.

Davis TL, Yang GJ, McCarrey JR and Bartolomei MS (2000) The H19 methylation imprint is erased and re-established differentially on the parental alleles during male germ cell development. *Hum Mol Genet* 9, 2885–2894.

De La Fuente R, Viveiros MM, Wigglesworth K and Eppig JJ (2004) ATRX, a member of the SNF2 family of helicase/ATPases, is required for chromosome alignment and meiotic spindle organization in metaphase II stage mouse oocytes. *Dev Biol* 272, 1–14.

Dean W, Bowden L, Aitchison A, Klose J, Moore T, Meneses JJ, Reik W and Feil R (1998) Altered imprinted gene methylation and expression in completely ES cell-derived mouse fetuses: association with aberrant phenotypes. *Development* 125, 2273–2282.

Dennis K, Fan T, Geiman T, Yan Q and Muegge K (2001) Lsh, a member of the SNF2 family, is required for genome-wide methylation. *Genes Dev* 15, 2940–2944.

Ding F, Patel C, Ratnam S, McCarrey JR and Chaillet JR (2003) Conservation of Dnmt1o cytosine methyltransferase in the marsupial *Monodelphis domestica*. *Genesis* 36, 209–213.

Doerksen T and Trasler JM (1996) Developmental exposure of male germ cells to 5-azacytidine results in abnormal preimplantation development in rats. *Biol Reprod* 55, 1155–1162.

Doerksen T, Benoit G and Trasler JM (2000) Deoxyribonucleic acid hypomethylation of male germ cells by mitotic and meiotic exposure to 5-azacytidine is associated with altered testicular histology. *Endocrinology* 141, 3235–3244.

Doherty AS, Mann MR, Tremblay KD, Bartolomei MS and Schultz RM (2000) Differential effects of culture on imprinted H19 expression in the preimplantation mouse embryo. *Biol Reprod* 62, 1526–1535.

Driscoll DJ and Migeon BR (1990) Sex difference in methylation of single-copy genes in human meiotic germ cells: implications for X chromosome inactivation, parental imprinting, and origin of CpG mutations. *Somat Cell Mol Genet* 16, 267–282.

Egger G, Liang G, Aparicio A and Jones PA (2004) Epigenetics in human disease and prospects for epigenetic therapy. *Nature* 429, 457–463.

El Maarri O, Buiting K, Peery EG, Kroisel PM, Balaban B, Wagner K, Urman B, Heyd J, Lich C, Brannan CI *et al.* (2001) Maternal methylation imprints on human chromosome 15 are established during or after fertilization. *Nat Genet* 27, 341–344.

Fan T, Hagan JP, Kozlov SV, Stewart CL and Muegge K (2005) Lsh controls silencing of the imprinted Cdkn1c gene. *Development* 132, 635–644.

Feng Q and Zhang Y (2001) The MeCP1 complex represses transcription through preferential binding, remodeling, and deacetylating methylated nucleosomes. *Genes Dev* 15, 827–832.

Fenic I, Sonnack V, Failing K, Bergmann M and Steger K (2004) *In vivo* effects of histone-deacetylase inhibitor trichostatin-A on murine spermatogenesis. *J Androl* 25, 811–818.

Ferguson-Smith AC, Sasaki H, Cattanach BM and Surani MA (1993) Parental–origin-specific epigenetic modification of the mouse H19 gene. *Nature* 362, 751–755.

Fernandez-Capetillo O, Mahadevaiah SK, Celeste A, Romanienko PJ, Camerini-Otero RD, Bonner WM, Manova K, Burgoyne P and Nussenzweig A (2003) H2AX is required for chromatin remodeling and inactivation of sex chromosomes in male mouse meiosis. *Dev Cell* 4, 497–508.

Frevel MA, Hornberg JJ and Reeve AE (1999) A potential imprint control element: identification of a conserved 42 bp sequence upstream of H19. *Trends Genet* 15, 216–218.

Frommer M, McDonald LE, Millar DS, Collis CM, Watt F, Grigg GW, Molloy PL and Paul CL (1992) A genomic sequencing protocol that yields a positive display of 5-methylcytosine residues in individual DNA strands. *Proc Natl Acad Sci USA* 89, 1827–1831.

Gabbara S and Bhagwat AS (1995) The mechanism of inhibition of DNA (cytosine-5-)-methyl-transferases by 5-azacytosine is likely to involve methyl transfer to the inhibitor. *Biochem J* 307 (Pt 1), 87–92.

Gazzoli I, Loda M, Garber J, Syngal S and Kolodner RD (2002) A hereditary nonpolyposis colorectal carcinoma case associated with hypermethylation of the MLH1 gene in normal tissue and loss of heterozygosity of the unmethylated allele in the resulting microsatellite instability-high tumor. *Cancer Res* 62, 3925–3928.

Geiman TM and Robertson KD (2002) Chromatin remodeling, histone modifications, and DNA methylation – How does it all fit together? *J Cell Biochem* 87, 117–125.

Geiman TM, Durum SK and Muegge K (1998) Characterization of gene expression, genomic structure, and chromosomal localization of Hells (Lsh). *Genomics* 54, 477–483.

Geiman TM, Tessarollo L, Anver MR, Kopp JB, Ward JM and Muegge K (2001) Lsh, a SNF2 family member, is required for normal murine development. *Biochim Biophys Acta* 1526, 211–220.

Geuns E, De Rycke M, Van Steirteghem A and Liebaers I (2003) Methylation imprints of the imprint control region of the SNRPN-gene in human gametes and preimplantation embryos. *Hum Mol Genet* 12, 2873–2879.

Geyer CB, Kiefer CM, Yang TP and McCarrey JR (2004) Ontogeny of a demethylation domain and its relationship to activation of tissue-specific transcription. *Biol Reprod* 71, 837–844.

Gibbons RJ, McDowell TL, Raman S, O'Rourke DM, Garrick D, Ayyub H and Higgs DR (2000) Mutations in ATRX, encoding a SWI/SNF-like protein, cause diverse changes in the pattern of DNA methylation. *Nat Genet* 24, 368–371.

Golding MC and Westhusin ME (2003) Analysis of DNA (cytosine 5) methyltransferase mRNA sequence and expression in bovine preimplantation embryos, fetal and adult tissues. *Gene Expr Patterns* 3, 551–558.

Goll MG and Bestor TH (2002) Histone modification and replacement in chromatin activation. *Genes Dev* 16, 1739–1742.

Goll MG and Bestor TH (2004) Eukaryotic cytosine methyltransferases. *Annu Rev Biochem* 74, 481–514.

Grewal SIS and Moazed D (2003) Heterochromatin and epigenetic control of gene expression. *Science* 301, 798–802.

Hajkova P, Erhardt S, Lane N, Haaf T, El Maarri O, Reik W, Walter J and Surani MA (2002) Epigenetic reprogramming in mouse primordial germ cells. *Mech Dev* 117, 15–23.

Hamatani T, Sasaki H, Ishihara K, Hida N, Maruyama T, Yoshimura Y, Hata J and Umezawa A (2001) Epigenetic mark sequence of the H19 gene in human sperm. *Biochim Biophys Acta* 1518, 137–144.

Handel MA (2004) The XY body: a specialized meiotic chromatin domain. *Exp Cell Res* 296, 57–63.

Hanel ML and Wevrick R (2001) Establishment and maintenance of DNA methylation patterns in mouse Ndn: implications for maintenance of imprinting in target genes of the imprinting center. *Mol Cell Biol* 21, 2384–2392.

Hark AT, Schoenherr CJ, Katz DJ, Ingram RS, Levorse JM and Tilghman SM (2000) CTCF mediates methylation-sensitive enhancer-blocking activity at the H19/Igf2 locus. *Nature* 405, 486–489.

Hata K, Okano M, Lei H and Li E (2002) Dnmt3L cooperates with the Dnmt3 family of *de novo* DNA methyltransferases to establish maternal imprints in mice. *Development* 129, 1983–1993.

Hayward BE, De Vos M, Judson H, Hodge D, Huntriss J, Picton HM, Sheridan E and Bonthron DT (2003) Lack of involvement of known DNA methyltransferases in familial hydatidiform mole implies the involvement of other factors in establishment of imprinting in the human female germline. *BMC Genet* 4, 2.

Hendrich B and Bickmore W (2001) Human diseases with underlying defects in chromatin structure and modification. *Hum Mol Genet* 10, 2233–2242.

Hermann A, Schmitt S and Jeltsch A (2003) The human Dnmt2 has residual DNA-(cytosine-C5) methyltransferase activity. *J Biol Chem* 278, 31717–31721.

Hermann A, Gowher H and Jeltsch A (2004) Biochemistry and biology of mammalian DNA methyltransferases. *Cell Mol Life Sci* 61, 2571–2587.

Holliday R and Pugh JE (1975) DNA modification mechanisms and gene activity during development. *Science* 187, 226–232.

Howell CY, Bestor TH, Ding F, Latham KE, Mertineit C, Trasler JM and Chaillet JR (2001) Genomic imprinting disrupted by a maternal effect mutation in the Dnmt1 gene. *Cell* 104, 829–838.

Howlett SK and Reik W (1991) Methylation levels of maternal and paternal genomes during preimplantation development. *Development* 113, 119–127.

Hsu DW, Lin MJ, Lee TL, Wen SC, Chen X and Shen CK (1999) Two major forms of DNA (cytosine-5) methyltransferase in human somatic tissues. *Proc Natl Acad Sci USA* 96, 9751–9756.

Humpherys D, Eggan K, Akutsu H, Hochedlinger K, Rideout III WM, Biniszkiewicz D, Yanagimachi R and Jaenisch R (2001) Epigenetic instability in ES cells and cloned mice. *Science* 293, 95–97.

Huntriss J, Daniels R, Bolton V and Monk M (1998) Imprinted expression of SNRPN in human preimplantation embryos. *Am J Hum Genet* 63, 1009–1014.

Huntriss J, Hinkins M, Oliver B, Harris SE, Beazley JC, Rutherford AJ, Gosden RG, Lanzendorf SE and Picton HM (2004) Expression of mRNAs for DNA methyltransferases and methyl-CpG-binding proteins in the human female germ line, preimplantation embryos, and embryonic stem cells. *Mol Reprod Dev* 67, 323–336.

Ishida C, Ura K, Hirao A, Sasaki H, Toyoda A, Sakaki Y, Niwa H, Li E and Kaneda Y (2003) Genomic organization and promoter analysis of the Dnmt3b gene. *Gene* 310, 151–159.

Jeanpierre M, Turleau C, Aurias A, Prieur M, Ledeist F, Fischer A and Viegas-Pequignot E (1993) An embryonic-like methylation pattern of classical satellite DNA is observed in ICF syndrome. *Hum Mol Genet* 2, 731–735.

Jiang YH, Bressler J and Beaudet AL (2004) Epigenetics and human disease. *Annu Rev Genomics Hum Genet* 5, 479–510.

Jinno Y, Sengoku K, Nakao M, Tamate K, Miyamoto T, Matsuzaka T, Sutcliffe JS, Anan T, Takuma N, Nishiwaki K *et al.* (1996) Mouse/human sequence divergence in a region with a paternal-specific methylation imprint at the human H19 locus. *Hum Mol Genet* 5, 1155–1161.

Jones PL, Veenstra GJC, Wade PA, Vermaak D, Kass SU, Landsberger N, Strouboulis J and Wolffe AP (1998) Methylated DNA and MeCP2 recruit histone deacetylase to repress transcription. *Nat Genet* 19, 187–191.

Judson H, Hayward BE, Sheridan E and Bonthron DT (2002) A global disorder of imprinting in the human female germ line. *Nature* 416, 539–542.

Jue K, Bestor TH and Trasler JM (1995a) Regulated synthesis and localization of DNA methyltransferase during spermatogenesis. *Biol Reprod* 53, 561–569.

Jue K, Benoit G, Alcivar-Warren AA and Trasler JM (1995b) Developmental and hormonal regulation of DNA methyltransferase in the rat testis. *Biol Reprod* 52, 1364–1371.

Kafri T, Ariel M, Brandeis M, Shemer R, Urven L, McCarrey J, Cedar H and Razin A (1992) Developmental pattern of gene-specific DNA methylation in the mouse embryo and germ line. *Genes Dev* 6, 705–714.

Kanai Y, Ushijima S, Nakanishi Y, Sakamoto M and Hirohashi S (2003) Mutation of the DNA methyltransferase (DNMT) 1 gene in human colorectal cancers. *Cancer Lett* 192, 75–82.

Kanduri C, Pant V, Loukinov D, Pugacheva E, Qi CF, Wolffe A, Ohlsson R and Lobanenkov VV (2000) Functional association of CTCF with the insulator upstream of the H19 gene is parent of origin-specific and methylation-sensitive. *Curr Biol* 10, 853–856.

Kane MF, Loda M, Gaida GM, Lipman J, Mishra R, Goldman H, Jessup JM and Kolodner R (1997) Methylation of the hMLH1 promoter correlates with lack of expression of hMLH1 in sporadic colon tumors and mismatch repair-defective human tumor cell lines. *Cancer Res* 57, 808–811.

Kaneda M, Okano M, Hata K, Sado T, Tsujimoto N, Li E and Sasaki H (2004) Essential role for *de novo* DNA methyltransferase Dnmt3a in paternal and maternal imprinting. *Nature* 429, 900–903.

Kato Y, Rideout III WM, Hilton K, Barton SC, Tsunoda Y and Surani MA (1999) Developmental potential of mouse primordial germ cells. *Development* 126, 1823–1832.

Kawasaki H and Taira K (2004) Induction of DNA methylation and gene silencing by short interfering RNAs in human cells. *Nature* 431, 211–217.

Kelly TL, Li E and Trasler JM (2003) 5-aza-2′-deoxycytidine induces alterations in murine spermatogenesis and pregnancy outcome. *J Androl* 24, 822–830.

Kelly TL, Neaga OR, Schwahn BC, Rozen R and Trasler JM (2005) Infertility in 5,10-methylenetetrahydrofolate reductase (MTHFR)-deficient male mice is partially alleviated by lifetime dietary betaine supplementation. *Biol Reprod* 72, 667–677.

Kerjean A, Dupont JM, Vasseur C, Le Tessier D, Cuisset L, Paldi A, Jouannet P and Jeanpierre M (2000) Establishment of the paternal methylation imprint of the human H19 and MEST/PEG1 genes during spermatogenesis. *Hum Mol Genet* 9, 2183–2187.

Khalil AM, Boyar FZ and Driscoll DJ (2004) Dynamic histone modifications mark sex chromosome inactivation and reactivation during mammalian spermatogenesis. *Proc Natl Acad Sci USA* 101, 16583–16587.

Khosla S, Dean W, Brown D, Reik W and Feil R (2001) Culture of preimplantation mouse embryos affects fetal development and the expression of imprinted genes. *Biol Reprod* 64, 918–926.

Kimura Y and Yanagimachi R (1995) Development of normal mice from oocytes injected with secondary spermatocyte nuclei. *Biol Reprod* 53, 855–862.

Kimura Y, Tateno H, Handel MA and Yanagimachi R (1998) Factors affecting meiotic and developmental competence of primary spermatocyte nuclei injected into mouse oocytes. *Biol Reprod* 59, 871–877.

Ko YG, Nishino K, Hattori N, Arai Y, Tanaka S and Shiota K (2005) Stage-by-stage change in DNA methylation status of DNA methyltransferase 1 (Dnmt1) locus during mouse early development. *J Biol Chem* 280, 9627–9634.

Kondo T, Bobek MP, Kuick R, Lamb B, Zhu X, Narayan A, Bourc'his D, Viegas-Pequignot E, Ehrlich M and Hanash SM (2000) Whole-genome methylation scan in ICF syndrome: hypomethylation of non-satellite DNA repeats D4Z4 and NBL2. *Hum Mol Genet* 9, 597–604.

Kono T, Obata Y, Yoshimzu T, Nakahara T and Carroll J (1996) Epigenetic modifications during oocyte growth correlates with extended parthenogenetic development in the mouse. *Nat Genet* 13, 91–94.

Kroft TL, Jethanandani P, McLean DJ and Goldberg E (2001) Methylation of CpG dinucleotides alters binding and silences testis-specific transcription directed by the mouse lactate dehydrogenase C promoter. *Biol Reprod* 65, 1522–1527.

La Salle S, Mertineit C, Taketo T, Moens PB, Bestor TH and Trasler JM (2004) Windows for sex-specific methylation marked by DNA methyltransferase expression profiles in mouse germ cells. *Dev Biol* 268, 403–415.

Lane N, Dean W, Erhardt S, Hajkova P, Surani A, Walter J and Reik W (2003) Resistance of IAPs to methylation reprogramming may provide a mechanism for epigenetic inheritance in the mouse. *Genesis* 35, 88–93.

Lee J, Inoue K, Ono R, Ogonuki N, Kohda T, Kaneko-Ishino T, Ogura A and Ishino F (2002) Erasing genomic imprinting memory in mouse clone embryos produced from day 11.5 primordial germ cells. *Development* 129, 1807–1817.

Lees-Murdock DJ, De Felici M and Walsh CP (2003) Methylation dynamics of repetitive DNA elements in the mouse germ cell lineage. *Genomics* 82, 230–237.

Lehnertz B, Ueda Y, Derijck AAHA, Braunschweig U, Perez-Burgos L, Kubicek S, Chen TP, Li E, Jenuwein T and Peters AHFM (2003) Suv39h-mediated histone H3 lysine 9 methylation directs DNA methylation to major satellite repeats at pericentric heterochromatin. *Curr Biol* 13, 1192–1200.

Lei H, Oh SP, Okano M, Juttermann R, Goss KA, Jaenisch R and Li E (1996) *De novo* DNA cytosine methyltransferase activities in mouse embryonic stem cells. *Development* 122, 3195–3205.

Li E (2002) Chromatin modification and epigenetic reprogramming in mammalian development. *Nat Rev Genet* 3, 662–673.

Li E, Bestor TH and Jaenisch R (1992) Targeted mutation of the DNA methyltransferase gene results in embryonic lethality. *Cell* 69, 915–926.

Li E, Beard C and Jaenisch R (1993) Role for DNA methylation in genomic imprinting. *Nature* 366, 362–365.

Li JY, Lees-Murdock DJ, Xu GL and Walsh CP (2004) Timing of establishment of paternal methylation imprints in the mouse. *Genomics* 84, 952–960.

Lippman Z and Martienssen R (2004b) The role of RNA interference in heterochromatic silencing. *Nature* 431, 364–370.

Lucifero D, Mertineit C, Clarke HJ, Bestor TH and Trasler JM (2002) Methylation dynamics of imprinted genes in mouse germ cells. *Genomics* 79, 530–538.

Lucifero D, Mann MR, Bartolomei MS and Trasler JM (2004a) Gene-specific timing and epigenetic memory in oocyte imprinting. *Hum Mol Genet* 13, 839–849.

Lucifero D, Chaillet JR and Trasler JM (2004b) Potential significance of genomic imprinting defects for reproduction and assisted reproductive technology. *Hum Reprod Update* 10, 3–18.

Ludwig M, Katalinic A, Gross S, Sutcliffe A, Varon R and Horsthemke B (2005) Increased prevalence of imprinting defects in patients with Angelman syndrome born to subfertile couples. *J Med Genet* 42, 289–291.

MacLean JA and Wilkinson MF (2005) Gene regulation in spermatogenesis. *Curr Top Dev Bio*, in press.

Marahrens Y, Panning B, Dausman J, Strauss W and Jaenisch R (1997) Xist-deficient mice are defective in dosage compensation but not spermatogenesis. *Genes Dev* 11, 156–166.

Margot JB, Ehrenhofer-Murray AE and Leonhardt H (2003) Interactions within the mammalian DNA methyltransferase family. *BMC Mol Biol* 4, 7.

Marques CJ, Carvalho F, Sousa M and Barros A (2004) Genomic imprinting in disruptive spermatogenesis. *Lancet* 363, 1700–1702.

Mayer W, Niveleau A, Walter J, Fundele R and Haaf T (2000) Demethylation of the zygotic paternal genome. *Nature* 403, 501–502.

McCarrey JR and Dilworth DD (1992) Expression of Xist in mouse germ cells correlates with X-chromosome inactivation. *Nat Genet* 2, 200–203.

McCarrey JR, Berg WM, Paragioudakis SJ, Zhang PL, Dilworth DD, Arnold BL and Rossi JJ (1992) Differential transcription of Pgk genes during spermatogenesis in the mouse. *Dev Biol* 154, 160–168.

McCarrey JR, Watson C, Atencio J, Ostermeier GC, Marahrens Y, Jaenisch R and Krawetz SA (2002) X-chromosome inactivation during spermatogenesis is regulated by an Xist/Tsix-independent mechanism in the mouse. *Genesis* 34, 257–266.

McDowell TL, Gibbons RJ, Sutherland H, O'Rourke DM, Bickmore WA, Pombo A, Turley H, Gatter K, Picketts DJ, Buckle VJ et al. (1999) Localization of a putative transcriptional regulator (ATRX) at pericentromeric heterochromatin and the short arms of acrocentric chromosomes. *Proc Natl Acad Sci USA* 96, 13983–13988.

Mertineit C, Yoder JA, Taketo T, Laird DW, Trasler JM and Bestor TH (1998) Sex-specific exons control DNA methyltransferase in mammalian germ cells. *Development* 125, 889–897.

Moglabey YB, Kircheisen R, Seoud M, El Mogharbel N, Van dV I and Slim R (1999) Genetic mapping of a maternal locus responsible for familial hydatidiform moles. *Hum Mol Genet* 8, 667–671.

Monk M, Boubelik M and Lehnert S (1987) Temporal and regional changes in DNA methylation in the embryonic, extraembryonic and germ-cell lineages during mouse embryo development. *Development* 99, 371–382.

Morgan HD, Sutherland HG, Martin DI and Whitelaw E (1999) Epigenetic inheritance at the agouti locus in the mouse. *Nat Genet* 23, 314–318.

Morris KV, Chan SWL, Jacobsen SE and Looney DJ (2004) Small interfering RNA-induced transcriptional gene silencing in human cells. *Science* 305, 1289–1292.

Nan XS, Ng HH, Johnson CA, Laherty CD, Turner BM, Eisenman RN and Bird A (1998) Transcriptional repression by the methyl-CpG-binding protein MeCP2 involves a histone deacetylase complex. *Nature* 393, 386–389.

Ng HH, Zhang Y, Hendrich B, Johnson CA, Turner BM, Erdjument-Bromage H, Tempst P, Reinberg D and Bird A (1999) MBD2 is a transcriptional repressor belonging to the MeCP1 histone deacetylase complex. *Nat Genet* 23, 58–61.

O'Carroll D, Scherthan H, Peters AH, Opravil S, Haynes AR, Laible G, Rea S, Schmid M, Lebersorger A, Jerratsch M *et al.* (2000) Isolation and characterization of Suv39h2, a second histone H3 methyltransferase gene that displays testis-specific expression. *Mol Cell Biol* 20, 9423–9433.

O'Neill RJ, O'Neill MJ and Graves JA (1998) Undermethylation associated with retroelement activation and chromosome remodelling in an interspecific mammalian hybrid. *Nature* 393, 68–72.

Oakeley EJ (1999) DNA methylation analysis: a review of current methodologies. *Pharmacol Ther* 84, 389–400.

Obata Y and Kono T (2002) Maternal primary imprinting is established at a specific time for each gene throughout oocyte growth. *J Biol Chem* 277, 5285–5289.

Obata Y, Kaneko-Ishino T, Koide T, Takai Y, Ueda T, Domeki I, Shiroishi T, Ishino F and Kono T (1998) Disruption of primary imprinting during oocyte growth leads to the modified expression of imprinted genes during embryogenesis. *Development* 125, 1553–1560.

Ohhata T, Tachibana M, Tada M, Tada T, Sasaki H, Shinkai Y and Sado T (2004) X-inactivation is stably maintained in mouse embryos deficient for histone methyl transferase G9a. *Genesis* 40, 151–156.

Okano M, Xie S and Li E (1998) Cloning and characterization of a family of novel mammalian DNA (cytosine-5) methyltransferases. *Nat Genet* 19, 219–220.

Okano M, Bell DW, Haber DA and Li E (1999) DNA methyltransferases Dnmt3a and Dnmt3b are essential for *de novo* methylation and mammalian development. *Cell* 99, 247–257.

Olek A and Walter J (1997) The pre-implantation ontogeny of the H19 methylation imprint. *Nat Genet* 17, 275–276.

Onyango P, Jiang S, Uejima H, Shamblott MJ, Gearhart JD, Cui H and Feinberg AP (2002) Monoallelic expression and methylation of imprinted genes in human and mouse embryonic germ cell lineages. *Proc Natl Acad Sci USA* 99, 10599–10604.

Oswald J, Engemann S, Lane N, Mayer W, Olek A, Fundele R, Dean W, Reik W and Walter J (2000) Active demethylation of the paternal genome in the mouse zygote. *Curr Biol* 10, 475–478.

Panning B and Jaenisch R (1996) DNA hypomethylation can activate Xist expression and silence X-linked genes. *Genes Dev* 10, 1991–2002.

Panning B and Jaenisch R (1998) RNA and the epigenetic regulation of X chromosome inactivation. *Cell* 93, 305–308.

Peters AH, O'Carroll D, Scherthan H, Mechtler K, Sauer S, Schofer C, Weipoltshammer K, Pagani M, Lachner M, Kohlmaier A *et al.* (2001) Loss of the Suv39h histone methyltransferases impairs mammalian heterochromatin and genome stability. *Cell* 107, 323–337.

Raabe EH, Abdurrahman L, Behbehani G and Arceci RJ (2001) An SNF2 factor involved in mammalian development and cellular proliferation. *Dev Dyn* 221, 92–105.

Rakyan VK, Preis J, Morgan HD and Whitelaw E (2001) The marks, mechanisms and memory of epigenetic states in mammals. *Biochem J* 356, 1–10.

Rakyan VK, Chong S, Champ ME, Cuthbert PC, Morgan HD, Luu KV and Whitelaw E (2003) Transgenerational inheritance of epigenetic states at the murine Axin(Fu) allele occurs after maternal and paternal transmission. *Proc Natl Acad Sci USA* 100, 2538–2543.

Ratnam S, Mertineit C, Ding F, Howell CY, Clarke HJ, Bestor TH, Chaillet JR and Trasler JM (2002) Dynamics of Dnmt1 methyltransferase expression and intracellular localization during oogenesis and preimplantation development. *Dev Biol* 245, 304–314.

Reik W and Walter J (2001) Genomic imprinting: parental influence on the genome. *Nat Rev Genet* 2, 21–32.

Reik W, Dean W and Walter J (2001) Epigenetic reprogramming in mammalian development. *Science* 293, 1089–1093.

Rice JC and Allis CD (2001) Histone methylation versus histone acetylation: new insights into epigenetic regulation. *Curr Opin Cell Biol* 13, 263–273.

Rice JC, Briggs SD, Ueberheide B, Barber CM, Shabanowitz J, Hunt DF, Shinkai Y and Allis CD (2003) Histone methyltransferases direct different degrees of methylation to define distinct chromatin domains. *Mol Cell* 12, 1591–1598.

Riggs AD (1975) X inactivation, differentiation, and DNA methylation. *Cytogenet Cell Genet* 14, 9–25.

Rougeulle C and Heard E (2002) Antisense RNA in imprinting: spreading silence through Air. *Trends Genet* 18, 434–437.

Rougier N, Bourc'his D, Gomes DM, Niveleau A, Plachot M, Paldi A and Viegas-Pequignot E (1998) Chromosome methylation patterns during mammalian preimplantation development. *Genes Dev* 12, 2108–2113.

Saito Y, Kanai Y, Sakamoto M, Saito H, Ishii H and Hirohashi S (2002) Overexpression of a splice variant of DNA methyltransferase 3b, DNMT3b4, associated with DNA hypomethylation on pericentromeric satellite regions during human hepatocarcinogenesis. *Proc Natl Acad Sci USA* 99, 10060–10065.

Sakai Y, Suetake I, Itoh K, Mizugaki M, Tajima S and Yamashina S (2001) Expression of DNA methyltransferase (Dnmt1) in testicular germ cells during development of mouse embryo. *Cell Struct Funct* 26, 685–691.

Sakai Y, Suetake I, Shinozaki F, Yamashina S and Tajima S (2004) Co-expression of de novo DNA methyltransferases Dnmt3a2 and Dnmt3L in gonocytes of mouse embryos. *Gene Expr Patterns* 5, 231–237.

Salido EC, Yen PH, Mohandas TK and Shapiro LJ (1992) Expression of the X-inactivation-associated gene XIST during spermatogenesis. *Nat Genet* 2, 196–199.

Sanford JP, Clark HJ, Chapman VM and Rossant J (1987) Differences in DNA methylation during oogenesis and spermatogenesis and their persistence during early embryogenesis in the mouse. *Genes Dev* 1, 1039–1046.

Santos F and Dean W (2004) Epigenetic reprogramming during early development in mammals. *Reproduction* 127, 643–651.

Santos F, Hendrich B, Reik W and Dean W (2002) Dynamic reprogramming of DNA methylation in the early mouse embryo. *Dev Biol* 241, 172–182.

Sapienza C (2002) Imprinted gene expression, transplantation medicine, and the 'other' human embryonic stem cell. *Proc Natl Acad Sci USA* 99, 10243–10245.

Sasagawa I, Kuretake S, Eppig JJ and Yanagimachi R (1998) Mouse primary spermatocytes can complete two meiotic divisions within the oocyte cytoplasm. *Biol Reprod* 58, 248–254.

Schmidt JV, Matteson PG, Jones BK, Guan XJ and Tilghman SM (2000) The Dlk1 and Gtl2 genes are linked and reciprocally imprinted. *Genes Dev* 14, 1997–2002.

Shamanski FL, Kimura Y, Lavoir MC, Pedersen RA and Yanagimachi R (1999) Status of genomic imprinting in mouse spermatids. *Hum Reprod* 14, 1050–1056.

Shiraishi M, Oates AJ and Sekiya T (2002) An overview of the analysis of DNA methylation in mammalian genomes. *Biol Chem* 383, 893–906.

Smit AF (1996) The origin of interspersed repeats in the human genome. *Curr Opin Genet Dev* 6, 743–748.

Sofikitis N, Mantzavinos T, Loutradis D, Yamamoto Y, Tarlatzis V and Miyagawa I (1998) Ooplasmic injections of secondary spermatocytes for non-obstructive azoospermia. *Lancet* 351, 1177–1178.

Spahn L and Barlow DP (2003) An ICE pattern crystallizes. *Nat Genet* 35, 11–12.

Stoger R, Kubicka P, Liu CG, Kafri T, Razin A, Cedar H and Barlow DP (1993) Maternal-specific methylation of the imprinted mouse Igf2r locus identifies the expressed locus as carrying the imprinting signal. *Cell* 73, 61–71.

Suetake I, Shinozaki F, Miyagawa J, Takeshima H and Tajima S (2004) DNMT3L stimulates the DNA methylation activity of Dnmt3a and Dnmt3b through a direct interaction. *J Biol Chem* 279, 27816–27823.

Suter CM, Martin DI and Ward RL (2004) Germline epimutation of MLH1 in individuals with multiple cancers. *Nat Genet* 36, 497–501.

Szabo PE and Mann JR (1995) Biallelic expression of imprinted genes in the mouse germ line: implications for erasure, establishment, and mechanisms of genomic imprinting. *Genes Dev* 9, 1857–1868.

Szabo PE, Hubner K, Scholer H and Mann JR (2002) Allele-specific expression of imprinted genes in mouse migratory primordial germ cells. *Mech Dev* 115, 157–160.

Tachibana M, Sugimoto K, Nozaki M, Ueda J, Ohta T, Ohki M, Fukuda M, Takeda N, Niida H, Kato H *et al.* (2002) G9a histone methyltransferase plays a dominant role in euchromatic histone H3 lysine 9 methylation and is essential for early embryogenesis. *Genes Dev* 16, 1779–1791.

Takada S, Tevendale M, Baker J, Georgiades P, Campbell E, Freeman T, Johnson MH, Paulsen M and Ferguson-Smith AC (2000) Delta-like and gtl2 are reciprocally expressed, differentially methylated linked imprinted genes on mouse chromosome 12. *Curr Biol* 10, 1135–1138.

Takada S, Paulsen M, Tevendale M, Tsai CE, Kelsey G, Cattanach BM and Ferguson-Smith AC (2002) Epigenetic analysis of the Dlk1-Gtl2 imprinted domain on mouse chromosome 12: implications for imprinting control from comparison with Igf2-H19. *Hum Mol Genet* 11, 77–86.

Tesarik J, Guido M, Mendoza C and Greco E (1998) Human spermatogenesis *in vitro*: respective effects of follicle-stimulating hormone and testosterone on meiosis, spermiogenesis, and Sertoli cell apoptosis. *J Clin Endocrinol Metab* 83, 4467–4473.

Tesarik J, Bahceci M, Ozcan C, Greco E and Mendoza C (1999) Restoration of fertility by *in-vitro* spermatogenesis. *Lancet* 353, 555–556.

Trasler JM, Hake LE, Johnson PA, Alcivar AA, Millette CF and Hecht NB (1990) DNA methylation and demethylation events during meiotic prophase in the mouse testis. *Mol Cell Biol* 10, 1828–1834.

Trasler JM, Alcivar AA, Hake LE, Bestor T and Hecht NB (1992) DNA methyltransferase is developmentally expressed in replicating and non-replicating male germ cells. *Nucleic Acids Res* 20, 2541–2545.

Tremblay KD, Saam JR, Ingram RS, Tilghman SM and Bartolomei MS (1995) A paternal-specific methylation imprint marks the alleles of the mouse H19 gene. *Nat Genet* 9, 407–413.

Tremblay KD, Duran KL and Bartolomei MS (1997) A 5′ 2-kilobase-pair region of the imprinted mouse H19 gene exhibits exclusive paternal methylation throughout development. *Mol Cell Biol* 17, 4322–4329.

Tsai MC, Takeuchi T, Bedford JM, Reis MM, Rosenwaks Z and Palermo GD (2000) Alternative sources of gametes: reality or science fiction? *Hum Reprod* 15, 988–998.

Turner JM, Mahadevaiah SK, Elliott DJ, Garchon HJ, Pehrson JR, Jaenisch R and Burgoyne PS (2002) Meiotic sex chromosome inactivation in male mice with targeted disruptions of Xist. *J Cell Sci* 115, 4097–4105.

Tycko B and Morison IM (2002) Physiological functions of imprinted genes. *J Cell Physiol* 192, 245–258.

Ueda T, Yamazaki K, Suzuki R, Fujimoto H, Sasaki H, Sakaki Y and Higashinakagawa T (1992) Parental methylation patterns of a transgenic locus in adult somatic tissues are imprinted during gametogenesis. *Development* 116, 831–839.

Ueda T, Abe K, Miura A, Yuzuriha M, Zubair M, Noguchi M, Niwa K, Kawase Y, Kono T, Matsuda Y *et al.* (2000) The paternal methylation imprint of the mouse H19 locus is acquired in the gonocyte stage during foetal testis development. *Genes Cells* 5, 649–659.

Verona RI, Mann MR and Bartolomei MS (2003) Genomic imprinting: intricacies of epigenetic regulation in clusters. *Annu Rev Cell Dev Biol* 19, 237–259.

Viegas-Pequignot E and Dutrillaux B (1976) Segmentation of human chromosomes induced by 5-ACR (5-azacytidine). *Hum Genet* 34, 247–254.

Wade PA, Gegonne A, Jones PL, Ballestar E, Aubry F and Wolffe AP (1999) Mi-2 complex couples DNA methylation to chromatin remodelling and histone deacetylation. *Nat Genet* 23, 62–66.

Walsh CP, Chaillet JR and Bestor TH (1998) Transcription of IAP endogenous retroviruses is constrained by cytosine methylation. *Nat Genet* 20, 116–117.

Watanabe D, Suetake I, Tada T and Tajima S (2002) Stage- and cell-specific expression of Dnmt3a and Dnmt3b during embryogenesis. *Mech Dev* 118, 187–190.

Watanabe D, Suetake I, Tajima S and Hanaoka K (2004) Expression of Dnmt3b in mouse hematopoietic progenitor cells and spermatogonia at specific stages. *Gene Expr Patterns* 5, 43–49.

Waterland RA and Jirtle RL (2003) Transposable elements: targets for early nutritional effects on epigenetic gene regulation. *Mol Cell Biol* 23, 5293–5300.

Webster KE, O'Bryan MK, Fletcher S, Crewther PE, Aapola U, Craig J, Harrison DK, Aung H, Phutikanit N, Lyle R *et al.* (2005) Meiotic and epigenetic defects in Dnmt3L-knockout mouse spermatogenesis. *Proc Natl Acad Sci USA* 102, 4068–4073.

Weisenberger DJ, Velicescu M, Preciado-Lopez MA, Gonzales FA, Tsai YC, Liang G and Jones PA (2002) Identification and characterization of alternatively spliced variants of DNA methyltransferase 3a in mammalian cells. *Gene* 298, 91–99.

Weisenberger DJ, Velicescu M, Cheng JC, Gonzales FA, Liang G and Jones PA (2004) Role of the DNA methyltransferase variant DNMT3b3 in DNA methylation. *Mol Cancer Res* 2, 62–72.

Wolff GL, Kodell RL, Moore SR and Cooney CA (1998) Maternal epigenetics and methyl supplements affect agouti gene expression in Avy/a mice. *FASEB J* 12, 949–957.

Wylie AA, Murphy SK, Orton TC and Jirtle RL (2000) Novel imprinted DLK1/GTL2 domain on human chromosome 14 contains motifs that mimic those implicated in IGF2/H19 regulation. *Genome Res* 10, 1711–1718.

Xie S, Wang Z, Okano M, Nogami M, Li Y, He WW, Okumura K and Li E (1999) Cloning, expression and chromosome locations of the human DNMT3 gene family. *Gene* 236, 87–95.

Xin Z, Tachibana M, Guggiari M, Heard E, Shinkai Y and Wagstaff J (2003) Role of histone methyltransferase G9a in CpG methylation of the Prader–Willi syndrome imprinting center. *J Biol Chem* 278, 14996–15000.

Xu GL, Bestor TH, Bourc'his D, Hsieh CL, Tommerup N, Bugge M, Hulten M, Qu X, Russo JJ and Viegas-Pequignot E (1999) Chromosome instability and immunodeficiency syndrome caused by mutations in a DNA methyltransferase gene. *Nature* 402, 187–191.

Yamazaki Y, Mann MR, Lee SS, Marh J, McCarrey JR, Yanagimachi R and Bartolomei MS (2003) Reprogramming of primordial germ cells begins before migration into the genital ridge, making these cells inadequate donors for reproductive cloning. *Proc Natl Acad Sci USA* 100, 12207–12212.

Yan Q, Huang J, Fan T, Zhu H and Muegge K (2003) Lsh, a modulator of CpG methylation, is crucial for normal histone methylation. *EMBO J* 22, 5154–5162.

Yanagisawa Y, Ito E, Yuasa Y and Maruyama K (2002) The human DNA methyltransferases DNMT3A and DNMT3B have two types of promoters with different CpG contents. *Biochim Biophys Acta* 1577, 457–465.

Yoder JA and Bestor TH (1998) A candidate mammalian DNA methyltransferase related to pmt1p of fission yeast. *Hum Mol Genet* 7, 279–284.

Yoder JA, Walsh CP and Bestor TH (1997) Cytosine methylation and the ecology of intragenomic parasites. *Trends Genet* 13, 335–340.

Yoon BJ, Herman H, Sikora A, Smith LT, Plass C and Soloway PD (2002) Regulation of DNA methylation of Rasgrf1. *Nat Genet* 30, 92–96.

Zhang Y, Ng HH, Erdjument-Bromage H, Tempst P, Bird A and Reinberg D (1999) Analysis of the NuRD subunits reveals a HDACs core complex and a connection with DNA methylation. *Genes Dev* 13, 1924–1935.

12

The *DAZ* gene family and human germ cell development from embryonic stem cells

Mark S. Fox, Renee A. Reijo Pera and Amander T. Clark

Program in Human Embryonic Stem Cell Biology; Center for Reproductive Sciences; Departments of Obstetrics, Gynecology and Reproductive Sciences, Physiology and Urology, and Programs in Developmental and Stem Cell Biology and Human Genetics; University of California; San Francisco, CA, USA

12.1 Introduction

Ten to fifteen percent of couples are infertile (Hull *et al.*, 1985). Yet, very little is known of the genetics of infertility in men or women. Given the heavy reliance upon technology in Western countries to bypass germ cell defects, it is timely that we begin to understand the genetics of infertility and the outcomes to the reproductive and somatic development of children that are conceived. Here we discuss studies that led to a greater understanding of one gene family implicated in human germ cell development, the *DAZ* (*Deleted in AZoospermia*) gene family and then review findings of experiments aimed at establishing an *in vitro* genetic system to study human germ cell formation and early differentiation. These studies provide the framework for building the genetic tools that are required to probe the functional genetics of germ cell development in men and women. With time, we expect that the availability of a system to assay the complex functions of human genes and gene variants *in vitro* will result in increased ability to design rational therapeutics for germ cell defects, to accurately assess outcomes of infertility treatments, to minimize risks associated with use of assisted reproduction and to develop useful genetic tests to aid infertile couples.

12.1.1 Specification of the germ cell lineage *in vivo* in model organisms

Two divergent developmental programs are associated with specification of the germ cell lineage in model organisms. In non-mammalian species such as worms, flies and frogs, germ cells of both males and females are specified via the inheritance of germ plasm, microscopically distinct oocyte cytoplasm that is particularly rich in RNAs and RNA-binding proteins; cells that inherit germ plasm upon cell division are destined to be germ cells (Houston and King, 2000b; Saffman and Lasko, 1999).

Some of the RNAs and RNA-binding proteins that are components of germ plasm, such as Pumilio, Nanos and Dazl (*DAZ-Like*), are highly conserved between organisms that specify germ cells via germ plasm inheritance and those that specify germ cells via a second mechanism (Jaruzelska *et al.*, 2003; Moore *et al.*, 2003; Saffman and Lasko, 1999; Tsuda *et al.*, 2003).

In mammalian species such as the mouse, microscopic germ plasm has not been observed early in development; instead, male and female germ cells are specified independently of germ plasm as a result of inductive signaling (Saffman and Lasko, 1999). Studies that map the fate of regional tissues in the pre-implantation mouse have revealed that mouse germ cells are specified in the proximal epiblast just after blastocyst formation or prior to gastrulation (Tam and Zhou, 1996), in response to signals from the neighboring extraembryonic ectodermal tissue (Fujiwara *et al.*, 2001). However, development of germ cells from the proximal epiblast is not hardwired as transplantation of other tissues, such as the distal epiblast to contact the extraembryonic ectoderm, also results in germ cell formation (Tam and Zhou, 1996). Thus, it is the extraembryonic ectoderm that provides one of the first signals for, or induces, germ cell specification in the epiblast. Following this inductive signaling, germ cells are then first recognized at embryonic day (E) 7.2 as cluster of extraembryonic cells that express distinctive marker RNAs and proteins such as tissue non-specific alkaline phosphatase (*TNAP*), Oct4 and *stella*, at the base of the allantois following gastrulation (Chiquoine, 1954; Saitou *et al.*, 2002; Scholer *et al.*, 1990a, b).

During the time of germ cell formation at gastrulation, the epiblast cells which give rise to germ cells will migrate through a region of the embryo termed the primitive streak. However, recent studies have demonstrated that there is not a requirement for the physical act of migration in order to promote the germ cell versus somatic cell fate (Pesce *et al.*, 2002; Ying *et al.*, 2001; Yoshimizu *et al.*, 2001). Growth of isolated epiblast at E6.0 on fibroblast feeder layers can specify primordial germ cell (PGC) differentiation from the epiblast explant (Yoshimizu *et al.*, 2001). Furthermore, just half a day earlier at E5.5, epiblast explants grown on fibroblast feeder layers are not capable of producing PGCs, unless co-cultured with extraembryonic ectoderm (Yoshimizu *et al.*, 2001). Thus, two conclusions regarding germ cell formation in mice can be made from these studies. First, the physical act of gastrulation is not necessary for germ cell specification and second, E5.5 epiblast cells that have not received signals from the extraembryonic ectoderm do not produce germ cells.

The embryological period equivalent to mouse E5.5–E7.2 in human embryo development occurs shortly after implantation. Thus, the analysis of human germ cell specification *in vivo* is impracticable due to ethical considerations regarding research during this period. However, recent studies in mice and humans have shown that embryonic stem cells (ESCs) (derived from the inner cell mass (ICM) of the blastocyst prior to epiblast formation) are capable of differentiating into female and male germ cells *in vitro*, thus providing a potential system to study germ cell development in its earliest stages, at the 'birth of germ cells' (Clark *et al.*, 2004a; Geijsen *et al.*, 2004; Hubner *et al.*, 2003; Toyooka *et al.*, 2003). Together these studies indicated that ESCs are capable of spontaneously forming germ cells *in vitro* and allowed comparisons between the mouse and human systems (Geijsen *et al.*, 2004; Hubner *et al.*, 2003; Toyooka *et al.*, 2003). We discuss this data in more detail below.

12.1.2 The relationship of ESCs and germ cells

Several novel findings are emerging from recent studies of ESC-derived germ cells. To review, mammalian ESCs, including human ESCs (hESCs), are derived from the ICM of blastocysts (Buehr and Smith, 2003; Evans and Hunter, 2002; Thomson *et al.*, 1998). In light of this fact, it might be logical to assume that cells of the ICM and ESCs are closely related or equivalent. However, recent data, discussed below, suggests strongly that ESCs and ICM cells are not equivalent and that hESCs are most closely related to PGCs (Clark *et al.*, 2004a; Evans and Hunter, 2002; Zwaka and Thomson, 2005). This observation has the practical implication that studies of ESCs and PGCs may have more in common than originally anticipated.

12.1.3 Justification for studying human germ cell development

Given the existence of excellent model systems to probe the genetics of germ cell development, one could question the need to specifically understand human germ cell development as it undoubtedly shares similarity with that of the mouse. However, as noted briefly above, there are many unique aspects to human germ cell development including the following: First, several human X and Y chromosome genes are expressed in different dosages or even absent in mice (Reijo *et al.*, 1995, 1996a; Skaletsky *et al.*, 2003; Vogt *et al.*, 1996; Zinn *et al.*, 1993). Thus, complete understanding of development of germ cells is difficult on a genetic background that lacks key regulators. Second, reproductive genes and proteins are known to evolve more rapidly than somatic genes (Hendry *et al.*, 2000; Swanson and Vacquier, 2002). For example, the amino acid sequences of the human genes that we recently identified, *STELLAR*, *GDF3* and *NANOG* are only 30% identical to the mouse homologs and have distinct differences in expression (Clark *et al.*, 2004b; Saitou *et al.*, 2002). Third, humans are remarkably infertile compared to other species, with nearly half of all infertility cases linked to faulty germ cell development (Menken and Larsen, 1994). Fourth, humans are remarkably imprecise in aspects of germ cell development that are reportedly highly conserved. For example, meiotic chromosome missegregation occurs in yeast in approximately 1/10,000 cells. In flies, missegregation occurs in 1/1000 to 1/2000 cells and in mice in fewer than 1/100. In humans, meiotic missegregation occurs in 5–20% of cells depending on sex and age

(Hunt and Hassold, 2002). Observations such as these are indicative of fundamental differences in the biology of human germ cells and highlight the necessity for exploration of the genetics of human germ cell biology directly.

12.2 The *DAZ* gene family and human germ cell development

12.2.1 DAZ, DAZL and interacting proteins

One of the best characterized gene families implicated in human germ cell development is the *DAZ* gene family (Agulnik *et al.*, 1998; Bielawski and Yang, 2001; Bienvenu *et al.*, 2001; Brekhman *et al.*, 2000; Carani *et al.*, 1997; Chai *et al.*, 1997; Cheng *et al.*, 1998; Cooke *et al.*, 1996; Dai *et al.*, 2001; Delbridge *et al.*, 1997; Dorfman *et al.*, 1999; Foresta *et al.*, 1997; Glaser *et al.*, 1998; Gromoll *et al.*, 1999; Habermann *et al.*, 1998; Houston and King, 2000a; Houston *et al.*, 1998; Johnson AD *et al.*, 2001; Karashima *et al.*, 2000; Kent-First *et al.*, 1996; Maegawa *et al.*, 1999; Maines and Wasserman, 1999; Maiwald *et al.*, 1996; McGuinness and Orth, 1992; Menke *et al.*, 1997; Mita and Yamashita, 2000; Mulhall *et al.*, 1997; Neiderberger *et al.*, 1997; Reijo *et al.*, 1995, 1996b, 2000; Ruggiu and Cooke, 2000; Ruggiu *et al.*, 1997; Saxena *et al.*, 1996, 2000; Schrans-Stassen *et al.*, 2001; Seboun *et al.*, 1997; Shan *et al.*, 1996; Shinka and Nakahori, 1996; Simoni *et al.*, 1997; Slee *et al.*, 1999; Stuppia *et al.*, 1996; Tsai *et al.*, 2000; Tsui *et al.*, 2000a,b; Venables *et al.*, 2001; Vereb *et al.*, 1997; Vries *et al.*, 2002; Yen *et al.*, 1996, 1997). The founding member of this family, *DAZ*, was identified in the mid-1990's in experiments aimed at exploring the hypothesis that a gene or genes on the human Y chromosome was required for production of sperm in men (Reijo *et al.*, 1995). This hypothesis, that there was a gene or gene cluster that was required for spermatogenesis on the Y chromosome, was first introduced in 1976 in a classic human genetics study (Tiepolo and Zuffardi, 1976). In this work, Tiepolo and Zuffardi karyotyped 1170 azoospermic men (with no sperm in the ejaculate) and oligospermic men (with less than 20 million sperm per ml) and found that six azoospermic men had microscopic deletions of the long arm of the Y chromosome and where tested, their fathers did not (Tiepolo and Zuffardi, 1976). Numerous studies confirmed these findings, but it was not until the mid-1990's that smaller, interstitial deletions of the Y chromosome were identified, following the complete mapping of the Y chromosome with PCR-based markers (Foote *et al.*, 1992; Reijo *et al.*, 1995; Vollrath *et al.*, 1992). Analysis of blood DNA from azoospermic men indicated that 13% of men who completely lacked all germ cells carried deletions of an *AZF* (*AZoospermia Factor*) region that encompassed a novel cluster of genes that we called the *DAZ* genes, whereas their fathers had intact Y chromosomes (Reijo *et al.*, 1995). With further analysis, it was demonstrated that approximately 6% of severely oligospermic men (with counts less than 1 million/ml) carried similar *de novo* deletions (Reijo *et al.*, 1996a). Subsequent studies identified two additional and less-frequent deletions linked to azoospermia and oligospermia (Vogt *et al.*, 1996). Still later, finer-structure genetic mapping and sequencing of the Y chromosome demonstrated that the human Y chromosome holds 156 transcription units that encode 27 distinct proteins (Skaletsky *et al.*, 2003). The most commonly deleted region of the Y chromosome, the *AZFc* region that encompasses the *DAZ* genes, encodes 11 apparently intact genes including the *RBMY1*, *PRY*, *BPY2*, *CDY1* and *DAZ* genes (Kuroda-Kawaguchi *et al.*, 2001; Lahn and Page, 1997). Yet, the contribution of these genes to azoospermia in men cannot be readily assessed given that Y chromosome homologs are only found in primates (Skaletsky *et al.*, 2003), whereas, autosomal homologs (called the *DAZ-Like* (*DAZL*) and *BOULE* (*BOL*) genes) are widely conserved and universally function in germ cell development to determine fertility (Brekhman *et al.*, 2000; Carani *et al.*, 1997; Cheng *et al.*, 1998; Cooke *et al.*, 1996; Dorfman *et al.*, 1999; Houston and King, 2000a; Houston *et al.*, 1998; Howley and Ho, 2000; Johnson AD *et al.*, 2001; Karashima *et al.*, 2000; Maegawa *et al.*, 1999; Menke *et al.*, 1997; Mita and Yamashita, 2000; Reijo *et al.*, 2000; Rocchietti-March *et al.*, 2000; Ruggiu *et al.*, 1997; Tsai *et al.*, 2000; Tsui *et al.*, 2000b; Yen *et al.*, 1996). Thus, two general approaches have been used to explore the function of the human *DAZ* gene family: (1) identification and characterization of proteins and RNAs which interact with *DAZ* family members and (2) construction of an *in vitro* system to directly probe gene function during germ cell development by silencing, overexpressing or mutating human genes directly.

12.2.2 Identification and characterization of a new member of the DAZ family in humans reconciles variant phenotypes in diverse organisms

As reported in Moore *et al.*, we identified 20 genes that encode proteins that potentially interacted with human DAZ/DAZL proteins via a yeast two-hybrid screen (Fig. 12.1) (Moore *et al.*, 2003). Seven proteins, encoded by six genes (DZIP 1 and 2 are isoforms), interacted by strict criteria. Several observations suggested that we identified legitimate partners. First, five interacting proteins, like DAZ/DAZL, are

Gene	Expression	Motif(s)
PUM2	Male/female germ cells and ES cells	PUF repeat
hQK3	Upregulated in ovary and testis	None
BOL	Male germ cells	RRM, DAZ repeat
DZIP1	Testis and specific tissues	Zinc finger
DZIP2	Male germ cells	Zinc finger
DZIP3	Unknown	None
DAZL	Male/female germ cells	RRM, DAZ repeat

Figure 12.1   Genes that encode proteins that interact with the members of the DAZ protein family (see text for further discussion)

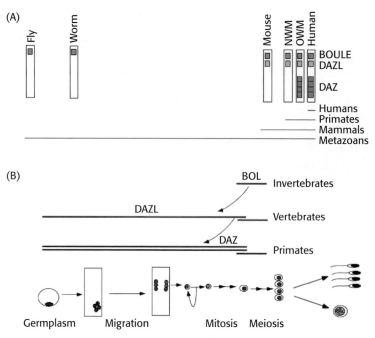

Figure 12.2 (A) *BOL* genes are conserved in all metazoans and gave rise to a gene family that contains *DAZL* and *DAZ*. Invertebrates such as flies and worms contain a single member of the *DAZ/BOL* gene family, non-primate vertebrates contain two members, and primates alone have *DAZ* genes themselves on the Y chromosome. (B) Expression and functional analyses suggest that *BOL* functions in meiosis, whereas *DAZ* and *DAZL* genes are required for novel vertebrate functions beginning in the earliest germ cells

predicted to bind RNA; thus, these proteins may function together to regulate translation. Second, four are homologs of proteins required for germ cell development in model organisms (Chubb, 1992; Eberhart *et al.*, 1996; Forbes and Lehmann, 1998; Ruggiu *et al.*, 1997). Third, five proteins demonstrated biochemical interaction, passing stringent tests of interaction.

Surprisingly, in sorting through potential interacting proteins a new member of the human *DAZ* gene family was identified (Fig. 12.2). However, the protein encoded by this gene was more similar to *Drosophila* Boule, the proposed fly ortholog of DAZ, than to human DAZ or DAZL (Eberhart *et al.*, 1996; Xu *et al.*, 2001). We called this newly identified gene, human *BOULE* (*BOL*). The extensive similarity shared by the RNA-binding domains of fly Boule, human BOL, DAZ and DAZL distinguished these proteins as a unique germ cell protein family (Xu *et al.*, 2001). We further characterized human *BOL* as reported. Notably, comparison of the expression of human and mouse *BOL* indicates that they share features with *DAZ/DAZL* but are divergent. For example, expression of all of these proteins is restricted to germ cells, with no expression in somatic cells (Cooke *et al.*, 1996; Dorfman *et al.*, 1999; Houston *et al.*, 1998; Maiwald *et al.*, 1996; Menke *et al.*, 1997; Mita and Yamashita, 2000; Reijo *et al.*,

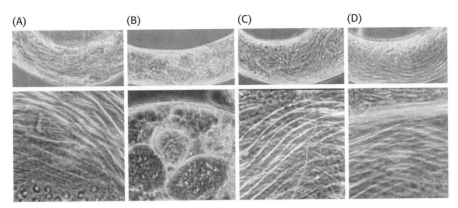

Figure 12.3   A human *BOL* transgene can rescue the meiotic arrest of infertile flies with a fly *boule* mutation. Shown is the testes of a (A) wildtype, (B) *boule* mutant, (C) *boule* mutant with a human transgene (tg) and (D) *boule* mutant with a fly tg. The lower panels are a higher magnification of the upper panels. Note the presence of long, filamentous sperm tails in all flies except the *boule* mutant with no transgene

1996b, 2000; Ruggiu *et al.*, 1997; Shan *et al.*, 1996; Yen *et al.*, 1996). Yet, DAZ and DAZL are expressed early in germ cell development and throughout development of adult germ cells (Dorfman *et al.*, 1999; Reijo *et al.*, 2000). In contrast, expression of BOL is restricted to meiotic cells in a pattern identical to fly *boule* (Cheng *et al.*, 1998; Maines and Wasserman, 1999; Xu *et al.*, 2001). Thus, given the similarity in expression of the human and fly genes, we tested whether human BOL could complement a fly *boule* mutation (Xu *et al.*, 2003). Remarkably, we found that progression of meiosis in mutant flies carrying a human BOL transgene was indistinguishable from that observed with the fly transgene (Fig. 12.3) (Xu *et al.*, 2003).

Results from studies briefly described above, along with previous studies on *DAZL* homologs in frogs and mice, suggested a resolution to the divergent functions of *DAZ* homologs. Essentially, *BOL* genes are found in all animals where, to date, they are known to function in meiosis; in contrast, *DAZL* genes only occur in vertebrates where they function in early germ cell development (Eberhart *et al.*, 1996; Houston and King, 2000a; Houston *et al.*, 1998; Karashima *et al.*, 2000; Ruggiu *et al.*, 1997). Finally, Y chromosome *DAZ* genes only occur in primates where expression and genetic data suggest they also function in early germ cell development (Reijo *et al.*, 1995, 1996a; Simoni *et al.*, 1997).

12.2.3 Identification and characterization of PUM2, a conserved stem cell factor that interacts with DAZ and DAZL

Another protein that interacts with DAZ and DAZL and has been well characterized is PUMILIO-2 (PUM2) (Moore *et al.*, 2003). PUM2 is a human homolog of fly Pumilio, a translational repressor that is required for embryonic axis determination and germ cell development, especially maintenance of germ line stem cells (Asaoka-Taguchi *et al.*, 1999; Crittenden *et al.*, 2002; Eckmann *et al.*, 2002; Forbes and Lehmann, 1998; Lehmann and Nusslen-Volhard, 1987; Lin and Spradling, 1997; Moore *et al.*, 2003; Murata and Wharton, 1995; Parisi and Lin, 1999; Wharton *et al.*, 1998). Identity between Pumilio proteins in diverse organisms was especially striking, with 80% identity over more than 280 amino acids that encode the RNA-binding domains (Moore *et al.*, 2003).

As outlined in several publications, data indicates that of the following:

(1) DAZ/DAZL and PUM2 interact in two-hybrid assays, pulldown assays from yeast, coimmunoprecipitation from mammalian cells overexpressing the proteins and in coimmunoprecipitation from testis extracts.

(2) DAZ/DAZL and PUM2 proteins colocalize to the nucleus and cytoplasm of PGCs, gonocytes and spermatogonia and the cytoplasm of spermatocytes.

(3) Specific regions of DAZ/DAZL protein were required for interaction with PUM2 protein, and vice versa.

(4) DAZ/DAZL and PUM2 can interact and bind the same RNA molecule.

(5) Interaction occurs through the functional domain of PUM2, required for complementation in flies.

(6) PUM2 interacts with DAZ, DAZL and also with the newest member of the family, BOL (Urano *et al.*, 2005).

These data suggest that human and mouse PUM2 plays a role similar to that of Pumilio in other organisms: First, the RNA-binding region, required to regulate translation during fly germ line development, is 80% identical to that of humans (Moore *et al.*, 2003). Moreover, our studies indicate that the RNA-binding domain is required for interaction of PUM2 with DAZ (Edwards *et al.*, 2001). Second, PUM2 protein can bind the NRE (Nanos Regulatory Element) sequence which is necessary for translational repression of some specific transcripts in *Drosophila*. This suggests that human PUM2 may also regulate translation. Finally, the pattern of PUM2 expression in embryonic cells and germ cells suggests that it functions in these cells. Based on these studies, we hypothesized that PUM2 may function as a translational regulator with DAZL in the formation and/or maintenance of early human germ cell populations. This hypothesis is consistent with reports that indicate translational repression by Pumilio homologs is a widespread mechanism for maintenance of germ line stem cells (Crittenden *et al.*, 2002; Wickens *et al.*, 2002). A model for how PUM2 and DAZ/DAZL may function in germ cell formation and/or maintenance of early germ cell populations is shown (Fig. 12.4).

12.2.4 Identification and characterization of RNAs to which DAZ/DAZL bind

We next identified and characterized RNA substrates potentially regulated by our protein complex. Since DAZL and PUM2 can interact and form a complex on the same RNA (Moore *et al.*, 2003), we sought to identify cellular target mRNAs to

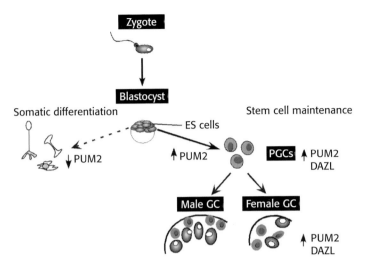

Figure 12.4   Model for the function of the DAZ family of proteins and interacting factors in the stem
cell populations of the embryo and germ line

Regulated by DAZL	Regulated by DAZL and PUM2
• Transition protein 1 • TRF2 – TBP-like protein • GRSF1 – cytoplasmic RNA binding protein • RNA binding motif protein 6 • Nuclear ribonucleoprotein U • Neural polypyrimidine tract binding protein • Guanine nucleotide binding protein • SWI/SNF related • Developmentally regulated GTP-binding protein 1 • NREBP, SON DNA binding protein • GAGE • XAGE-1 • Calmegin • Numerous ESTs/hypothetical genes	• Poly A-binding protein 1 • Protamine 2 • Enhancer of rudimentary (Drosophila) homolog (ERH) • Polymerase (DNA directed) iota or RAD30 • Nuclear domain 10 protein • Suv39h2 – histone H3 methyltransferase • Testis specific bromodomain protein • Numerous ESTs/hypothetical genes • RNF2: Ring finger protein 2 • PhD domain protein

Figure 12.5   mRNAs identified by co-immunoprecipitation with DAZL or DAZL and PUM2 protein
attached to inert beads that are potentially regulated by DAZL and/or DAZL and PUM2;
further analysis is required to confirm interactions *in vivo* (see text for further explanation)

which both proteins bind in order to minimize capture of non-specific targets. We
used tagged proteins crosslinked to beads to co-precipitate human testis mRNAs.
Complexes bound by either DAZL or PUM2 were extracted and amplified via
reverse transcriptase polymerase chain reaction (RT-PCR). Serial immunoprecip-
itations were performed to minimize background; resulting products were labeled
and used to screen for clones that were bound by both DAZL and PUM2 in at least
two rounds of screening (Fig. 12.5). Our results and those of Jiao and colleagues

overlapped (Jiao *et al.*, 2002); both groups obtained transcripts of transition protein 1, XAGE and GAGE mRNAs, as well as unique transcripts.

12.2.5 The PUM2 recognition sequence

Previously, we demonstrated that PUM2 binds the *Drosophila* NRE with or without DAZL (Moore *et al.*, 2003). In order to define the nucleotide requirements of this sequence, we used mutational analysis to determine if binding was specific and to define a minimal recognition sequence. As shown (Fig. 12.6), single nucleotide changes to the NRE sequence completely abolished PUM2 binding. Thus, with a PUM2 recognition sequence in hand, we determined which mRNAs from Figure 12.5 contained the sequence. Although 21 NRE elements were identified in 13 transcripts, only one mRNA, FLJ10498, was recruited by both DAZL and PUM2 and a subset of the other interacting proteins in the three-hybrid assay. We tentatively called the gene that encodes FLJ10498, *DAZ-Regulated* (*DAZR*). It is expressed at low levels in several tissues and abundantly in testis.

Box A					N N N N N	Box B						*Dros* pum	PUM2	PUM1
G	U	U	G	U	– – – – –	A	U	U	G	U	A	+	+	+
U	U	U	U	U	– – – – –	A	U	U	U	U	A	–	–	–
U	U	U	U	U	– – – – –	A	U	U	G	U	A	–	–	+
U	U	U	G	U	– – – – –	A	U	U	G	U	A	+	–	+
G	G	U	G	U	– – – – –	A	U	U	G	U	A	+	+	?
G	U	G	G	U	– – – – –	A	U	U	G	U	A	–	+	+
G	U	U	U	U	– – – – –	A	U	U	G	U	A	–	+	+
G	U	U	G	G	– – – – –	A	U	U	G	U	A	–	+	?
G	U	U	G	U	– – – – –	C	U	U	G	U	A	+	+	+
G	U	U	G	U	– – – – –	A	G	U	G	U	A	+	+	+
G	U	U	G	U	– – – – –	A	U	G	G	U	A	–	–	–
G	U	U	G	U	– – – – –	A	U	U	U	U	A	–	–	–
G	U	U	G	U	– – – – –	A	U	U	G	G	A	–	–	–
G	U	U	G	U	– – – – –	A	U	U	G	U	C	–	–	–

Figure 12.6 The human PUM2 protein specifically recognizes the NRE sequence that was identified as the sequence that confers regulation to the *nanos* gene by Pumilio protein in *Drosophila*. Note that several mutant mRNAs with single nucleotide changes were constructed; changes of single nucleotides can completely abolish binding of Pumilio proteins to the NRE sequences. Shown are results for a subset of mutant sequences and binding of *Drosophila* Pumilio, the human PUM2 protein and a closely related human homolog, PUM1

12.2.6 Identification of PUM2 and DAZL response elements

We defined the PUM2 *cis*-element via 5′ and 3′ deletion constructs that formed over-lapping 90 bp fragments and analyzed ability to support binding of PUM2. In this way, we mapped sequences required for PUM2 to 20 bps in *DAZR* (bases 178 and 198). This region contains a PUM2 recognition sequence as defined above. Furthermore comparison of sequences that DAZL binds in our analysis (the region at basepairs 0–90 of *DAZR*) to those obtained by Jiao *et al.* yields a consensus recognition sequence of UAUGUAGUUAUUAAAAAUUUUUAAAUCA (Jiao *et al.*, 2002). Gel shift assays were performed to confirm binding constraints for interactions between DAZL and the 0–90 sequence and PUM2 and the 128–218 sequence (Fox *et al.*, 2005). We found that both proteins recognized their putative sequences and were competed with spe-cific but not non-specific competitors (Fox *et al.*, 2005). In addition, as diagrammed below, we identified sequences in *DAZR* that may be bound by proteins that interact with DAZ and DAZL (Fig. 12.7, Color plate 11).

12.2.7 DAZL and PUM2 and the DAZR transcript

To date then, we had identified a complex of proteins that are predicted to bind RNA. We next wished to explore the function of *PUM2*, *DAZL* and *DAZR* in RNA metab-olism in order to address questions such as: Is there evidence that *PUM2* may act as a translational repressor in mammals, as it does in other organisms? Thus, we con-structed a reporter gene that contained the *DAZR* regulatory sequences and then silenced the genes in a spermatogonial stem cell line that was recently derived by Dym and colleagues (Feng *et al.*, 2002). Silencing was verified as shown (Fig. 12.8A). When we examined the action of *DAZR* sequences on a luciferase reporter, we found that addition of *DAZL* recognition sequences from 0 to 90 in the 3′UTR increased luciferase activity (Fig. 12.8B). This increase was abolished when DAZL was silenced (Fig. 12.8C). In contrast, PUM2 recognition sequences from 128 to 218 in the 3′UTR resulted in decreased luciferase activity (Fig. 12.8B) and silencing of PUM2 abolished the decrease (Fig. 12.8D). The mechanism of this regulation via mRNA stability

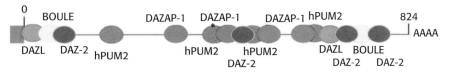

Figure 12.7   Screening of the *DAZR* 3′UTR (UnTranslated Region) for binding of multiple RNA-binding proteins. Diagrammed are results of binding assays with PUM2, BOULE, DAZL, DAZ2, DAZAP1 and DZIP1 proteins. The strongest reaction in the three-hybrid system was observed for sequences bound by PUM2 and DAZL. Binding by other proteins has not been investigated further. DAZAP1 was previously identified in the laboratory of Dr. Pauline Yen (Tsui *et al.*, 2000a) (see Color plate 11)

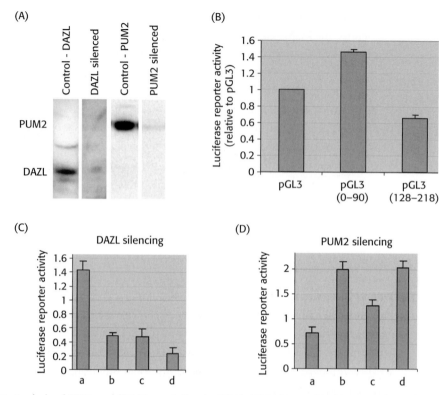

Figure 12.8   Analysis of DAZL and PUM2 regulation by RNAi. (A) PUM2 and DAZL were silenced. Oligos: DAZL, GATCCCgttcaccagttcaggtcatTTCAAGAGAatgacctgaactggtgaacTTTTTTGGAAA; PUM2, GATCCCgcactaacctgcagtctaaTTCAAGAGAttagactgcaggttagtgcTTTTTTTGGAAA under control of U6 promoter system. Control cells express significantly more PUM2 and DAZL than silenced cells. (B) The sequences at the 3′UTR regulate luciferase activity from a pGL3 reporter construct. (C) Silencing of *DAZL* leads to a significant reduction in luciferase activity (b–d) compared to controls (A). (D) Silencing of *PUM2* leads to a significant increase in luciferase activity (b–d) compared to controls (a). This suggests that DAZL protein may upregulate expression via modulation of mRNA stability or translation at the nucleotides 0–90 of the 3′UTR. In contrast, PUM2 may act to repress translation at the nucleotides 128–218 of the 3′UTR

and/or translational modulation is currently under study. Nonetheless, these data are compatible with the hypothesis that PUM2 functions as a repressor whereas, DAZL is stimulatory.

12.2.8 Conclusions from identification and characterization of DAZ, DAZL and interacting proteins and RNAs

As noted, an RNA termed *DAZR* was identified as an RNA bound by DAZ, DAZL and several interacting proteins (Fox *et al.*, 2005). Although the function of this RNA is

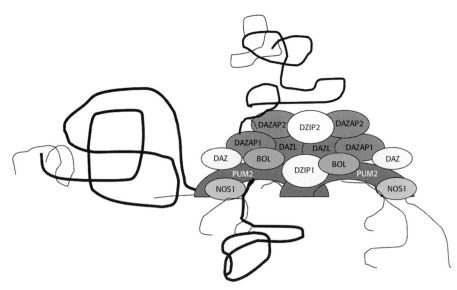

Figure 12.9 Protein interactions specific to germ cells. The putative structure of a germ cell particle which may specifically define the cytoplasm of germ cells, as distinct from somatic cells

not known, the observation of multiple partners binding the same RNA molecule suggests potential for coordinate regulation of RNAs and the presence of a complex of proteins and RNAs that is definitive of germ cells (Fig. 12.9). Furthermore, as shown in our and others' work, the *DAZ* gene family has homologs in diverse organisms from flies and worms to humans. Yet, the genetic composition of the gene family in primates differs from that of all other organisms making direct extrapolation of function difficult. For example, based on studies from model organisms, we cannot predict whether the Y chromosome *DAZ* genes have functions redundant with the autosomal *DAZL* gene or unique functions. Thus, we explored whether hESCs differentiation might allow genetic analysis of human germ cell development (Clark *et al.*, 2004a).

12.3 Differentiation of hESCs to the germ cell lineage

Since very little was known about gene expression in multiple human ES cell lines, we compared gene expression in three hESC lines prior to differentiating these three hESC lines to embryoid bodies (Ebs) and assaying germ cell development as described below.

12.3.1 Gene expression analysis in hESCs

Global gene expression analysis is useful for examining expression profiles that are shared between, and specific to, distinct cell types (Smith and Greenfield, 2003). In

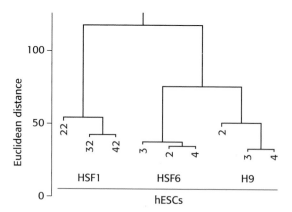

Figure 12.10   Hierarchical clustering of gene expression in independently derived hESC lines using Euclidean distance and complete linkage. Microarray analysis and probe generation were as described (Abeyta *et al.*, 2004)

most studies, 10–20% of genes and expressed sequence tags (ESTs) are reported to be expressed in any one cell type (Warrington *et al.*, 2000). In contrast, gene expression in stem cells is slightly elevated; yet, by no means are most or all genes expressed as popular lore may suggest. In one study, the number of genes expressed in three different stem cell types was tallied and it was found that approximately 60% of the genes and ESTs probed were expressed in these three stem cell types together (or approximately 20% in each type of cell; embryonic, neural and hematopoietic stem cells) (Ramalho-Santos *et al.*, 2002). In a second study, approximately 30% of the sequences on oligonucleotide arrays were expressed in cultured neural stem cells (Wright *et al.*, 2003). In Abeyta *et al.* (2004), the first comparison of global gene expression between independent hESC lines was reported (Fig. 12.10) (Abeyta *et al.*, 2004). Similar to results with other stem cell types, 31% of the total gene and EST sequences on the oligoarrays were expressed in at least one cell line; just 16% were expressed in all three lines examined, including genes such as *OCT4* and others required for ES cell pluripotency (Abeyta *et al.*, 2004). Thus, hESCs express many genes and ESTs, but clearly not the majority (Abeyta *et al.*, 2004). In addition, this work demonstrated that each independently derived hESC line analyzed possessed a unique gene expression signature (Abeyta *et al.*, 2004).

12.3.2 Search for the first expressed marker of human germ cells

In order to identify nascent germ cells as they differentiate, we searched for the earliest marker of human germ cells (Clark *et al.*, 2004b). Mouse *stella* was reported to be expressed only in early, lineage-restricted germ cells and not in somatic cells (Saitou *et al.*, 2002). Given the lack of known human genes with these properties, we identified and characterized a human *stella* homolog. We mapped a gene with structural similarity to chromosome 12 p and found that the region surrounding this

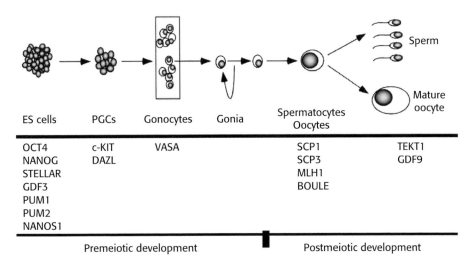

ES cells	PGCs	Gonocytes	Gonia	Spermatocytes Oocytes	
OCT4	c-KIT	VASA		SCP1	TEKT1
NANOG	DAZL			SCP3	GDF9
STELLAR				MLH1	
GDF3				BOULE	
PUM1					
PUM2					
NANOS1					

Premeiotic development	Postmeiotic development

Figure 12.11   Diagrammatic representation of the different stages of germ cell differentiation. We note the earliest expression of each gene that can be used to predict each stage of germ cell development. Most genes are specific to germ cells, though a subset such as *c-KIT* and the *PUM* genes are also expressed in somatic tissues. Expression in germ cells is described (Caricasole *et al.*, 1998; Castrillon *et al.*, 2000; Chambers *et al.*, 2003; Clark *et al.*, 2004b; Dong *et al.*, 1996; Edelmann *et al.*, 1996; Hansis *et al.*, 2000; Koprunner *et al.*, 2001; Larsson *et al.*, 2000; Lynn *et al.*, 2002; Matsui *et al.*, 1997; Mitsui *et al.*, 2003; Moore *et al.*, 2003; Niwa *et al.*, 2000; Pesce *et al.*, 1998; Reijo *et al.*, 2000; Saitou *et al.*, 2002; Xu *et al.*, 2001)

gene, which we called *STELLA-Related* (*STELLAR*), encoded two other genes, *GDF3* (*Growth and Differentiation Factor 3*) and *NANOG* (Clark *et al.*, 2004b). Although these syntenous genes are remarkably divergent from mice to humans, we expected that if the expression of human *STELLAR* was similar to that reported for mouse *stella*, it would mark nascent germ cells as they differentiate. Surprisingly, however, we found that *STELLAR*, *NANOG* and *GDF3*, were expressed highly in undifferentiated ES cells; expression was downregulated with ES cell differentiation in a manner identical to *OCT4* (Hansis *et al.*, 2000; Niwa *et al.*, 2000; Pesce and Scholer, 2000; Pesce *et al.*, 1998). Then, in the fetus and adult, expression was limited to germ cells (Clark *et al.*, 2004b).

12.3.3 Germ cell markers in undifferentiated hESC lines

Since we unexpectedly found that *STELLAR* is expressed in undifferentiated hESCs, we created a profile of expression of markers that might define development of the germ cell lineage (Fig. 12.11). We then examined expression of these potential markers in order to identify those that are expressed in human germ cells but not in three hESC lines. We observed expression not only of *OCT4*, *GDF3*, *NANOG* and *STELLAR*

Table 12.1. Mean normalized expression of genes in HSF1, H9 and HSF6 undifferentiated, hESC lines analyzed via quantitative PCR

Gene name	HSF1 ($\times 10^3$)	H9 ($\times 10^3$)	HSF6 ($\times 10^3$)
NCAM1	+	+	+
KDR	+	+	+
AFP	+	+	+
OCT4	+	+	+
GDF3	+	+	+
STELLAR	+	+	+
NANOG	+	+	+
NANOS	+	+	+
DAZL	+	+	+
KIT	+	+	+
PUM1	+	+	+
PUM2	+	+	+
VASA	−	−	−
SCP1	−	−	−
GDF9	−	−	−
TEKTIN1	−	−/+	−/+

Values were calculated, as described (Pfaffl *et al.*, 2002), and significance was calculated by ANOVA for each gene followed by a two-tailed *t*-test (see Clark *et al.*, 2004b for details) (Clark *et al.*, 2004b). Note that genes expressed are in bold type; those that were not expressed are in italics.

in undifferentiated ESCs as expected, but also *DAZL* (Table 12.1 also see Clark *et al.* for CT values) (Clark *et al.*, 2004b). Furthermore, all three lines of undifferentiated hESCs expressed the genes *cKIT, NANOS1, PUM1* and *PUM2*. In contrast to expression of these pre-meiotic genes, markers of later germ cell differentiation were at or below levels of detection including, *VASA*, a specific marker of germ cell migration, entry into the gonads and meiosis (Castrillon *et al.*, 2000), *SCP1*, a specific marker of meiosis in male and female germ cells (Lynn *et al.*, 2002), *GDF9*, a specific marker of meiotic and post-meiotic germ cell differentiation in oocytes (Dong *et al.*, 1996), and *TEKT1*, a specific marker of post-meiotic germ cell differentiation in haploid spermatids (Larsson *et al.*, 2000) (Table 12.1). None of these markers were expressed at detectable levels with the exception of the expression of *TEKT1* at background level in one of three samples of the HSF6 line.

12.3.4 Protein expression in hESC lines

Since undifferentiated hESCs apparently shared a pre-meiotic transcriptional expression profile with germ cells, we tested whether the corresponding germ cell specific

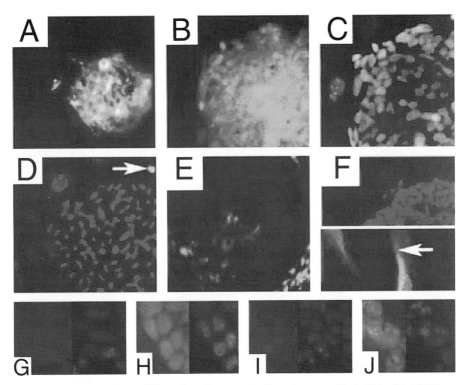

Figure 12.12   Protein expression in undifferentiated human (A–F) and mouse (G–J) ESCs. (A) SSEA3
(green) and TRA-1-81 (red) were used to assess status of hESC differentiation (orange
indicates co-localization). Immunofluorescence: DAZL (B) and DAPI (C). Merged images
of KDR and DAPI (D; white arrow shows positive cell); AFP (E) and NCAM1 (upper panel
of F). NCAM1 was only detected in differentiated EBs (lower panel; F); white arrow shows
cytoplasmic expression. mESC Immunofluorescence (G, I) Control preimmune for Dazl and
Dzip; (H, J) specific antisera for Dazl and Dzip proteins. Immunofluorescence (lefthand)
and DAPI (righthand panel) of G, I, H, J (see Color plate 12)

proteins were expressed. Our results indicated that not just RNAs, but proteins were
also expressed (Clark *et al.*, 2004a).

12.3.5 Immunohistochemistry in undifferentiated hESCs

We next addressed whether part or the entirety of the hESC population was expressing
proteins indicative of germ cell development via immunofluorescence (Fig. 12.12,
Color plate 12). We showed that undifferentiated hESCs expressed pluripotency
markers, as expected (Fig. 12.12A), and also STELLAR protein in nearly all cells (Clark
et al., 2004a). Most surprisingly, we also observed that DAZL was present in nearly all
hESCs (Fig. 12.12B, C), while, VASA was never detected in undifferentiated hESCs
(Clark *et al.*, 2004a). In contrast, somatic proteins were rarely expressed (Fig. 12.12D,
E); NCAM1 was only detected after differentiation (Fig. 12.12F). These results were

confirmed with mESCs as well (Fig. 12.12G–I). mESCs also expressed DAZL and an interacting protein, DZIP, in nearly all cells (Moore *et al.*, 2004).

We did not expect expression of *DAZL* mRNA and protein in the majority of hESCs, simply because in species of flies, worms, frogs, fish, salamanders, mice and non-human primates, as in humans, expression of *DAZ* gene homologs is restricted to germ cells (Brekhman *et al.*, 2000; Carani *et al.*, 1997; Cheng *et al.*, 1998; Cooke *et al.*, 1996; Dorfman *et al.*, 1999; Houston and King, 2000a; Houston *et al.*, 1998; Howley and Ho, 2000; Johnson AD *et al.*, 2001; Karashima *et al.*, 2000; Maegawa *et al.*, 1999; Menke *et al.*, 1997; Mita and Yamashita, 2000; Reijo *et al.*, 2000; Rocchietti-March *et al.*, 2000; Ruggiu *et al.*, 1997; Tsai *et al.*, 2000; Tsui *et al.*, 2000b; Yen *et al.*, 1996). Our observations suggested that of the following:

(1) Expression of 'germ cell' genes in undifferentiated hESCs may simply reflect random, unregulated gene expression. However, several reports, including from my laboratory, have documented that ES cells express approximately the same percentage of genes as other cells (Abeyta *et al.*, 2004; Hsiao *et al.*, 2001; Ivanova *et al.*, 2002; Ramalho-Santos *et al.*, 2002; Tanaka *et al.*, 2002; Warrington *et al.*, 2000). Moreover, if random expression were the case, we would expect expression of markers such as *VASA, SCP1, SCP3, BOULE, GDF9* and *TEKT1*. Yet, this was not the case. We observed expression of all pre-meiotic germ cell markers but no later germ cell markers.

(2) hESCs and germ cells may share aspects of a common molecular program and therefore express similar genes. In fact, expression of genes such as *OCT4, NANOG, STELLAR* and *GDF3* supports this possibility (Clark *et al.*, 2004b; Pesce *et al.*, 1998).

(3) Expression of genes such as *DAZL* may indicate spontaneous differentiation of part or all of the population of ESCs to germ cells.

12.3.6 DAZL is expressed in undifferentiated hESCs but not in ICM

To address these possibilities, we compared expression of several genes in the ICM (which is the source of ESCs) to that of cultured, undifferentiated hESC lines (Table 12.2). We found that human ICM cells expressed *NANOS1* but not *DAZL* or later germ cell markers such as *VASA* or *SCP1*, or somatic markers such as *NCAM1*. Due to limited availability of tissues, additional markers were not be assayed. Nevertheless, these results demonstrated that undifferentiated hESCs differed in *DAZL* and *NCAM1* transcription compared to their *in vivo* counterpart, ICM cells. This suggested that removal of the ICM from the blastocyst and subsequent culturing on feeder cells either resulted in transcription of markers which are normally not expressed in the ICM in ES cells or resulted in the preferential propagation of germ cell-like cells. If we focus on differentiation towards a germ cell-specific pathway, removal and culture of the ICM may result in spontaneous differentiation of cells

Table 12.2. Comparison of expression of a subset of genes in human ICM and undifferentiated hESCs (see text and Clark *et al.*, 2004a for further explanation)

Gene name	ICM	hESCs
NCAM1	−	+
OCT4	+	+
STELLAR	+	+
NANOS	+	+
DAZL	−	+
VASA	−	−
SCP1	−	−

towards the germ cell lineage. Thus, hESCs may be thought to be 'primed for germ cell development.' However, the next temporal marker of germ cell differentiation that we know, VASA, is not expressed. Similar results are observed with mouse ESCs (Moore *et al.*, 2003, 2004).

12.3.7 Meiotic and post-meiotic germ cell differentiation using hESCs

We next determined whether hESCs could form mature germ cells by differentiating hESCs and generating EBs. With differentiation, genes expressed predominantly or exclusively in pluripotent cell types should decrease as somatic lineages form. Thus, as expected, markers *OCT4*, *STELLAR*, *NANOG* and *GDF3* decreased as *NCAM1*, *AFP* and *KDR* increased with differentiation (Clark *et al.*, 2004a). However, by day 14 of differentiation, expression of both *NANOS1* and *DAZL* also decreased sharply. Conversely, there was a sharp increase in expression of later germ cell markers including *VASA*, *SCP1*, *GDF9* and *TEKT1* as EB differentiation progressed (Clark *et al.*, 2004a). Decreased *NANOS1* and *DAZL* expression suggested, as discussed below, that cells positive for these markers contribute to both somatic and germ cell lineages.

Given that RNAs indicative of germ cell development are expressed with differentiation, whether proteins diagnostic of germ cells were present in EBs was analyzed. At days 14 and 21, EBs were analyzed for VASA, STELLAR and DAZL. We found that all three proteins were expressed in distinct cells within EBs, frequently overlapping (Fig. 12.13A, B, Color plate 13). Also, examination of expression of the synaptonemal complex protein-3 (SCP3), revealed no SCP3-positive cells in undifferentiated hESCs (Fig. 12.13C, D, Color plate 13). In contrast, by day 14 of differentiation, we detected SCP3-positive cells throughout the EBs in nuclear structures (Fig. 12.13E, F, Color plate 13). We did not, detect MLH1 expression in recombination nodules; nor did studies with mESC-derived germ cells (Geijsen *et al.*, 2004; Hubner *et al.*, 2003), though their presence was not sought in the studies of

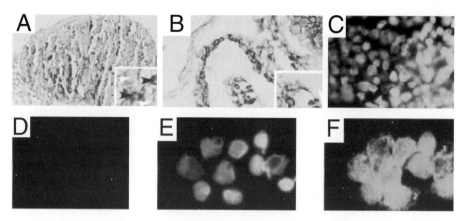

Figure 12.13   Immunohistochemistry and meiotic analysis of Day 14 EBs. See Clark *et al.*, for additional panels and controls. Day 14 EBs from HSF-6 and HSF-1 hESCs stained for VASA (A) and DAZL (B). Meiotic proteins (C–F). Undifferentiated hESCs stained with DAPI (C) and SCP3 antisera (D). Day 14 EBs stained for DAPI (E) and SCP3 (F) (see Color plate 13)

Toyooka *et al.* (2003) and results from Geijsen and colleagues indicated the presence of mature sperm from *in vitro* differentiation of mESC-derived germ cells. *DAZL as an early marker of the human germ cell lineage.*

12.2.8 Conclusions from hESC differentiation

hESC differentiation is a promising approach to dissect genetics of human germ cell specification and differentiation. We showed that undifferentiated hESCs expressed *STELLAR* and *DAZL* but not later germ cell markers such as *VASA*. Given this expression pattern and the observation that in diverse organisms including flies, worms, frogs, fish, mice and humans, *DAZL* expression is restricted to germ cells (Xu *et al.*, 2001). Along with additional data on embryonic expression of *DAZL* and *STELLAR*, we propose that *DAZL* is the earliest known marker of human germ cells. Construction of a *DAZL* promoter reporter system confirms expression from this promoter in hESCs and mESCs, as well as germ cells (Fig. 12.14). We expect that expression from the *DAZL* promoter will be maintained only in germ cells and not somatic cells upon differentiation.

Further consideration of the time course of expression of the genes *OCT4*, *NANOG*, *NANOS1*, *STELLAR* and *DAZL* in hESCs leads to two suggestions, also outlined in our model (Fig. 12.14): First, growth and propagation of a self-renewing population from ICM cells to form ES cells may lead to the spontaneous differentiation of all or a portion of cells to the germ cell lineage. Second, putative *DAZL*- and *STELLAR*-positive germ cells may differentiate to form both germ cells and somatic cells. These conclusions are supported by observations that the germ cell lineage is one of the first lineages to form in many organisms and does not require an intermediate embryonic precursor of ectoderm, endoderm or mesoderm lineages

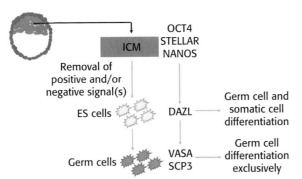

Figure 12.14   Model of the formation and differentiation of mammalian germ cells. We hypothesize that hESCs and early germ cells are equivalent cell types, as shown, that are distinct from cells of the ICM. Cells that are positive for expression of *OCT4*, *STELLAR*, *NANOS* and *DAZL* may contribute to both germ cell and somatic cell lineages. We hypothesize that with expression of later genes such as *VASA* or *SCP3* cells are committed to the germ cell lineage. Details are based on published results (Clark *et al.*, 2004a,b)

(Tsang *et al.*, 2001). Moreover, embryonic germ (EG) cell lines, derived from human PGCs in the gonadal ridge, share characteristics with ESC lines. Just as ESC lines, EG lines are pluripotent, able to self-renew and form EBs containing all major somatic lineages (Onyango *et al.*, 2002; Shamblott *et al.*, 1998, 2001). These observations suggest that even when PGCs are in the gonad of developing humans, their potential may not yet restricted to the germ cell lineage alone. Clearly under conditions of culture, they can form germ cells or somatic cells.

12.4 Summary

The ability to differentiate human ESCs to the germ cell lineage will ultimately allow the production of eggs and sperm, *in vitro*. This has both scientific and practical implications. On the basic side, for the first time, there may be the potential to develop a rigorous human genetic system that can be manipulated for investigation of specific genes implicated in germ cell development, such as those described above. In addition, from a practical point of view, the ability to produce eggs in vitro will allow reprogramming of nuclear DNA for somatic cell nuclear transfer (SCNT) without the need to obtain oocytes directly from women. Thus, there is a need to further explore the potential of hESCs in establishing germ cells.

REFERENCES

Abeyta M, Clark AT, Rodriguez R *et al.* (2004) Unique gene expression signatures of independently-derived human embryonic stem cell lines. *Human Mol Genet* 13, 601–608.

Agulnik AI, Zharkikh A, Tong HB *et al.* (1998) Evolution of the *DAZ* gene family suggests that Y-linked DAZ plays little, or a limited, role in spermatogenesis but underlines a recent African origin for human populations. *Human Molec Genet* 7, 1371–1377.

Asaoka-Taguchi M, Yamada M, Nakamura A *et al.* (1999) Maternal Pumilio acts together with Nanos in germline development in Drosophila embryos. *Nature Cell Biol* 1, 431–437.

Bielawski JP and Yang Z (2001) Positive and negative selection in the *DAZ* gene family. *Mol Biol Evol* 18, 523–429.

Bienvenu T, Patrat C, McElreavey K *et al.* (2001) Reduction in the *DAZ* gene copy number in two infertile men with impaired spermatogenesis. *Annales de Genet* 44, 125–128.

Brekhman V, Itskovitz-Eldor J, Yodko E *et al.* (2000) The *DAZL1* gene is expressed in human male and female embryonic gonads before meiosis. *Mol Human Reprod* 6, 465–468.

Buehr M and Smith A (2003) Genesis of embryonic stem cells. *Philos Trans R Soc Lond B Biol Sci* 358, 1397–1402.

Carani C, Gromoll J, Brinkworth MH *et al.* (1997) *cynDAZLA*: a cynomolgus monkey homologue of the human autosomal *DAZ* gene. *Mol Human Reprod* 3, 479–483.

Caricasole AA, van Schaik RH, Zeinstra LM *et al.* (1998) Human growth-differentiation factor 3 (*hGDF3*): developmental regulation in human teratocarcinoma cell lines and expression in primary testicular germ cell tumors. *Oncogene* 16, 95–103.

Castrillon DH, Quade BJ, Wang TY *et al.* (2000) The human *VASA* gene is specifically expressed in the germ cell lineage. *Proc Natl Acad Sci* 97, 9585–9590.

Chai NN, Phillips A, Fernandez A *et al.* (1997) A putative human male infertility gene *DAZLA*: genomic structure and methylation status. *Mol Human Reprod* 3, 705–708.

Chambers I, Colby D, Robertson M *et al.* (2003) Functional expression cloning of Nanog, a pluripotency sustaining factor in embryonic stem cells. *Cell* 113, 643–655.

Cheng MH, Maines JZ and Wasserman SA (1998) Biphasic subcellular localization of the DAZL-related protein Boule in *Drosophila* spermatogenesis. *Dev Biol* 204, 567–576.

Chiquoine A (1954) The identification, origin and migration of the primordial germ cells in the mouse embryo. *Anat Rec* 118, 135–146.

Chubb C (1992) Oligotriche and quaking gene mutations. Phenotypic effects on mouse spermatogenesis and testicular steroidogenesis. *J Androl* 13, 312–317.

Clark AT, Bodnar MS, Fox MS *et al.* (2004a) Spontaneous differentiation of germ cells from human embryonic stem cells *in vitro*. *Human Mol Genet* 13, 727–739.

Clark AT, Rodriguez R, Bodnar M *et al.* (2004b) Human *STELLAR, NANOG*, and GDF3 genes are expressed in pluripotent cells and map to chromosome 12p13, a hot-spot for teratocarcinoma. *Stem Cells* 22, 169–179.

Cooke HJ, Lee M, Kerr S *et al.* (1996) A murine homologue of the human *DAZ* gene is autosomal and expressed only in male and female gonads. *Human Mol Genet* 5, 513–516.

Crittenden SL, Bernstein D, Bachorik J *et al.* (2002) FBF and control of germline stem cells in *Caenorhabditis elegans*. *Nature* 417, 660–663.

Dai T, Vera Y, Salido EC *et al.* (2001) Characterization of the mouse *Dazap1* gene encoding an RNA-binding protein that interacts with infertility factors DAZ and DAZL. *BMC Genomics* 2, 6.

Delbridge ML, Harry JL, Toder R *et al.* (1997) A human candidate spermatogenesis gene, *RBM1*, is conserved and amplified on the marsupial Y chromosome. *Nat Genet* 15, 131–136.

Dong J, Albertini DF, Nishimori K *et al.* (1996) Growth differentiation factor-9 is required during ovarian folliculogenesis. *Nature* 383, 531–535.

Dorfman DM, Genest DR and Pera RAR (1999) Human *DAZL1* encodes a candidate fertility factor in women that localizes to the prenatal and postnatal germ cells. *Human Reprod* 14, 2531–2536.

Eberhart CG, Maines JZ and Wasserman SA (1996) Meiotic cell cycle requirement for a fly homologue of human *Deleted in AZoospermia*. *Nature* 381, 783–785.

Eckmann CR, Kraemer B, Wickens M *et al.* (2002) GLD-3, a bicaudal-C homolog that inhibits FBF to control germline sex determination in *C. elegans*. *Dev Cell* 3, 697–710.

Edelmann W, Cohen PE, Kane M *et al.* (1996) Meiotic pachytene arrest in *Mlh1*-deficient mice. *Cell* 85, 1125–1134.

Edwards TA, Pyle SE, Wharton RP *et al.* (2001) Structure of Pumilio reveals similarity between RNA and peptide binding motifs. *Cell* 105, 281–289.

Evans M and Hunter S (2002) Source and nature of embryonic stem cells. *C R Biol* 325, 1003–1007.

Feng LX, Chen Y, Dettin L *et al.* (2002) Generation and *in vitro* differentiation of a spermatogonial cell line. *Science* 297, 392–395.

Foote S, Vollrath D, Hilton A *et al.* (1992) The human Y chromosome: overlapping DNA clones spanning the euchromatic region. *Science* 258, 60–66.

Forbes A and Lehmann R (1998) *Nanos* and *Pumilio* have critical roles in the development and function of *Drosophila* germline stem cells. *Development* 125, 679–690.

Foresta C, Ferlin A, Garolla A *et al.* (1997) Y-chromosome deletions in idiopathic severe testiculopathies. *J Clin Endocrinol Metab* 82, 1075–1080.

Fox M, Urano J and Pera RR (2005) Identification and characterization of RNA sequences to which human PUMILIO-2 (PUM2) and Deleted in Azoospermia-Like (DAZL) bind. *Genomics* 85, 92–105.

Fujiwara T, Dunn NR and Hogan BL (2001) Bone morphogenetic protein 4 in the extraembryonic mesoderm is required for allantois development and the localization and survival of primordial germ cells in the mouse. *Proc Natl Acad Sci* 98, 13739–13744.

Geijsen N, Horoschak M, Kim K *et al.* (2004) Derivation of embryonic germ cells and male gametes from embryonic stem cells. *Nature* 427, 148–154.

Glaser B, Yen PH and Schempp W (1998) Fibre-fluorescence *in situ* hybridization unravels apparently seven *DAZ* genes or pseudogenes clustered within a Y-chromosome region frequently deleted in azoospermic males. *Chromosome Res* 6, 481–486.

Gromoll J, Weinbauer GF, Skaletsky H *et al.* (1999) The Old World monkey *DAZ* (*Deleted in AZoospermia*) gene yields insights into the evolution of the *DAZ* gene cluster on the human Y chromosome. *Human Mol Genet* 8, 2017–2024.

Habermann B, Mi HF, Edelmann A *et al.* (1998) *DAZ* (*Deleted in AZoospermia*) genes encode proteins located in human late spermatids and in sperm tails. *Human Reprod* 13, 363–369.

Hansis C, Grifo JA and Krey LC (2000) Oct-4 expression in inner cell mass and trophectoderm of human blastocysts. *Mol Human Reprod* 6, 999–1004.

Hendry AP, Wenburg JK, Bentzen P *et al.* (2000) Rapid evolution of reproductive isolation in the wild: evidence from introduced salmon. *Science* 290, 516–518.

Houston DW and King ML (2000a) A critical role for *Xdazl*, a germ plasm-localized RNA, in the differentiation of primordial germ cells in *Xenopus*. *Development* 127, 447–456.

Houston DW and King ML (2000b) Germ plasm and molecular determinants of germ cell fate. *Curr Top Dev Biol* 50, 155–181.

Houston DW, Zhang J, Maines JZ *et al.* (1998) A *Xenopus DAZ-Like* gene encodes an RNA component of germ plasm and is a functional homologue of *Drosophila boule*. *Development* 125, 171–180.

Howley C and Ho RK (2000) mRNA localization patterns in zebrafish oocytes. *Mech Dev* 92, 305–309.

Hsiao LL, Dangond F, Yoshida T *et al.* (2001) A compendium of gene expression in normal human tissues. *Physiol Genomics* 7, 97–104.

Hubner K, Fuhrmann G, Christenson L *et al.* (2003) Derivation of oocytes from mouse embryonic stem cells. *Science* 300, 1251–1256.

Hull MGR, Glazener CMA, Kelly NJ *et al.* (1985) Population study of causes, treatment, and outcome of infertility. *Br Med J* 291, 1693–1697.

Hunt PA and Hassold TJ (2002) Sex matters in meiosis. *Science* 296, 2181–2183.

Ivanova NB, Dimos JT, Schaniel C *et al.* (2002) A stem cell molecular signature. *Science* 298, 601–604.

Jaruzelska J, Kotecki M, Kusz K *et al.* (2003) Conservation of a Pumilio–Nanos complex from Drosophila germ plasm to human germ cells. *Dev Genes Evol* 213, 120–126.

Jiao X, Trifillis P and Kiledjian M (2002) Identification of target messenger RNA substrates for the murine Deleted in AZoospermia-Like RNA-binding protein. *Biol Reprod* 66, 475–485.

Johnson AD BR, Drum M, Masi T (2001) Expression of axolotl *dazl* rna, a marker of germ plasm: widespread maternal rna and onset of expression in germ cells approaching the gonad. *Dev Biol* 234, 402–415.

Karashima T, Sugimoto A and Yamamoto M (2000) *Caenorhabditis elegans* homologue of the human azoospermia factor *DAZ* is required for oogenesis but not for spermatogenesis. *Development* 127, 1069–1079.

Kent-First MG, Kol S, Muallem A *et al.* (1996) The incidence and possible relevance of Y-linked microdeletions in babies born after intractyoplasmic sperm injection and their infertile fathers. *Mol Human Reprod* 2, 943–950.

Koprunner M, Thisse C, Thisse B *et al.* (2001) A zebrafish nanos-related gene is essential for the development of primordial germ cells. *Genes Dev* 15, 2877–2885.

Kuroda-Kawaguchi T, Skaletsky H, Brown LG *et al.* (2001) The AZFc region of the Y chromosome features massive palindromes and uniform recurrent deletions in infertile men. *Nature Genet* 29, 279–286.

Lahn BT and Page DC (1997) Functional coherence of the human Y chromosome. *Science* 278, 675–680.

Larsson M, Norrander J, Graslund S *et al.* (2000) The spatial and temporal expression of Tekt1, a mouse tektin C homologue, during spermatogenesis suggest that it is involved in the development of the sperm tail basal body and axoneme. *Eur J Cell Biol* 79, 718–725.

Lehmann R and Nusslen-Volhard C (1987) Involvement of the *Pumilio* gene in the transport of an abdominal signal in the *Drosophila* embryo. *Nature* 329, 167–170.

Lin H and Spradling AC (1997) A novel group of *pumilio* mutations affects the asymmetric division of germline stem cells in the *Drosophila* ovary. *Development* 124, 2463–2476.

Lynn A, Koehler KE, Judis L *et al.* (2002) Covariation of synaptonemal complex length and mammalian meiotic exchange rates. *Science* 296, 2222–2225.

Maegawa S, Yasuda K and Inoue K (1999) Maternal mRNA localization of zebrafish *DAZ-like* gene. *Mech Dev* 81, 223–226.

Maines JZ and Wasserman SA (1999) Post-transcriptional regulation of the meiotic Cdc25 protein Twine by the Dazl orthologue Boule. *Nature Cell Biol* 1, 171–174.

Maiwald R, Luche RM and Epstein CJ (1996) Isolation of a mouse homolog of the human *DAZ* (*Deleted in AZoospermia*) gene. *Mamm Genome* 7, 628.

Matsui M, Ichibara H, Kobayashi S *et al.* (1997) Mapping of six germ cell-specific genes to mouse chromosomes. *Genome* 8, 873–874.

McGuinness MP and Orth JM (1992) Gonocytes of male rats resume migratory activity postnatally. *Eur J Cell Biol* 59, 196–210.

Menke DB, Mutter GL and Page DC (1997) Expression of *DAZ*, an azoospermia factor candidate, in human spermatogonia. *Am J Human Genet* 60, 237–241.

Menken J and Larsen U (1994) Estimating the incidence and prevalence and analyzing the correlates of infertility and sterility. *Ann NY Acad Sci* 709, 249–265.

Mita K and Yamashita M (2000) Expression of *Xenopus* Daz-like protein during gametogenesis and embryogenesis. *Mech Dev* 94, 251–255.

Mitsui K, Tokuzawa Y, Itoh H *et al.* (2003) The homeoprotein Nanog is required for maintenance of pluripotency in mouse epiblast and ES cells. *Cell* 113, 631–642.

Moore FL, Jaruzelska J, Fox MS *et al.* (2003) Human Pumilio-2 is expressed in embryonic stem cells and germ cells and interacts with DAZ (Deleted in AZoospermia) and DAZ-Like proteins. *Proc Natl Acad Sci* 100, 538–543.

Moore FL, Jaruzelska J, Dorfmann D *et al.* (2004) Identification of a novel gene, *DZIP* (*DAZ Interacting Protein*), that encodes a protein that interacts with DAZ and DAZL (Deleted in AZoospermia and DAZ-Like) and is expressed in embryonic stem cells and germ cells. *Genomics* 83, 834–843.

Mulhall JP, Reijo R, Alaggappan R *et al.* (1997) Azoospermic men with deletion of the *DAZ* gene cluster are capable of completing spermatogenesis: fertilization, normal embryonic development and pregnancy occur when retrieved testicular spermatozoa are used for intracytoplasmic sperm injection. *Human Reprod* 12, 503–508.

Murata Y and Wharton RP (1995) Binding of Pumilio to maternal hunchback mRNA is required for posterior patterning in *Drosophila* embryos. *Cell* 80, 747–756.

Neiderberger C, Agulnik AI, Cho Y *et al.* (1997) *In situ* hybridization shows that *Dazla* expression in mouse testis is restricted to premeiotic stages IV–VI of spermatogenesis. *Mamm Genome* 8, 277–278.

Niwa H, Miyazaki J and Smith AG (2000) Quantitative expression of Oct-3/4 defines differentiation, dedifferentiation or self-renewal of ES cells. *Nature Genet* 24, 372–376.

Onyango P, Jiang S, Uejima H *et al.* (2002) Monoallelic expression and methylation of imprinted genes in human and mouse embryonic germ cell lineages. *Proc Natl Acad Sci* 99, 10599–10604.

Parisi M and Lin H (1999) The *Drosophila Pumilio* gene encodes two functional protein isoforms that play multiple roles in germline development, gonadogenesis, oogenesis, and embryogenesis. *Genetics* 153, 235–250.

Pesce M and Scholer HR (2000) Oct4: Control of totipotency and germline determination. *Mol Reprod Dev* 55, 452–457.

Pesce M, Wang X, Wolgemuth DJ *et al.* (1998) Differential expression of the Oct-4 transcription factor during mouse germ cell differentiation. *Mech Dev* 71, 89–98.

Pesce M, Gioia-Klinger F and Felici MD (2002) Derivation in culture of primordial germ cells from cells of the mouse epiblast: phenotypic induction and growth control by Bmp4 signalling. *Mech Dev* 112, 15–24.

Pfaffl MW, Horgan GW and Dempfle L (2002) Relative expression software tool (REST) for group-wise comparison and statistical analysis of relative expression results in real-time PCR. *Nucl Acids Res* 30, e36.

Ramalho-Santos M, Yoon S, Matsuzaki Y *et al.* (2002) 'Stemness': transcriptional profiling of embryonic and adult stem cells. *Science* 298, 597–600.

Reijo R, Lee TY, Salo P *et al.* (1995) Diverse spermatogenic defects in humans caused by Y chromosome deletions encompassing a novel RNA-binding protein gene. *Nat Genet* 10, 383–393.

Reijo R, Alagappan RK, Patrizio P *et al.* (1996a) Severe oligospermia resulting from deletions of the *Azoospermia Factor* gene on the Y chromosome. *Lancet* 347, 1290–1293.

Reijo R, Seligman J, Dinulos MB *et al.* (1996b) Mouse autosomal homolog of DAZ, a candidate male sterility gene in humans, is expressed in male germ cells before and after puberty. *Genomics* 35, 346–352.

Reijo RA, Dorfman DM, Slee R *et al.* (2000) DAZ family proteins exist throughout male germ cell development and transit from nucleus to cytoplasm at meiosis in humans and mice. *Biol Reprod* 63, 1490–1496.

Rocchietti-March M, Weinbauer GF, Page DC *et al.* (2000) Dazl protein expression in adult rat testis is up-regulated at meiosis and not hormonally regulated. *Int J Androl* 23, 51–56.

Ruggiu M and Cooke H (2000) *In vivo* and *in vitro* analysis of homodimerisation activity of the mouse Dazl protein. *Gene* 252, 119–126.

Ruggiu M, Speed R, Taggart M *et al.* (1997) The mouse *Dazla* gene encodes a cytoplasmic protein essential for gametogenesis. *Nature* 389, 73–77.

Saffman EE and Lasko P (1999) Germline development in vertebrates and invertebrates. *Cell Mol Life Sci* 55, 1141–1163.

Saitou M, Barton SC and Surani MA (2002) A molecular programme for the specification of germ cell fate in mice. *Nature* 418, 293–300.

Saxena R, Brown LG, Hawkins T *et al.* (1996) The DAZ gene cluster on the human Y chromosome arose from an autosomal gene that was transposed, repeatedly amplified and pruned. *Nat Genet* 14, 292–299.

Saxena R, Vries JWAd, Repping S *et al.* (2000) Four *DAZ* genes in two clusters found in the *AZFc* region of the human Y chromosome. *Genomics* 67, 256–267.

Scholer H, Dressler G, Balling R *et al.* (1990a) Oct-4: a germ line specific transcription factor mapping to the mouse t-complex. *EMBO J* 9, 2185–2195.

Scholer H, Ruppert S, Suzuki N *et al.* (1990b) New type of POU domain in germ line-specific protein Oct-4. *Nature* 344, 435–439.

Schrans-Stassen BHGJ, Saunders PTK, Cooke HJ *et al.* (2001) Nature of the spermatogenic arrest in *Dazl* −/− mice. *Biol Reprod* 65, 771–776.

Seboun E, Barbaux S, Bourgeron T *et al.* (1997) Gene sequence, localization and evolution conservation of *DAZLA*, a candidate male sterility gene. *Genomics* 41, 227–235.

Shamblott MJ, Axelman J, Wang S *et al.* (1998) Derivation of pluirpotent stem cells from cultured human primordial germ cells. *Proc Natl Acad Sci* 95, 13726–13731.

Shamblott MJ, Axelman J, Littlefield JW *et al.* (2001) Human embryonic germ cell derivatives express a broad range of developmentally distinct markers and proliferate extensively *in vitro*. *Proc Natl Acad Sci* 98, 113–118.

Shan Z, Hirschmann P, Seebacher T *et al.* (1996) A SPGY copy homologous to the mouse gene *Dazla* and the *Drosophila* gene *boule* is autosomal and expressed only in the human male gonad. *Human Mol Genet* 5, 2005–2011.

Shinka T and Nakahori Y (1996) The azoospermic factor on the Y chromosome. *Acta Paediatr Jpn* 38, 399–404.

Simoni M, Gromoll J, Dworniczak B *et al.* (1997) Screening for deletions of the Y chromosome involving the *DAZ* (*Deleted in AZoospermia*) gene in azoospermia and severe oligozoospermia. *Fertil Steril* 67, 542–547.

Skaletsky H, Kuroda-Kawaguchi T, Minx PJ *et al.* (2003) The male-specific region of the human Y chromosome is a mosaic of discrete sequence classes. *Nature* 423, 825–837.

Slee R, Grimes B, Speed RM *et al.* (1999) A human *DAZ* transgene confers partial rescue of the mouse *Dazl* null phenotype. *Proc Natl Acad Sci* 96, 8040–8045.

Smith L and Greenfield A (2003) DNA microarrays and development. *Human Mol Genet* 12, R1–8.

Stuppia L, Calabrese G, Franchi PG *et al.* (1996) Widening of a Y-chromosome interval-6 deletion transmitted from a father to his infertile son accounts for an oligozoospermia critical region distal to the *RBM1* and *DAZ* genes. *Am J Human Genet* 59, 1393–1395.

Swanson WJ and Vacquier VD (2002) The rapid evolution of reproductive proteins. *Nature Rev, Genet* 3, 137–144.

Tam P and Zhou S (1996) The allocation of epiblast cells to ectodermal and germ-line lineages is influenced by position of the cells in the gastrulating mouse embryo. *Dev Biol* 178, 124–132.

Tanaka TS, Kunath T, Kimber WL *et al.* (2002) Gene expression profiling of embryo-derived stem cells reveals candidate genes associated with pluripotency and lineage specificity. *Genome Res* 12, 1921–1928.

Thomson J, J I-E, Shapiro S *et al.* (1998) Embryonic stem cell lines derived from human blastocysts. *Science* 282, 1145–1147.

Tiepolo L and Zuffardi O (1976) Localization of factors controlling spermatogenesis in the non-fluorescent portion of the human Y chromosome long arm. *Human Genet* 34, 119–124.

Toyooka Y, Tsunekawa N, Akasu R *et al.* (2003) Embryonic stem cells can form germ cells *in vitro*. *Proc Natl Acad Sci* 100, 11457–11462.

Tsai MY, Chang SY, Lo HY *et al.* (2000) The expression of DAZL1 in the ovary of the human female fetus. *Fertil Steril* 73, 627–630.

Tsang TE, Khoo P, Jamieson RV *et al.* (2001) The allocation and differentiation of mouse primordial germ cells. *Int J Dev Biol* 45, 549–555.

Tsuda M, Sasaoka Y, Kiso M *et al.* (2003) Conserved role of nanos proteins in germ cell development. *Science* 301, 1239–1241.

Tsui S, Dai T, Roettger S *et al.* (2000a) Identification of two novel proteins that interact with germ-cell specific RNA-binding proteins DAZ and DAZL1. *Genomics* 65, 266–273.

Tsui S, Dai T, Warren ST *et al.* (2000b) Association of the mouse infertility factor *DAZL1* with actively translating polyribosomes. *Biol Reprod* 62, 1655–1660.

Urano J, Fox M and Pera RR (2005) Interaction of the conserved meiotic regulators, BOULE (BOL) and PUMILIO-2 (PUM2). *Mol Reprod Dev* 71, 290–298.

Venables JP, Ruggiu M and Cooke HJ (2001) The RNA binding specificity of the mouse *Dazl* protein. Nucl Acids Res 29, 2479–2483.

Vereb M, Agulnik AI, Houston JT *et al.* (1997) Absence of DAZ gene mutations in cases of non-obstructed azoospermia. *Mol Human Reprod* 3, 55–59.

Vogt PH, Edelmann A, Kirsch S *et al.* (1996) Human Y chromosome azoospermia factors (AZF) mapped to different subregions in Yq11. *Human Mol Genet* 5, 933–943.

Vollrath D, Foote S, Hilton A *et al.* (1992) The human Y chromosome: a 43-interval map based on naturally occurring deletions. *Science* 258, 52–59.

Vries JWAd, Hoffer MJV, Repping S *et al.* (2002) Reduced copy number of *DAZ* genes in subfertile and infertile men. *Fertil Steril* 77, 68–75.

Warrington JA, Nair A, Mahadevappa M *et al.* (2000) Comparison of human adult and fetal expression and identification of 535 housekeeping/maintenance genes. *Physiol Genomics* 2, 143–147.

Wharton RP, Sonoda J, Lee T *et al.* (1998) The Pumilio RNA-binding domain is also a translational regulator. *Mol Cell* 1, 863–872.

Wickens M, Bernstein DS, Kimble J *et al.* (2002) A PUF family portrait: 3′UTR regulation as a way of life. *Trends Genet* 18, 150–157.

Wright LS, Li J, Caldwell MA *et al.* (2003) Gene expression in human neural stem cells: effects of leukemia inhibitory factor. *J Neurochem* 86, 179–195.

Xu EY, Lee DF, Klebes A *et al.* (2003) Human *BOULE* gene rescues meiotic defects in infertile flies. *Human Mol Genet* 12, 169–175.

Xu EY, Moore FL and Pera RAR (2001) A gene family required for human germ cell development evolved from an ancient meiotic gene conserved in all metazoans. *Proc Natl Acad Sci* 98, 7414–7419.

Yen PH, Chai NN and Salido EC (1996) The human autosomal gene DAZLA: testis specificity and a candidate for male infertility. *Human Mol Genet* 5, 2013–2017.

Yen PH, Chai NN and Salido EC (1997) The human *DAZ* genes, a putative male infertility factor on the Y chromosome, are highly polymorphic in the DAZ repeat regions. *Mamm Genome* 8, 756–759.

Ying Y, Qi X and Zhao G-Q (2001) Induction of primordial germ cells from murine epiblasts by synergistic action of BMP4 and BMP8B signaling pathways. *Proc Natl Acad Sci* 98, 7858–7862.

Yoshimizu T, Obinata M and Matsui Y (2001) Stage-specific tissue and cell interactions play key roles in mouse germ cell specification. *Development* 128, 481–490.

Zinn AR, Page DC and Fisher EMC (1993) Turner syndrome: the case of the missing sex chromosome. *Trends Genet* 9, 90–93.

Zwaka T and Thomson J (2005) A germ cell origin of embryonic stem cells? *Development* 132, 227–233.

Index